Gamal Eldin Swielim

Atlas Anatomy of the Horse

Gamal Eldin Swielim

Atlas Anatomy of the Horse

Noor Publishing

Imprint
Any brand names and product names mentioned in this book are subject to trademark, brand or patent protection and are trademarks or registered trademarks of their respective holders. The use of brand names, product names, common names, trade names, product descriptions etc. even without a particular marking in this work is in no way to be construed to mean that such names may be regarded as unrestricted in respect of trademark and brand protection legislation and could thus be used by anyone.

Cover image: www.ingimage.com

Publisher:
Noor Publishing
is a trademark of
Dodo Books Indian Ocean Ltd., member of the OmniScriptum S.R.L Publishing group
str. A.Russo 15, of. 61, Chisinau-2068, Republic of Moldova Europe
Printed at: see last page
ISBN: 978-620-0-06236-9

Atlas Anatomy of the Horse

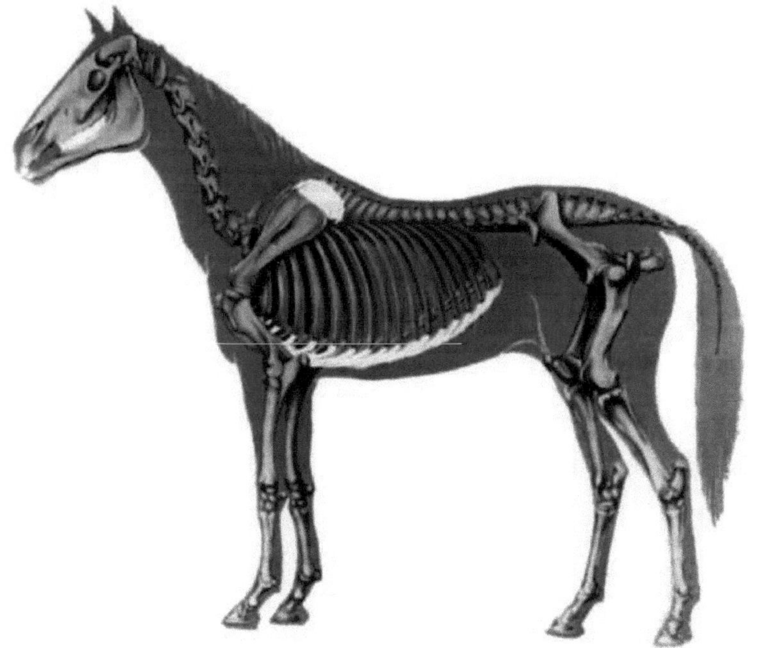

Prof.Dr. Gamal Eldin Abdelhakim Swielim

Professor of Anatomy, Faculty of Veterinary Medicine

Cairo University

Atlas
Anatomy of the Horse

Prof.Dr.Gamal Eldin Abdelhakim Swielim

Professor of Anatomy Faculty of Veterinary Medicine

Cairo University

Preface

This atlas is providing an idealized view of the horse anatomy. The classic illustrations are performed to be simple and sufficient for the needs of the preclinical students. Colored diagrams and illustrations, which profess considerable accuracy of details and emphasized the relationship of structures, were selected and drawn carefully to useful as possible to the students during the superficial and deep dissection. Many new schematic illustrations were added to this edition. All labeled illustrations were reviewed to ensure that they conform to the *Nomina Anatomica Veterinaria* (2017) and its annex. The atlas is also provided with tables summarizing the muscles, arteries and nerves of the different regions and structures of the horse body.

Finally, I would like to express my gratitude to my colleges in Anatomy Department, Faculty of Veterinary Medicine, Cairo University and I hope that they will give their advice for any improvements, additional terms or figures to be added to this work.

Gamal Eeldin Swielim

Contents

iv

List of tables

Part I

Figures and Diagrams

Chapter 1
The Body

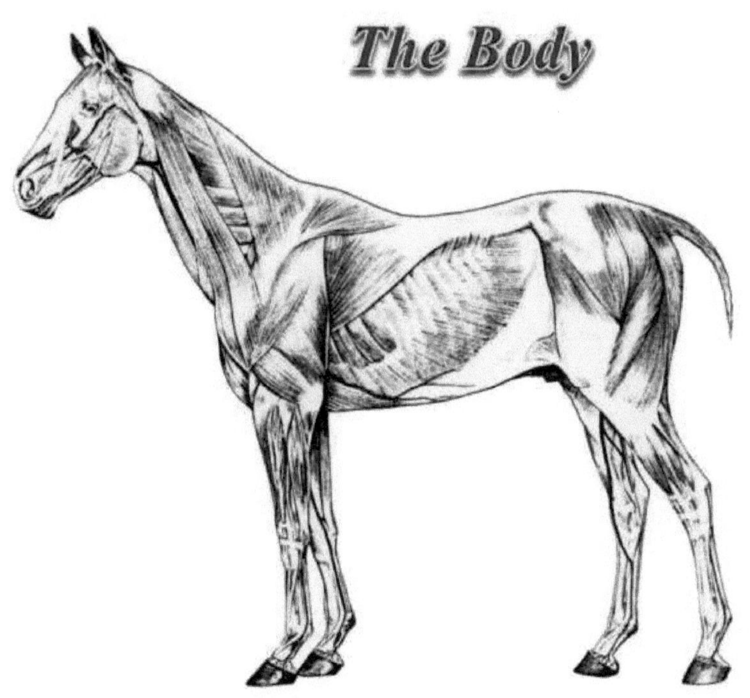

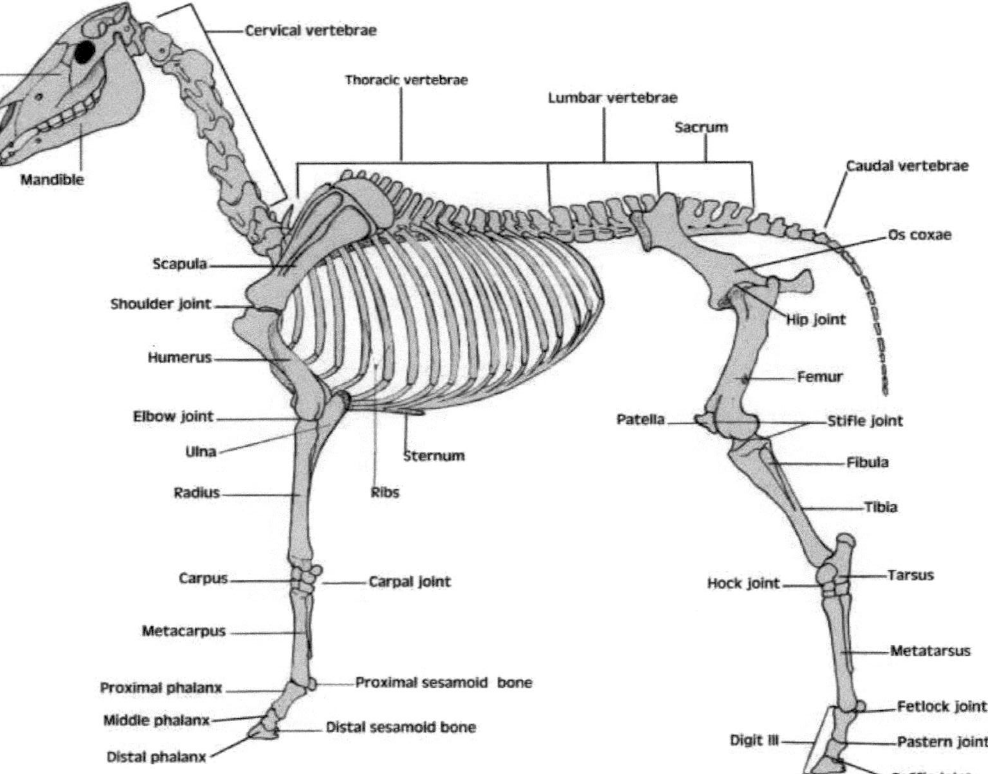

Fig.1. Skeleton ; left lateral view

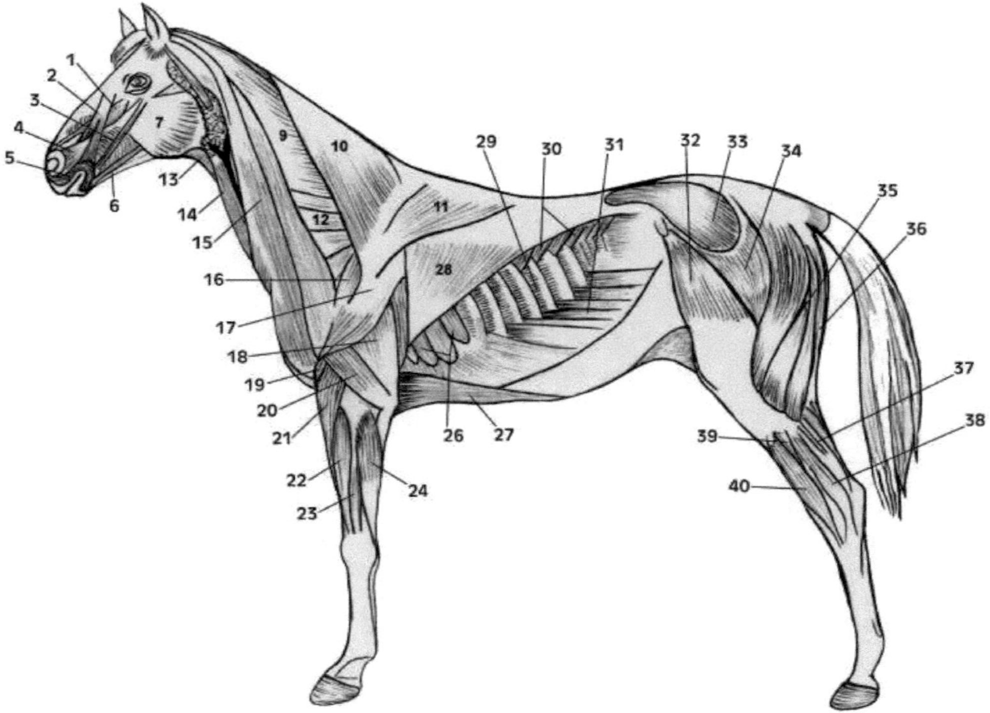

Fig.2. Superficial muscles of the body

Fig.2. Superficial muscles of the body

1. M. levator labii maxillaries
2. M. levator nasolabialis
3. M. zygomaticus
4. M. caninus
5. M. orbicularis oris
6. M. depressor labii mandibularis
7. M. masseter
8. M. rhomboideus cervicis
9. M. splenius
10. M. trapezius cervicis
11. M. trapezius thoracis
12. M. serratus ventralis cervicis
13. M. omohyoideus
14. M. sternocephalicus
15. M. brachiocephalicus
16. M. supraspinatus
17. M. deltoideus
18. Long head of M. triceps brachii
19. M. brachialis
20. Lateral head of M. triceps brachii
21. M. extensor carpi radialis
22. M. common digital extensor
23. M. extensor digitorum lateralis
24. M. ulnaris lateralis
25. Superficial digital extensor tendon
26. M. serratus ventralis thoracis
27. M. pectoralis ascendens
28. M. latissimus dorsi
29. M. intercostalis externus
30. M. serratus dorsalis caudalis
31. M. obliquus abdominis externus
32. M. tensor fasciae latae
33. M. gluteus medius
34. M. gluteus superficialis
35. M. biceps brachii
36. M. semitendinosus
37. M. soleus
38. M. flexor digitorum profundus
39. M. extensor digitorum superficialis
40. M. extensor digitorum longus

Chapter 2
Head and Neck

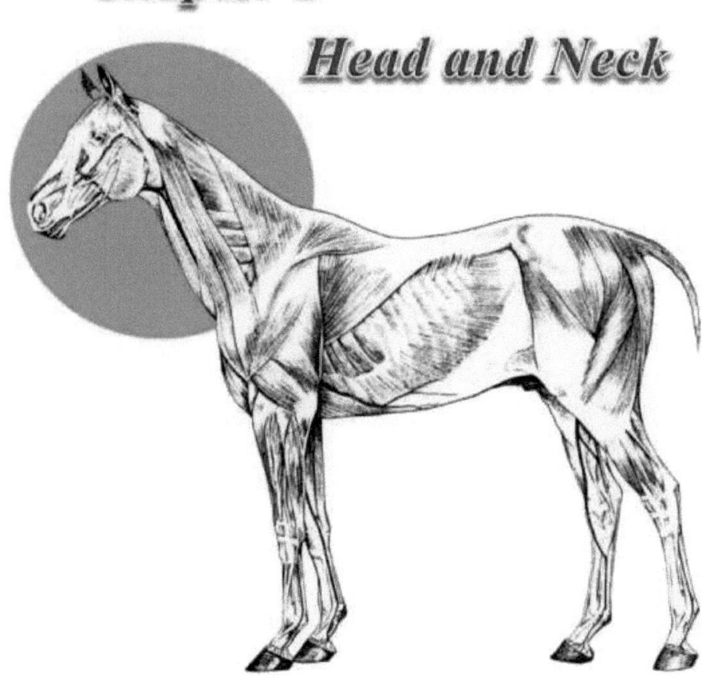

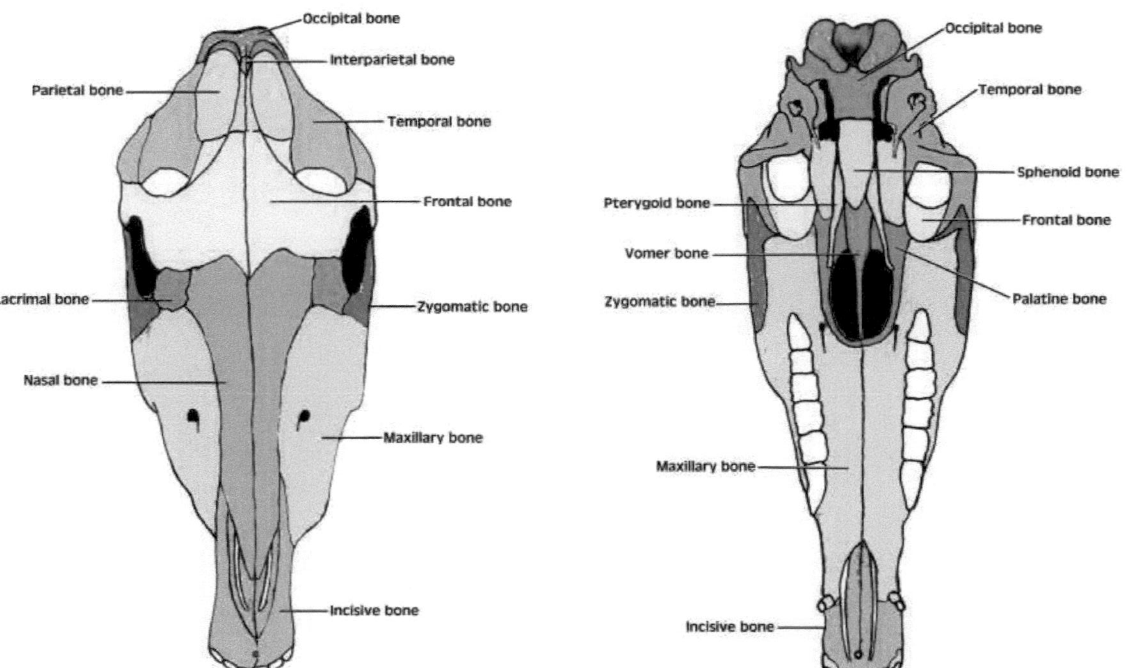

Fig.3.Bones of skull, dorsal view

Fig.4. Bones of skull, ventral view

11

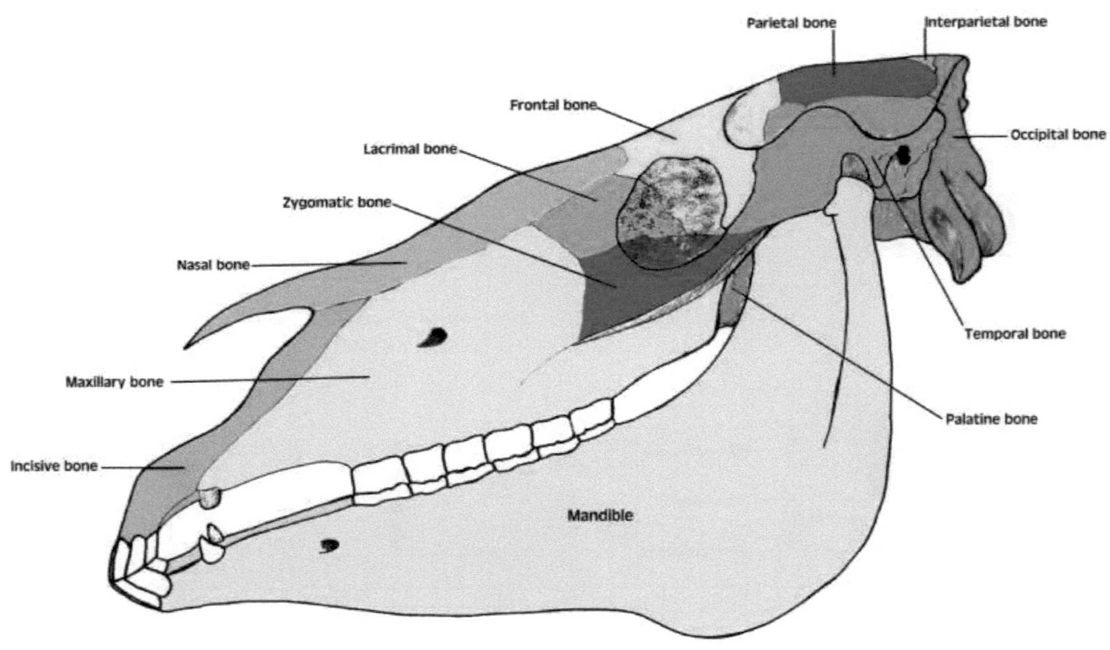

Fig.5. Bones of the skull and mandible , left lateral view

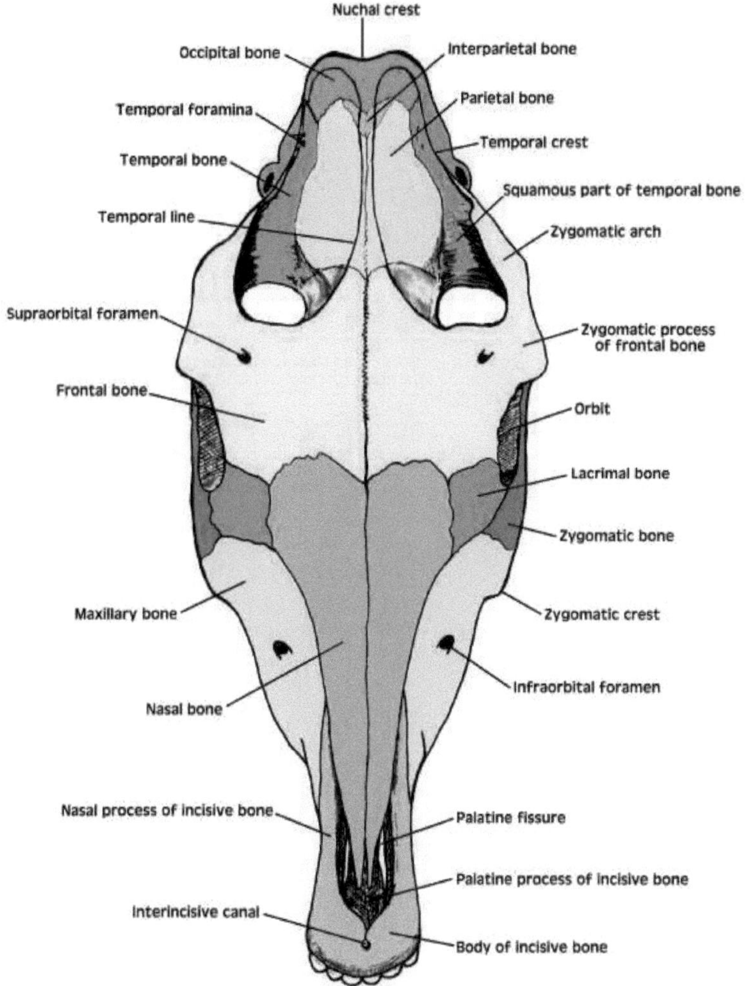

Fig.6. Skull ; dorsal surface

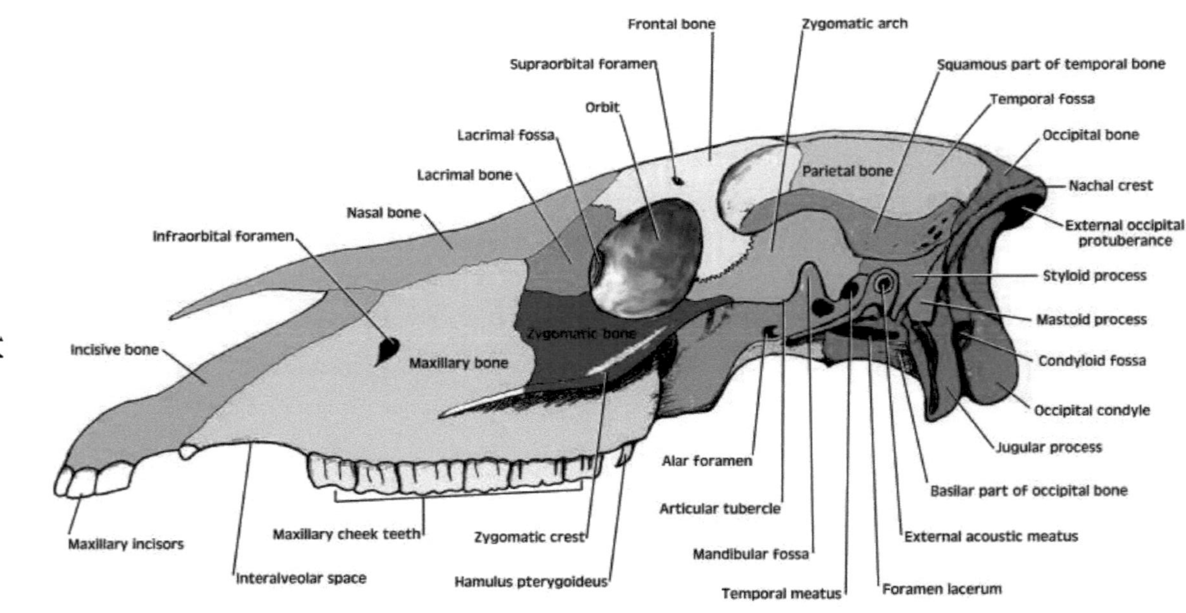

Fig.7. Skull ; lateral surface

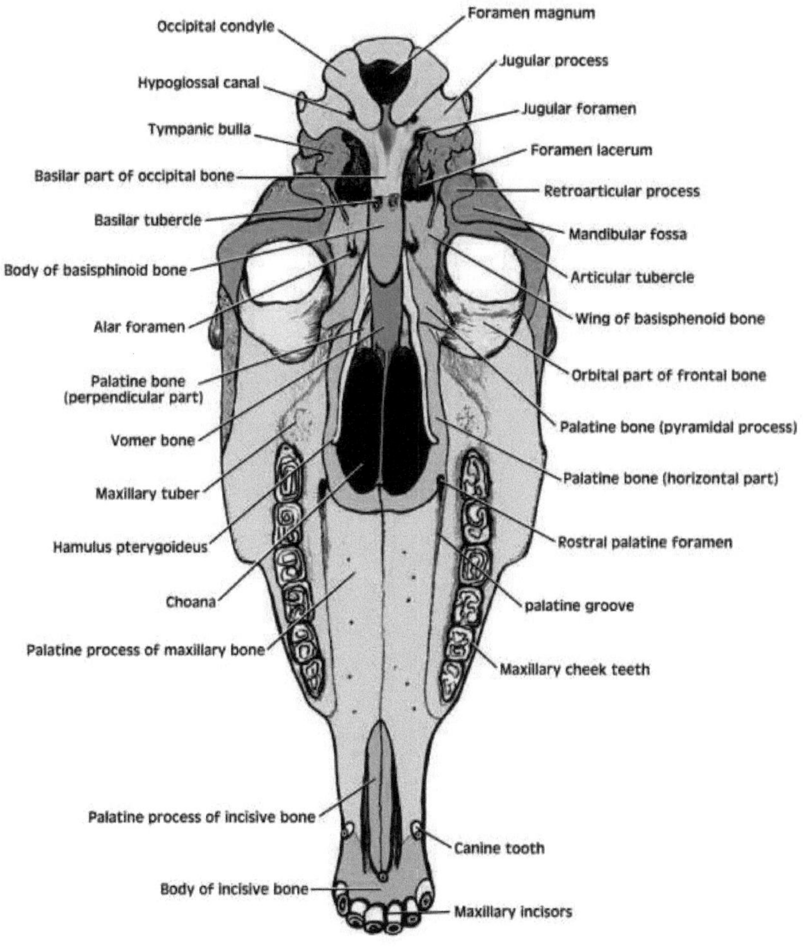

Fig.8. Skull , ventral surface

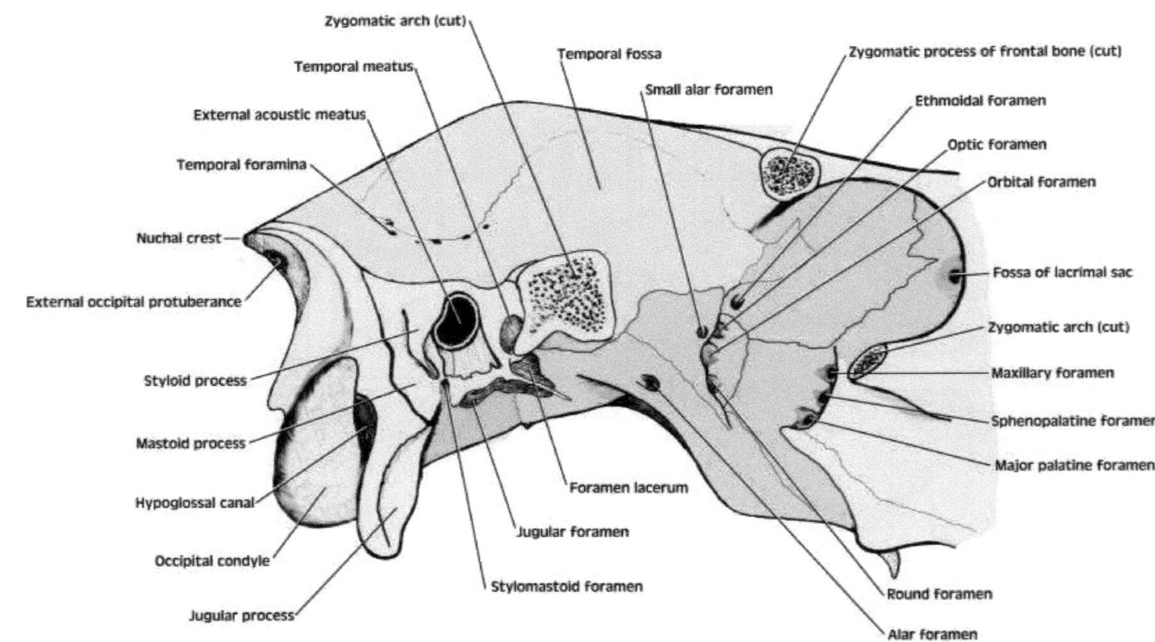

Fig 9. Cranial and orbital regions of the skull , zygomatic arch is cut

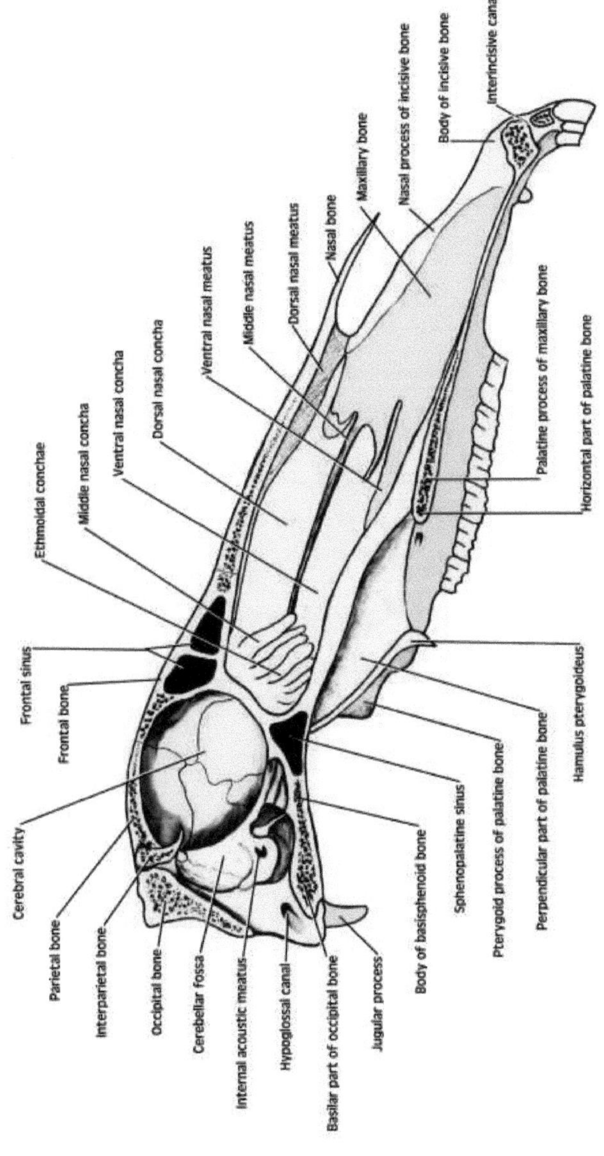

Fig.10. Sagittal section of the skull

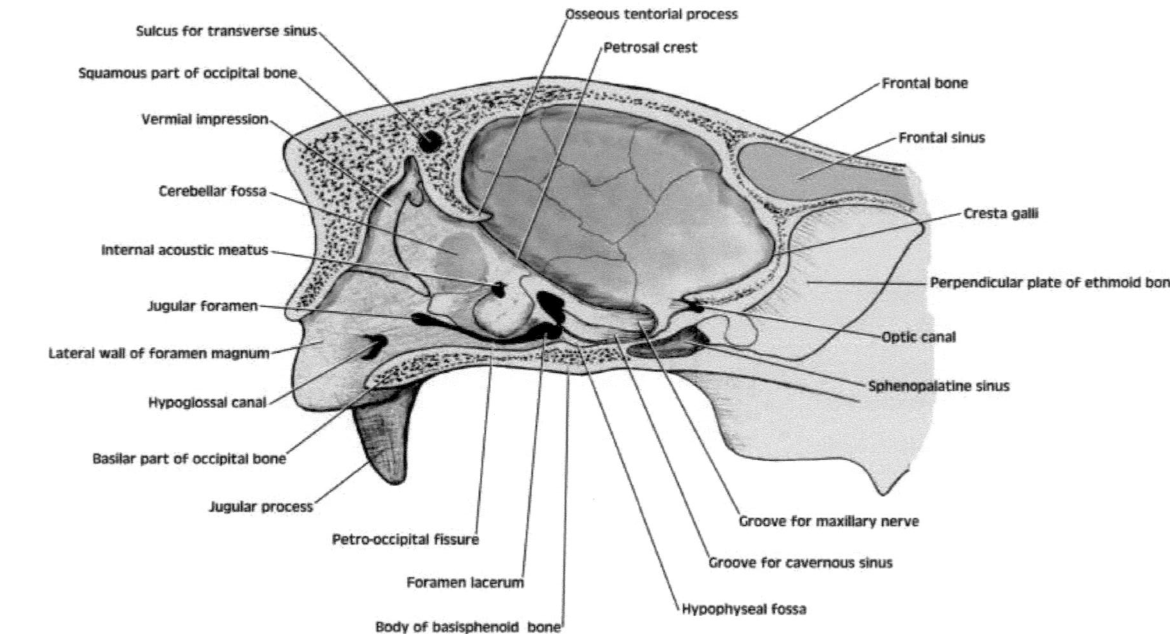

Fig.11. Sagittal section of the cranial cavity

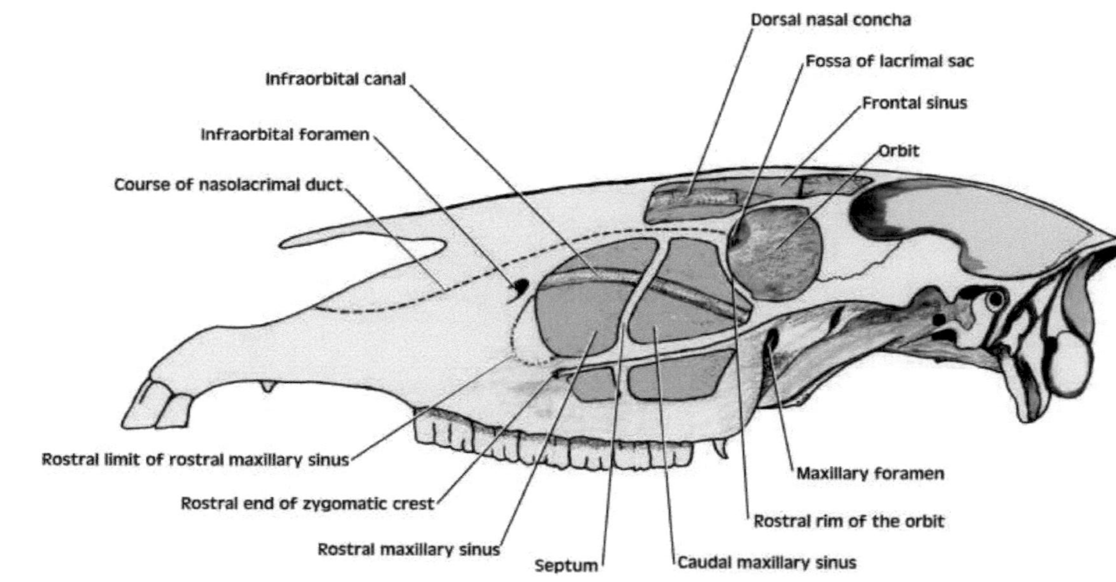

Fig.12. Skull with limited paranasal sinuses , lateral view

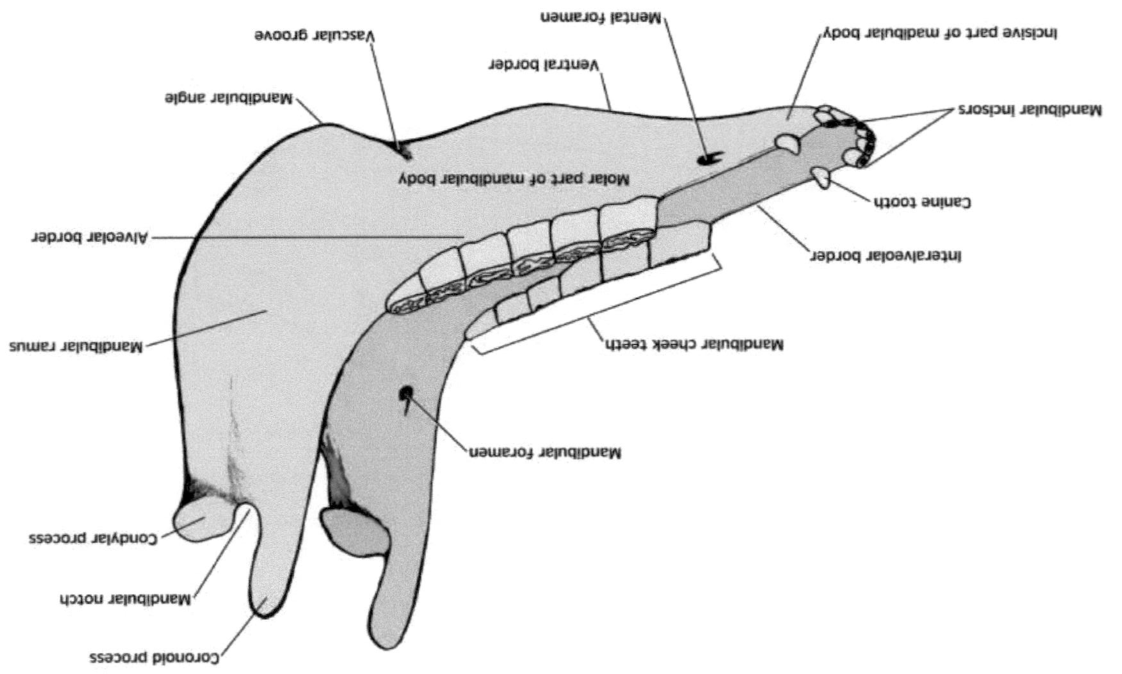

Fig.13. Mandible , left lateral view

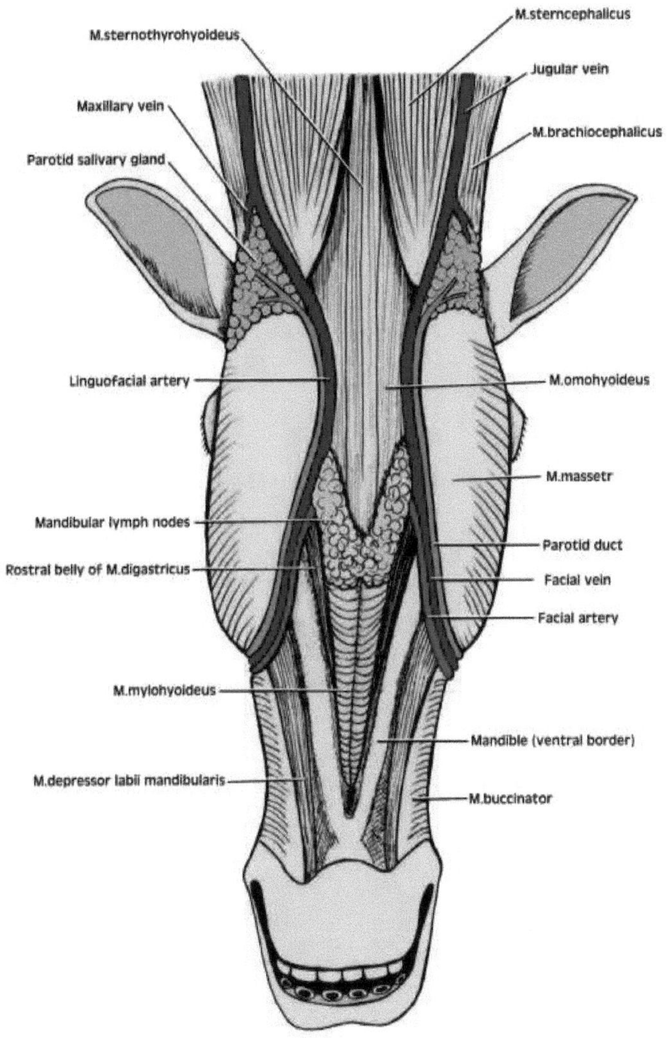

Fig.14. Dissection of intermandibular space and adjacent part of the neck

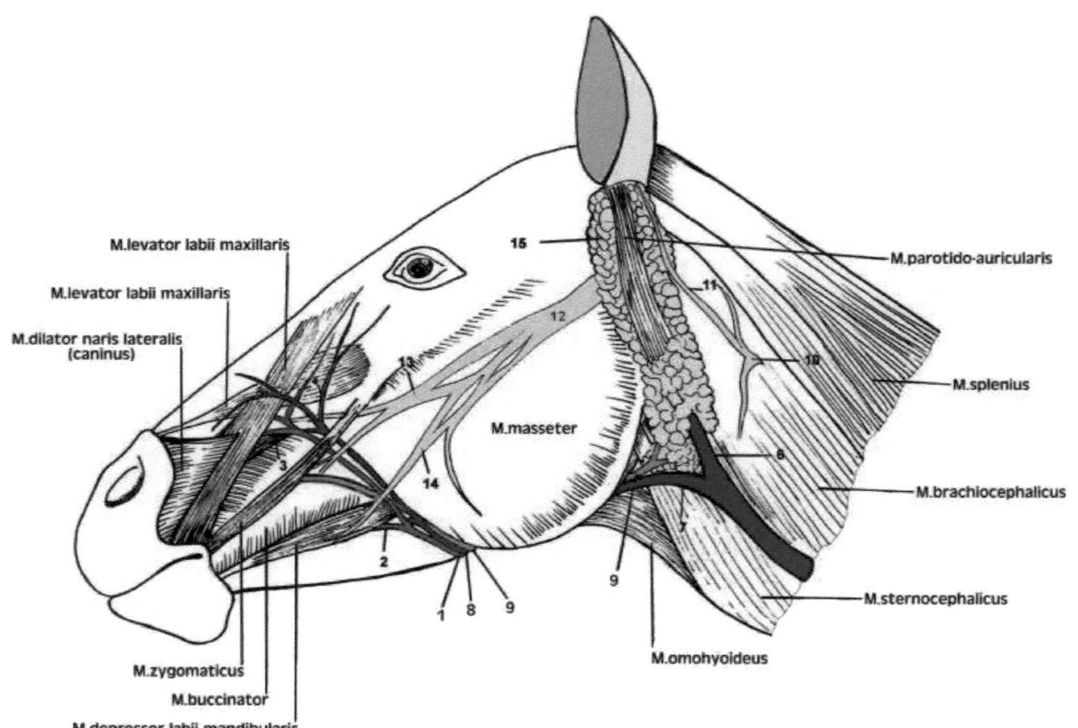

Fig.15.Dissection of the head , superficial layer ; lateral view

Fig.15. Dissection of the head, superficial layer; lateral view

1. Facial artery
2. Mandibular labial artery
3. Maxillary labial artery
4. Angularis oculi artery and vein
5. Jugular vein
6. Maxillary vein
7. Linguofacial vein
8. Facial vein
9. Parotid duct
10. Second cervical nerve
11. Great auricular vein
12. Facial nerve
13. Dorsal buccal branch
14. Ventral buccal branch
15. Parotid salivary

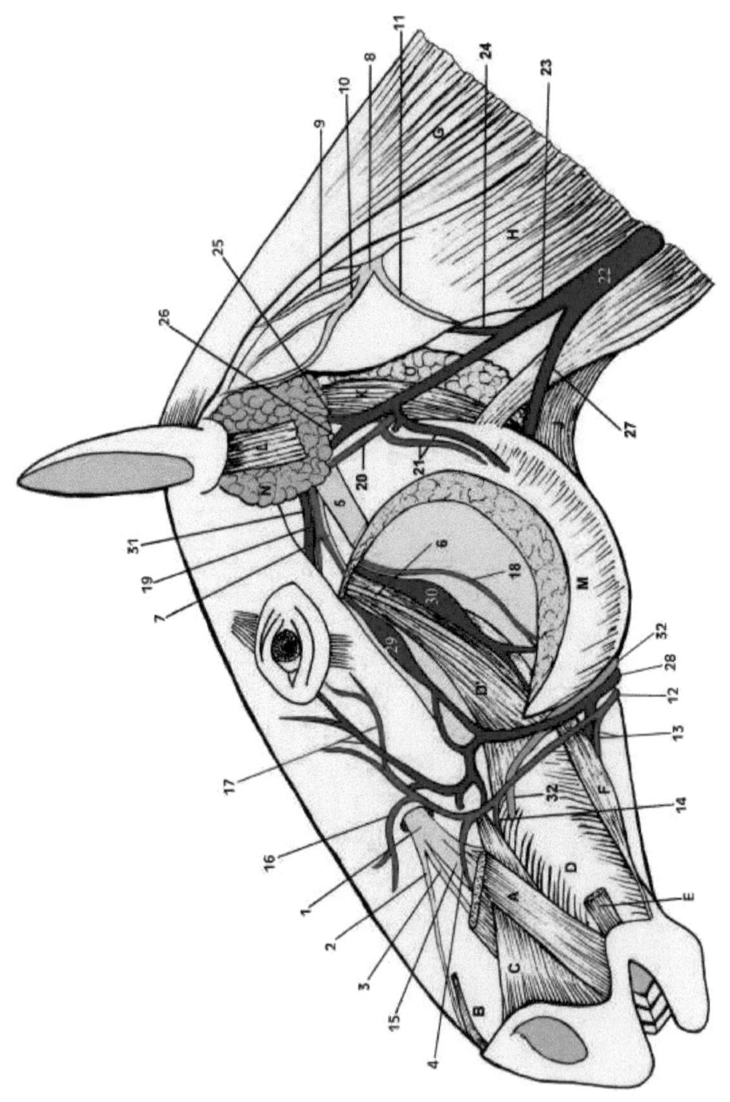

Fig.16. Dissection of head showing the vessels and nerves of the face ; lateral view

Fig.16. Dissection of the head muscles, vessels and nerves of the face

A. M. levator nasolabiali
B. M. levator labii maxillaries
C. M. caninus
D. M. buccinator (buucal part)
D` M. buccinator (molar part)
E. M. cutaneous faciei
F. M. depressor labii mandibularis
G. M. splenius
H. M. brachiocephalicus
I. M. sternocephalicus
J. M. omohyoideus
K. M. jugulomandibularis
L. M. parotidoauricularis
M. M. masseter
N. Parotid salivary gland
O. Mandibular salivary gland

1. Infraorbital nerve
2. External nasal branch
3. Internal nasal branch
4. Maxillary labial branches
5. Facial nerve
6. Buccinator nerve
7. Transverse facial nerve
8. Second cervical nerve
9. Dorsal branch of 8
10. Great auricular nerve
11. Transverse cervical nerve
12. Facial artery
13. Mandibular labial vessels
14. Maxillary labial artery
15. Lateral nasal artery
16. Dorsal nasal artery
17. Angularis oculi artery
18. Buccinator artery
19. Transverse facial artery
20. Superfacial temporal artery

21. Massetric artery and vein
22. Jugular vein
23. Maxillary vein
24. Occipital vein
25. Caudal auricular vein
26. Superficial temporal vein
27. Linguofacial vein
28. Facial vein
29. Deep facial vein
30. Buccinator vein
31. Transverse facial vein
32. Parotid duct

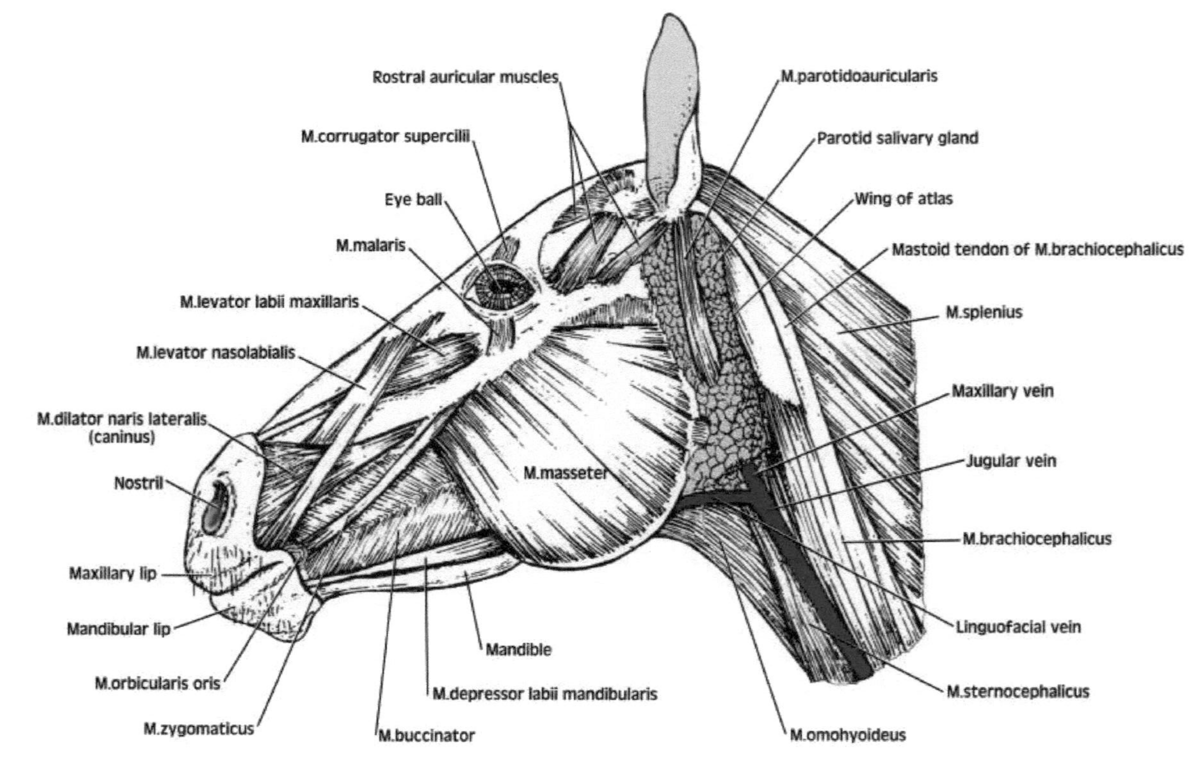

Fig.17. Superficial muscles of the head , lateral view

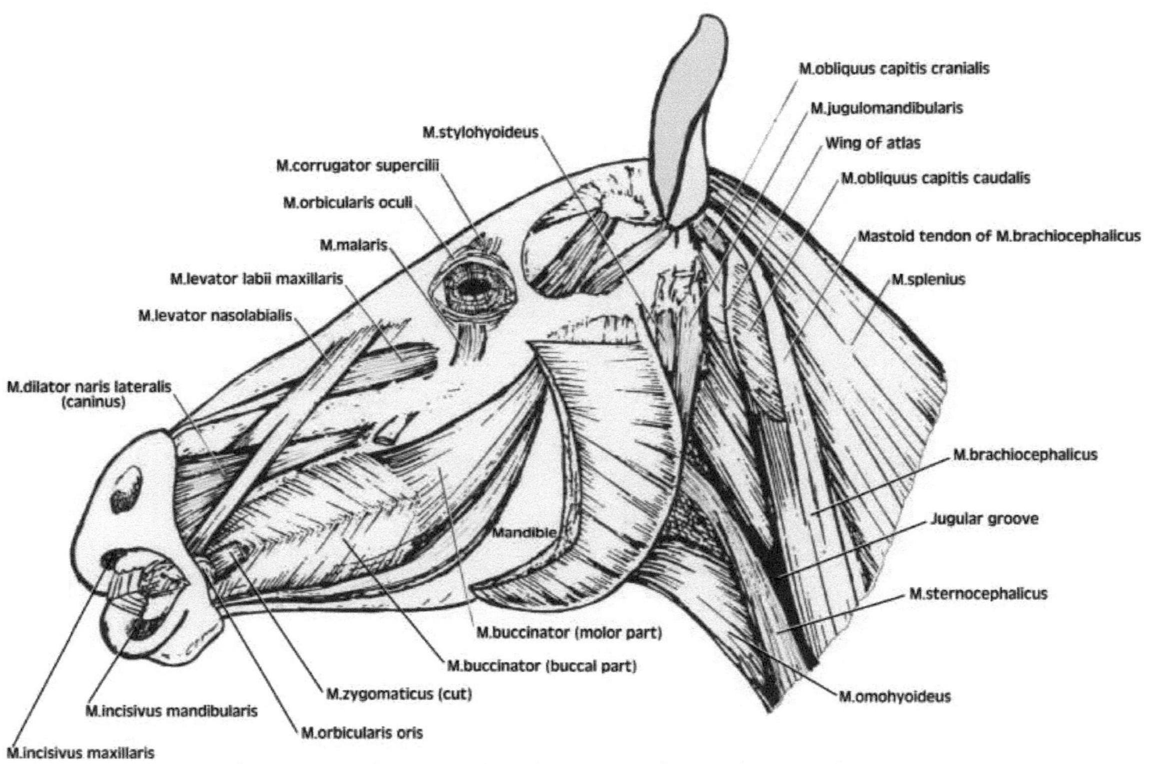

Fig.18. Muscles of the head , second layer : lateral view

27

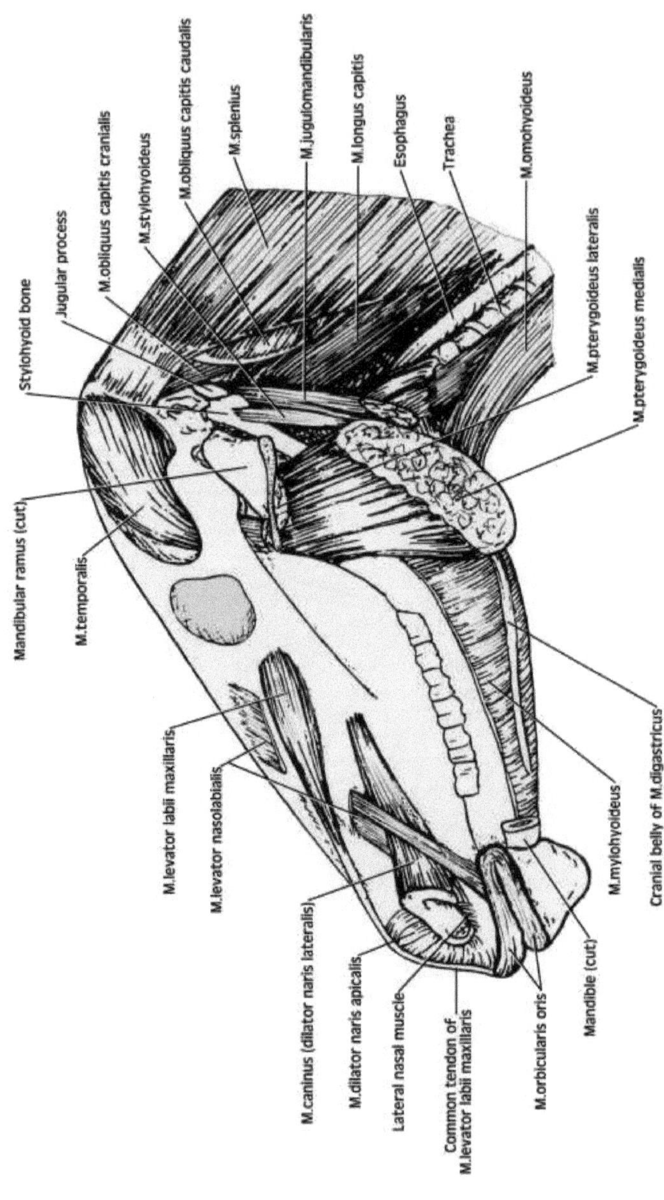

Fig.19. Dissection of the head after removal of mandible ; third layer

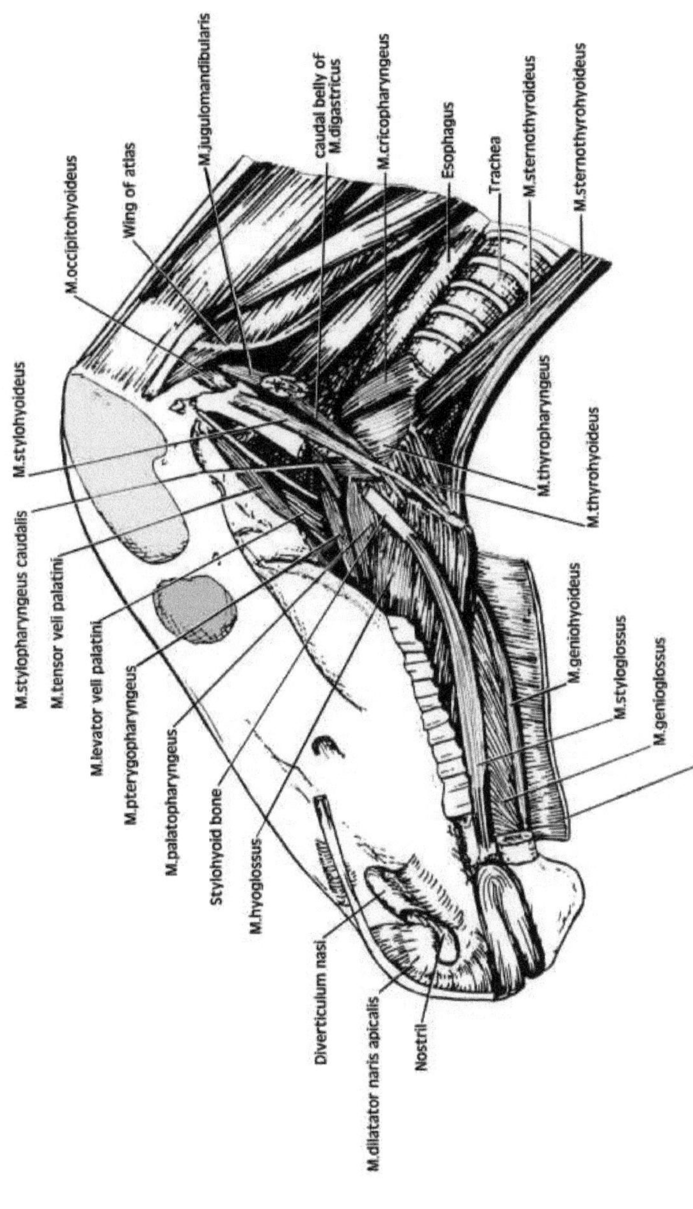

Fig.20. Dissection of the head ; fourth layer

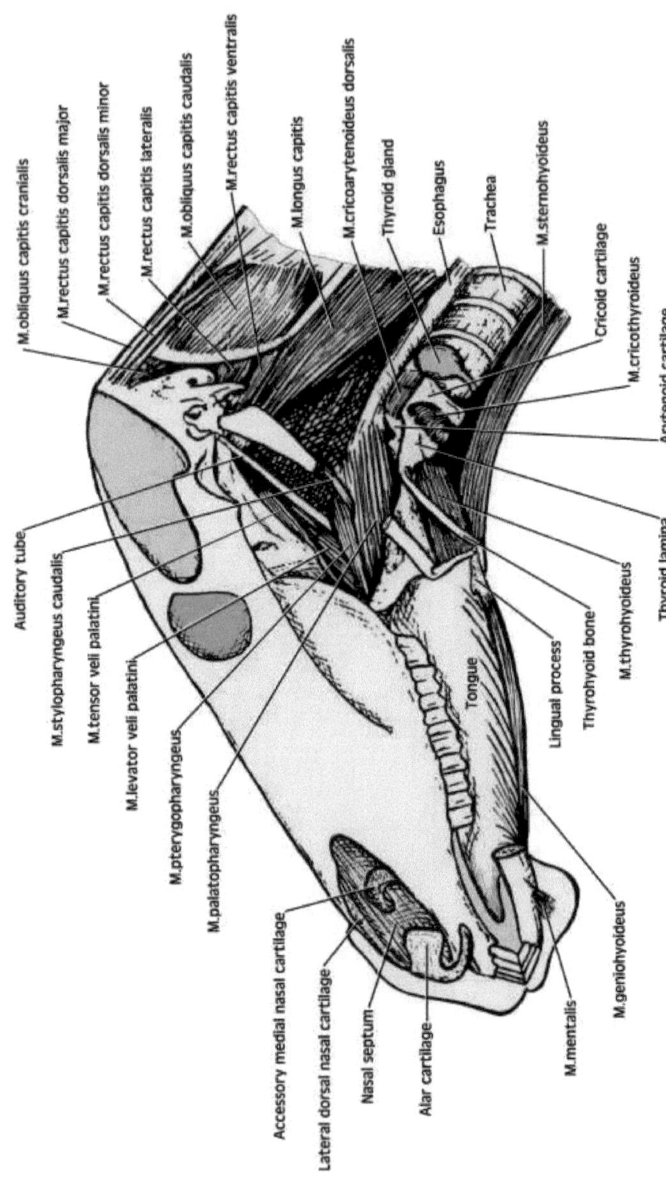

Fig.21. Dissection of the head ; the deepest layer

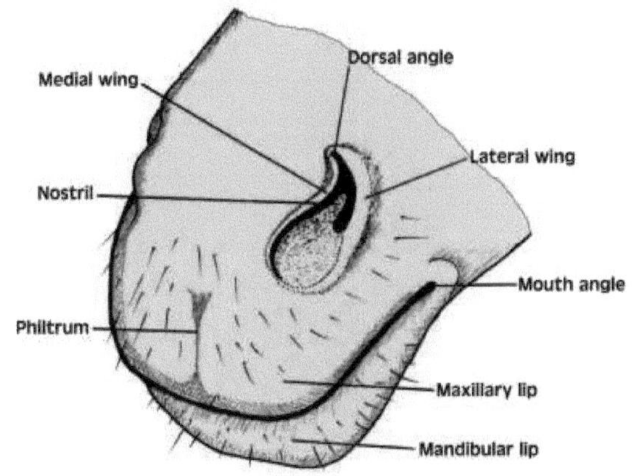

Fig.22. Nostril and lips

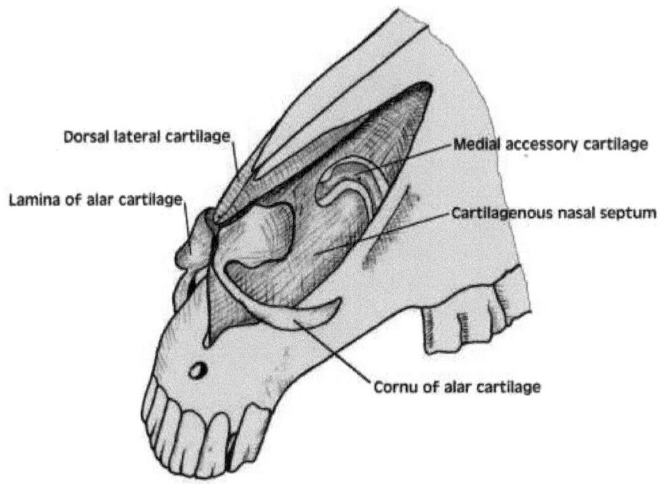

Fig. 23. Nasal cartilages

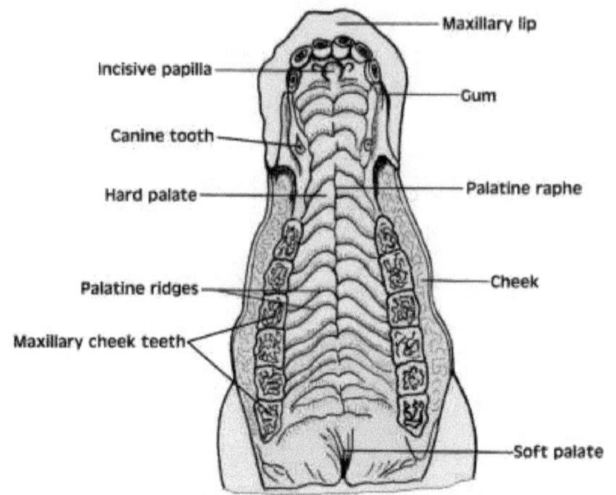

Fig.24. Hard palate and roof of oral cavity

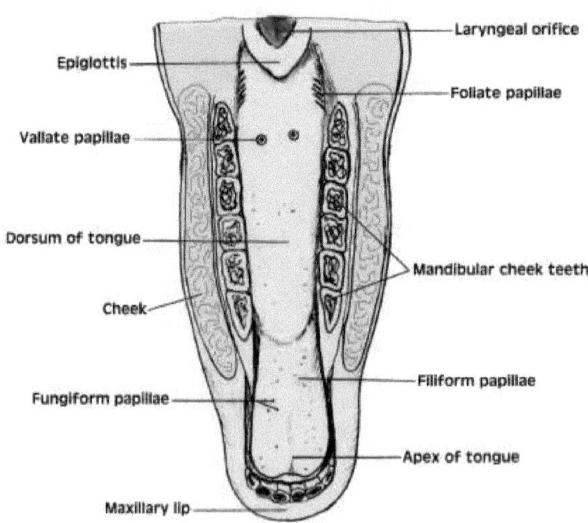

Fig.25. Tongue and floor of oral cavity

32

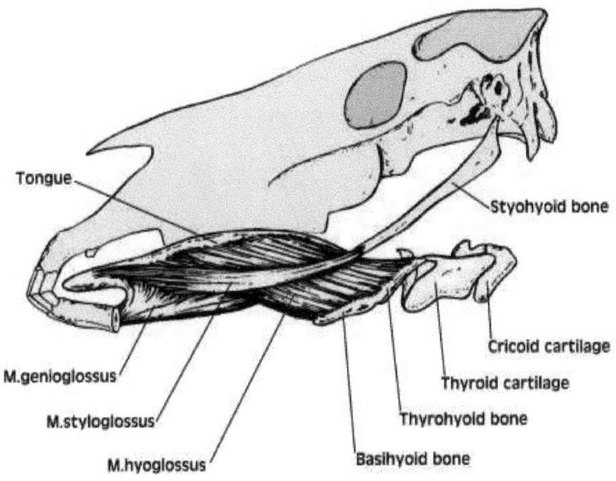

Fig.26. Muscles of tongue

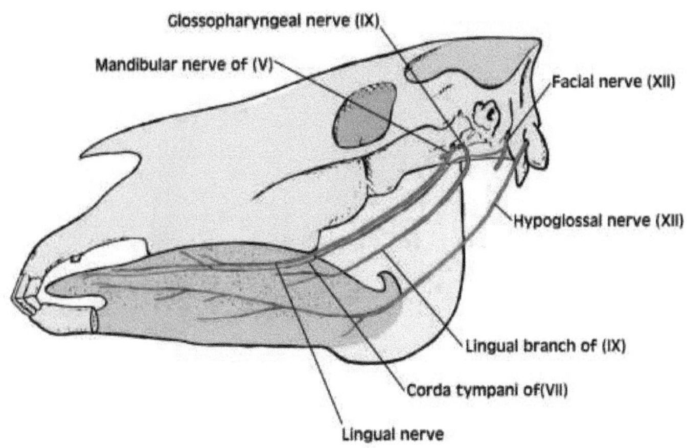

Fig.27. Nerve supply of tongue

33

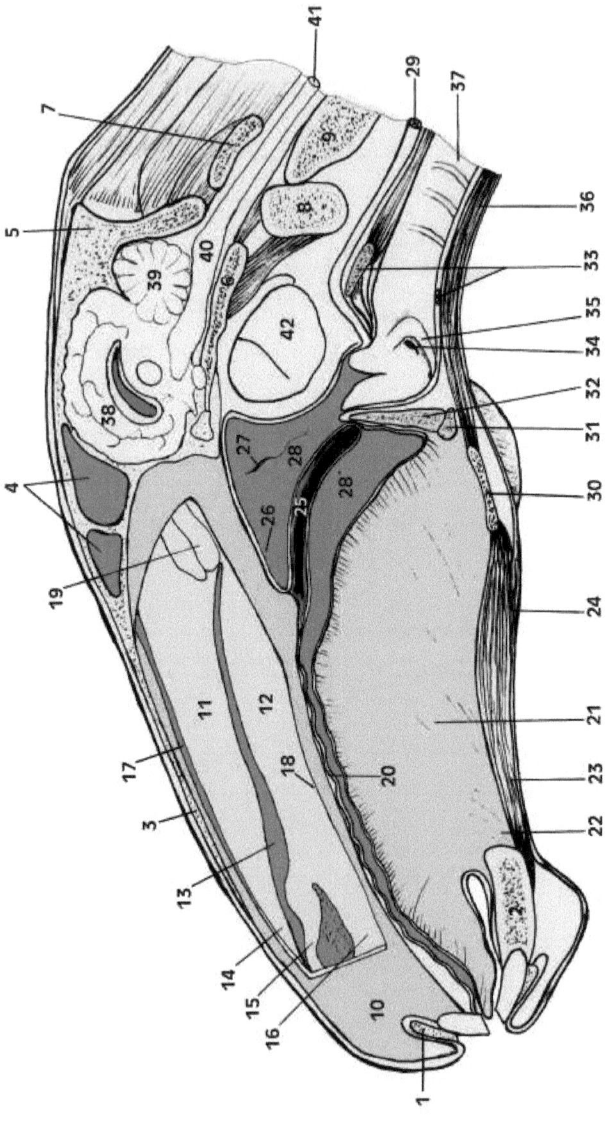

Fig. 28. Sagittal section in the head

Fig.28. Sagittal section in the head

1. Incisive bone
2. Body of mandible
3. Nasal bone
4. Frontal sinus
5. Squamous part of occipital bone
6. Basilar part of occipital bone
7. Dorsal arch of atlas
8. Ventral arch of atlas
9. Axis (second cervical vertebra)
10. Nasal septum
11. Dorsal nasal concha
12. Ventral nasal concha
13. Middle nasal meatus (sinus meatus)
14. Straight fold
15. Alar fold
16. Basal fold
17. Dorsal nasal meatus (olfactory meatus)
18. Ventral nasal meatus (respiratory meatus)
19. Ethmoidal conchae
20. Hard palate
21. Tongue
22. M. genioglossus
23. M. geniohyoideus
24. M. mylohyoideus
25. Soft palate
26. Nasopharyngeal orifice
27. Pharyngeal orifice of auditory tube
28. Nasopharynx
28 Oropharynx
29. Esophagus
30. Lingual process of hyoid bone
31. Body of thyroid cartilage
32. Epiglottis
33. Cricoid cartilage
34. Lateral ventricle
35. Vocal fold
36. M. sternohyoideus
37. Trachea
38. Cerebral hemisphere
39. Cerebellum
40. Medulla oblongata
41. Spinal cord
42. Diverticulum of auditory tube

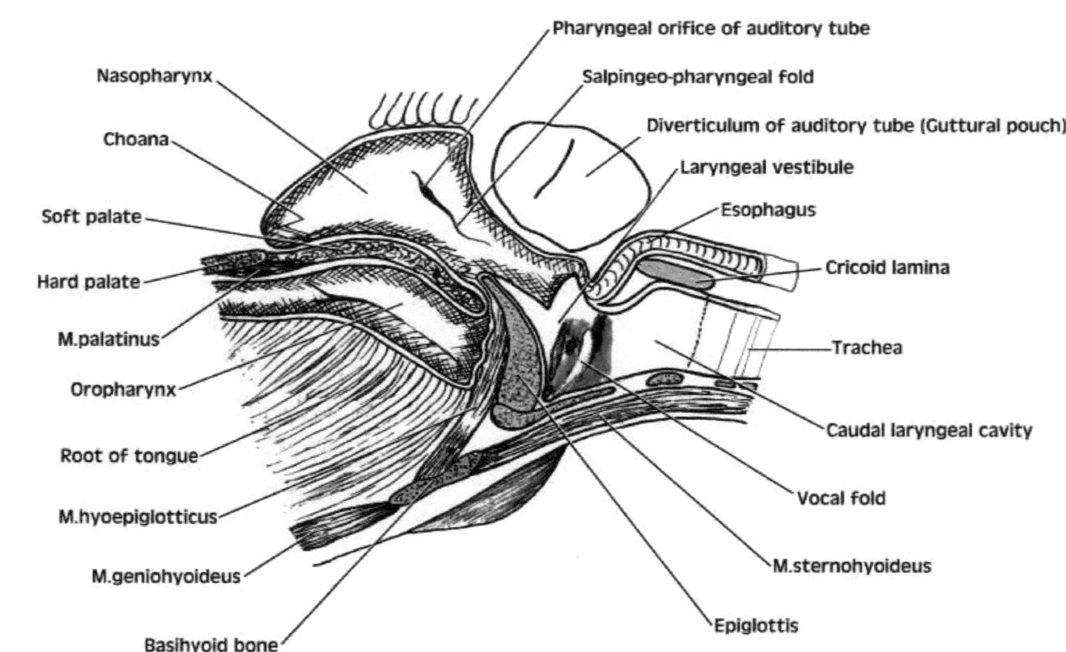

Fig.29.Pharyngeal cavity, soft palate and larynx ; sagittal section

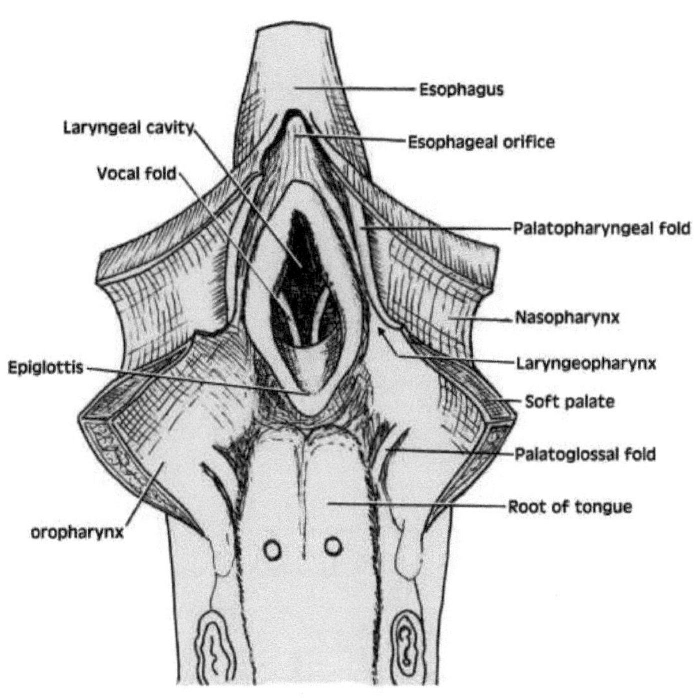

Fig.30. Pharynx and soft palate , dorsal view

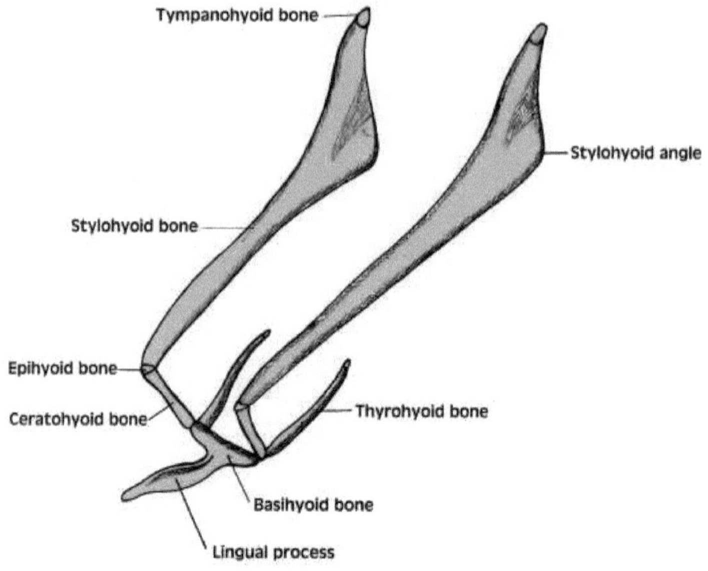

Fig.31. Hyoid bone , rostrolateral view

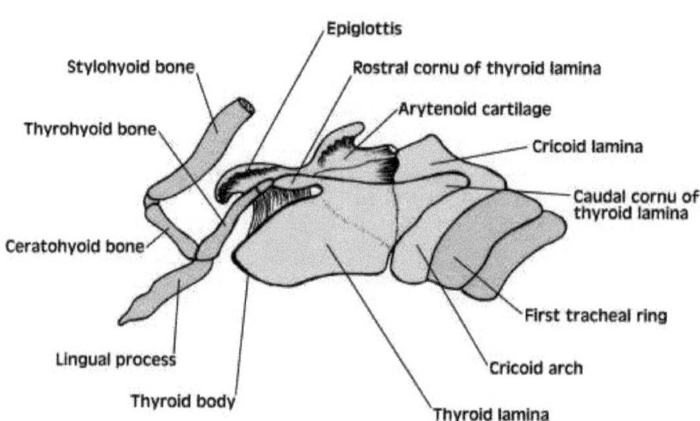

Fig.32. Hyoid bone and laryngeal cartilages

38

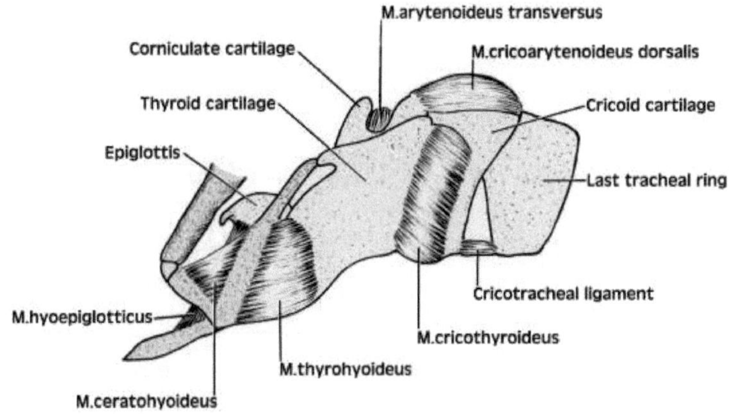

Laryngeal muscles ; left lateral view

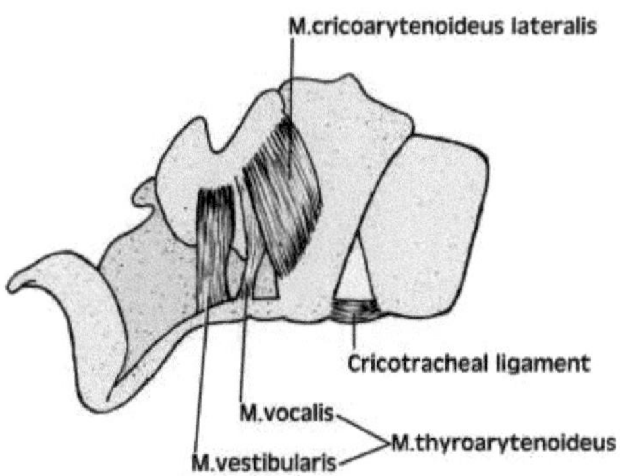

Longitudinal section in the larynx

Fig.33. Laryngeal muscles

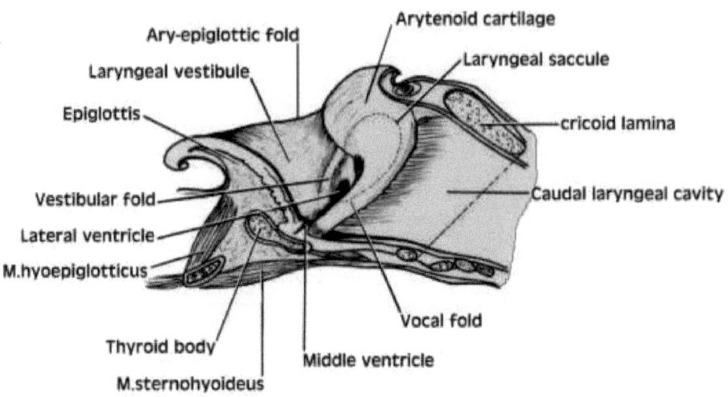

Median section of the Larynx

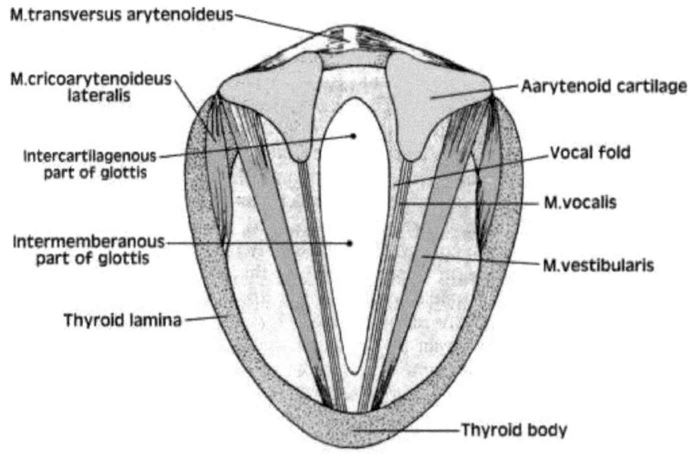

Cross section of the Larynx ; diagrammatic

Fig.34. Laryngeal cavity

40

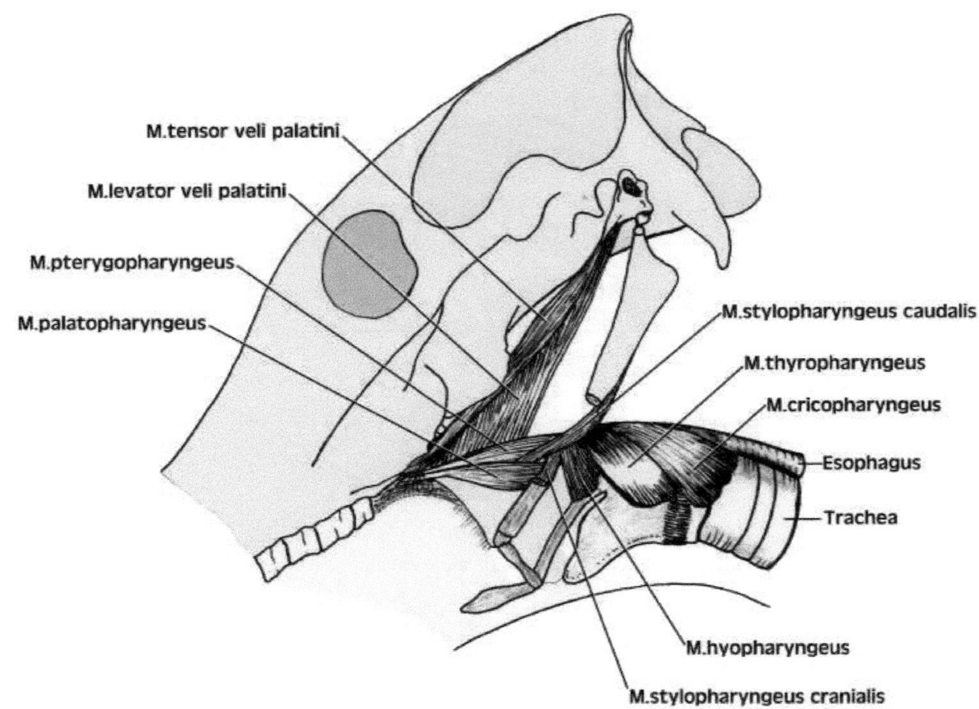

Fig.35. Muscles of soft palate and phrynx

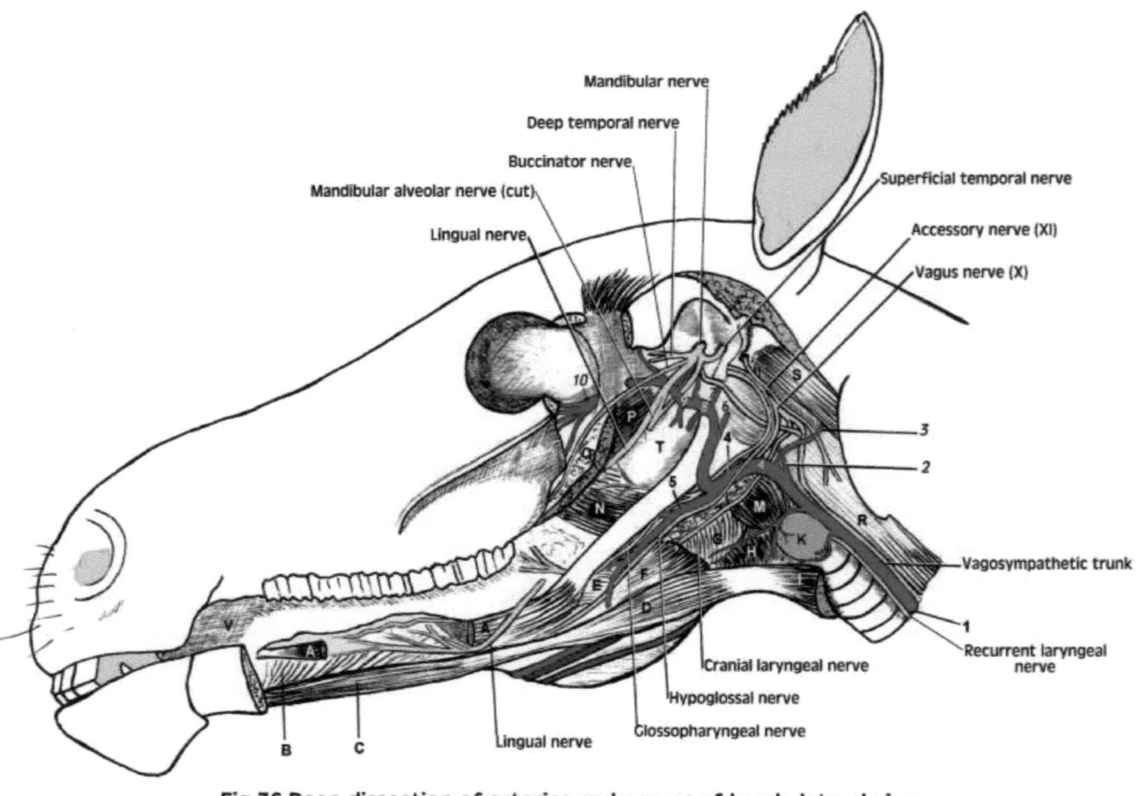

Fig.36.Deep dissection of arteries and nerves of head ; lateral view

42

Fig.36. Deep dissection of the head, lateral view

A. M. styloglossus
B. M. genioglossus
C. M. geniohyoideus
D. M. omohyoideus
E. M. ceratohyoideus
F. M. thyrohyoideus
G. M. thyropharyngeus
H. M. cricothyroideus
J. M. sternothyroideus
K. Thyroid gland
M. M. cricopharyngeus
N. M. palatopharyngeuS
O. M. pterygoideus lateralis
P. M. tensor veli palatine
Q. M. temporalis
R. M. longus capitis
S. M. obliquus capitis cranialis
T. Diverticulum of auditory tube
U. Stylohyoid bone
V. Tongue

1. Common carotid artery
2. Internal carotid artery
3. Occipital artery
4. External carotid artery
5. Linguofacial artery
6. Caudal auricular artery
7. Superficial temporal artery
8. Occipital artery
9. First part of maxillary artery
10. Third part of maxillary artery

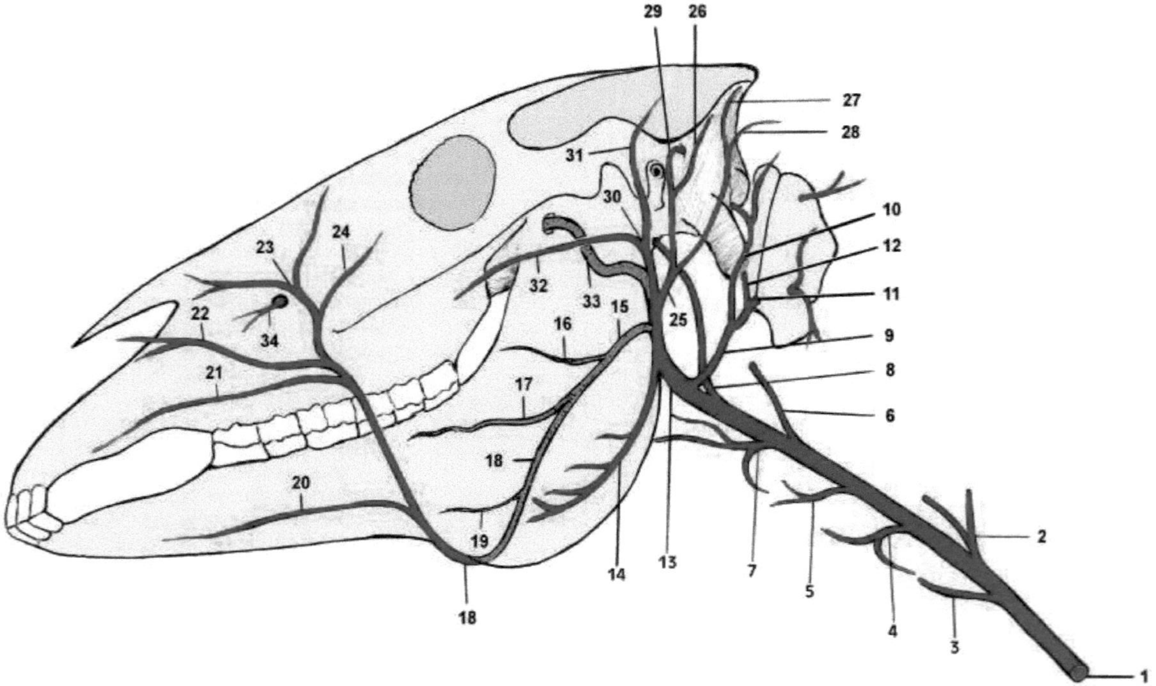

Fig.37. Branches of the common carotid artery ; diagrammatic

Fig.37. Branches of the common carotid artery; diagrammatic

1. Common carotid artery
2. Esophageal branch
3. Tracheal branch
4. Muscular branch
5. Caudal thyroid artery
6. Parotid branch
7. Cranial thyroid artery
8. Internal carotid artery
9. Occipital artery
10. Condyloid artery
11. Occipital branch of occipital artery
12. Caudal meningeal artery
13. External carotid artery
14. Massetric branch
15. Linguofacial artery
16. Ascending palatine artery
17. Lingual artery
18. Facial artery
19. Sublingual artery
20. Mandibular labial artery
21. Maxillary labial artery
22. Lateral nasal artery
23. Dorsal nasal artery
24. Angularis oculi artery
25. Caudal auricular artery
26. Lateral auricular branch
27. Intermediate auricular artery
28. Medial auricular artery
29. Deep auricular artery
30. Superficial temporal artery
31. Rostral auricular artery
32. Transverse facial artery
33. Maxillary artery
34. Infraorbital artery

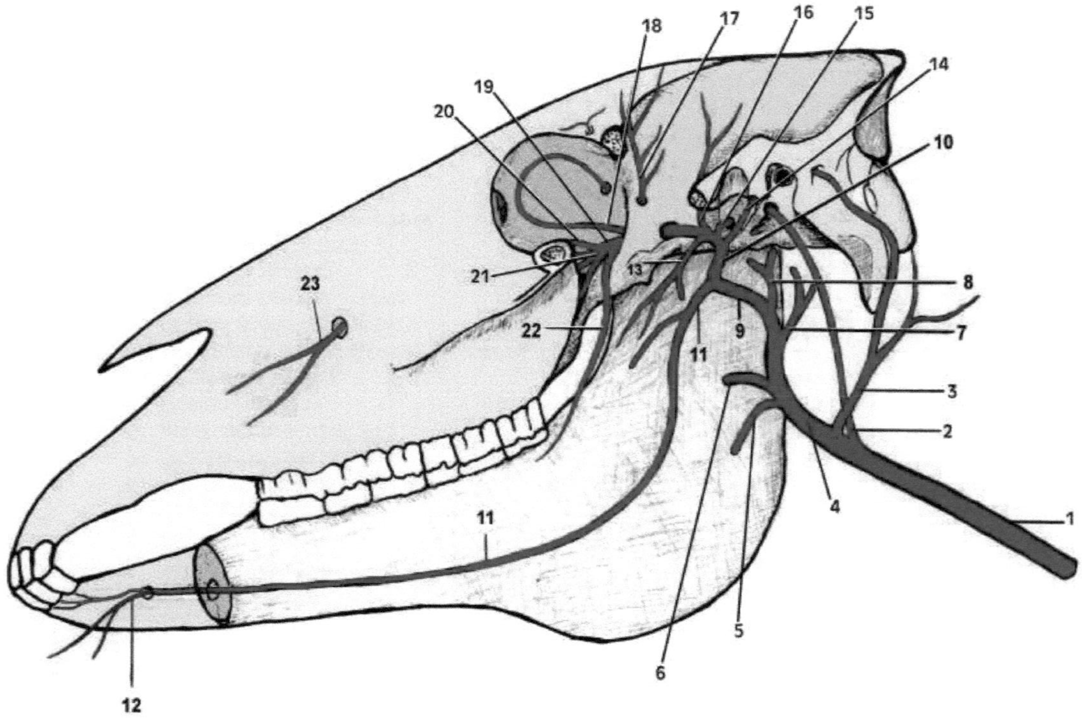

Fig.38. Terminal branches of common carotid artery ; diagrammatic

Fig.38. Terminal branches of common carotid artery; diagrammatic

1. Common carotid artery
2. Internal carotid artery
3. Occipital artery
4. External carotid artery
5. Massetric artery
6. Liguofacial artery
7. Caudal auricular artery
8. Superficial temporal artery
9. Maxillary artery
10. First part of maxillary artery
11. Mandibular alveolar artery
12. Mental artery
13. Pterygoid branches
14. Rostral tympanic artery
15. Middle meningeal artery
16. Caudal deep temporal artery
17. Rostral deep temporal artery
18. External ophthalmic artery
19. Third part of maxillary artery
20. Infraorbital artery
21. Descending palatine artery
22. Buccal artery (buccinator)
23. Infraorbital artery

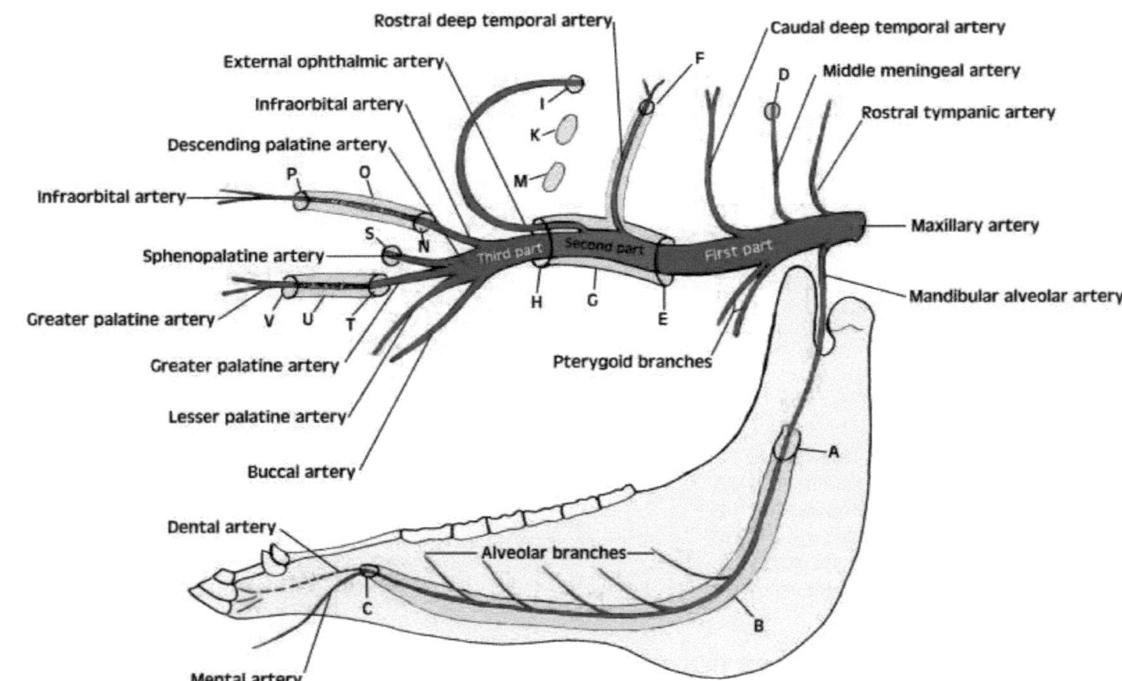

Fig.39. Branches of the maxillary artery, diagrammatic

Fig.39. Branches of the maxillary artery, diagrammatic

A. Mandibular foramen
B. Mandibular canal
C. Mental foramen
D. Foramen spinosum
E. Alar foramen
F. Small alar foramen
G. Alar canal
H. Round foramen
I. Ethmoidal foramen
K. Optic foramen
M. Orbital fissure
N. Maxillary foramen
O. Infraorbital canal
P. Infraorbital foramen
S. Sphenopalatine foramen
T. Greater palatine foramen
U. Greater palatine canal
V. Rostral palatine foramen

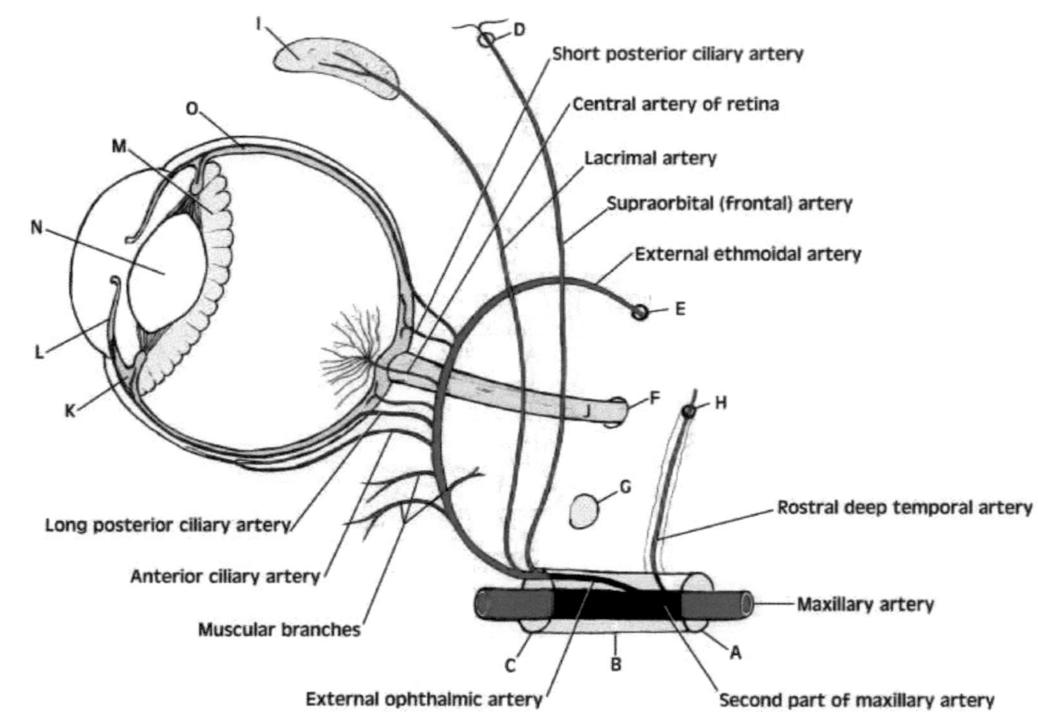

Fig.40. Branches of second part of maxillary artery , diagrammatic

Fig.40. Branches of second part of maxillary artery, diagrammatic

A. Alar foramen
B. Alar canal
C. Round foramen
D. Supraorbital foramen
E. Ethmoidal foramen
F. Optic foramen
G. Orbital fissure
H. Small alar foramen
I. Lacrimal gland
J. Optic nerve
K. Ciliary body
L. Iris
M. Ciliary processes
N. Lens
O. Choroid

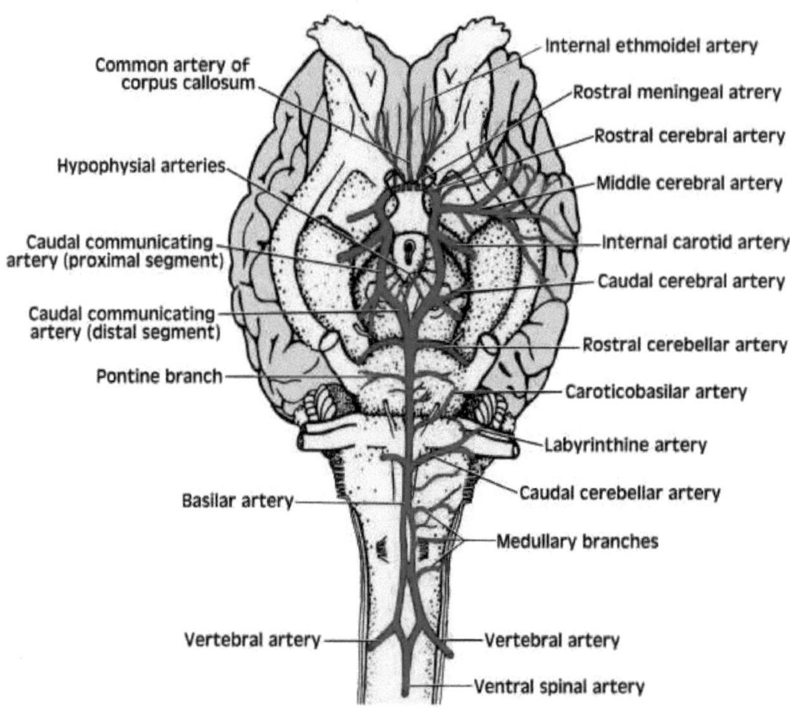

Fig.41. Arteries of brain , ventral view

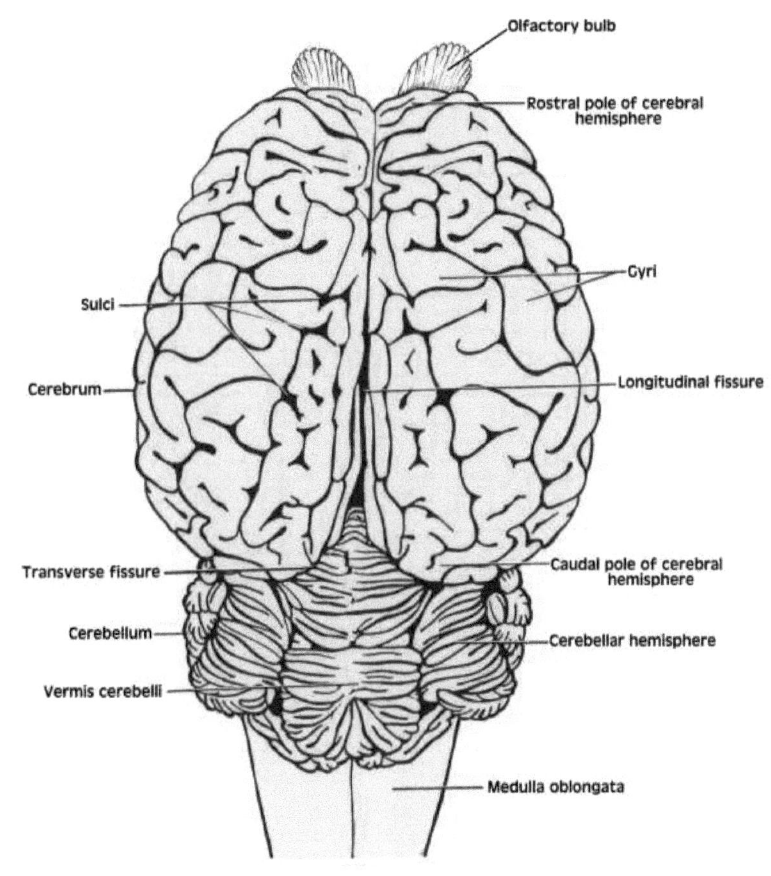

Fig.42. Brain , dorsal view

53

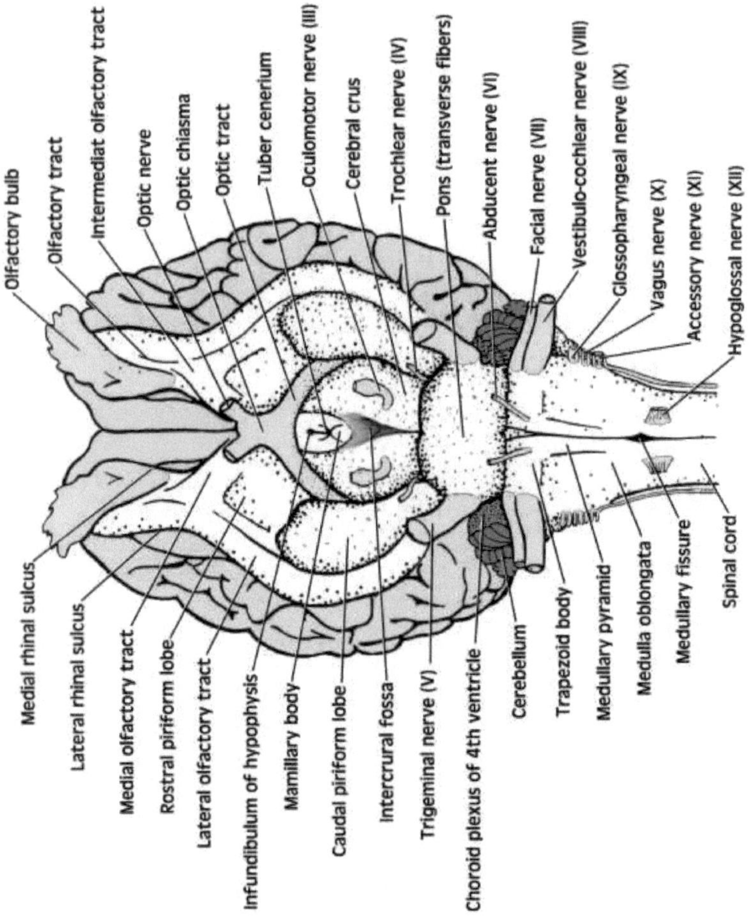

Olfactory bulb
Olfactory tract
Intermediat olfactory tract
Optic nerve
Optic chiasma
Optic tract
Tuber cenerium
Oculomotor nerve (III)
Cerebral crus
Trochlear nerve (IV)
Pons (transverse fibers)
Abducent nerve (VI)
Facial nerve (VII)
Vestibulo-cochlear nerve (VIII)
Glossopharyngeal nerve (IX)
Vagus nerve (X)
Accessory nerve (XI)
Hypoglossal nerve (XII)

Medial rhinal sulcus
Lateral rhinal sulcus
Medial olfactory tract
Rostral piriform lobe
Lateral olfactory tract
Infundibulum of hypophysis
Mamillary body
Caudal piriform lobe
Intercrural fossa
Trigeminal nerve (V)
Choroid plexus of 4th ventricle
Cerebellum
Trapezoid body
Medullary pyramid
Medulla oblongata
Medullary fissure
Spinal cord

Fig. 43. Brain, ventral view

54

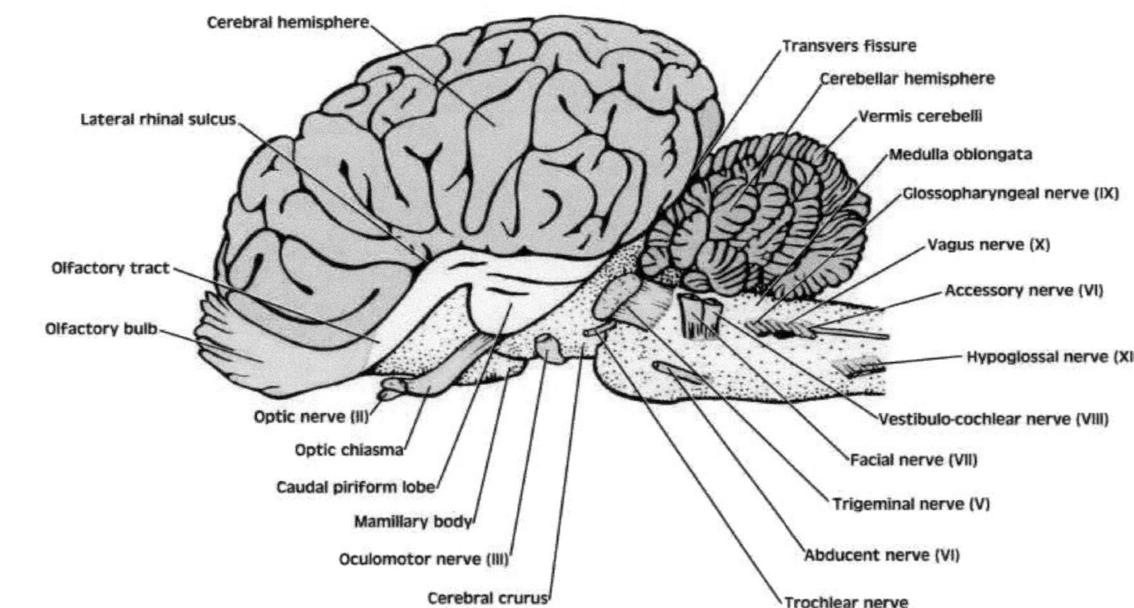

Fig.44. Brain , lateral view

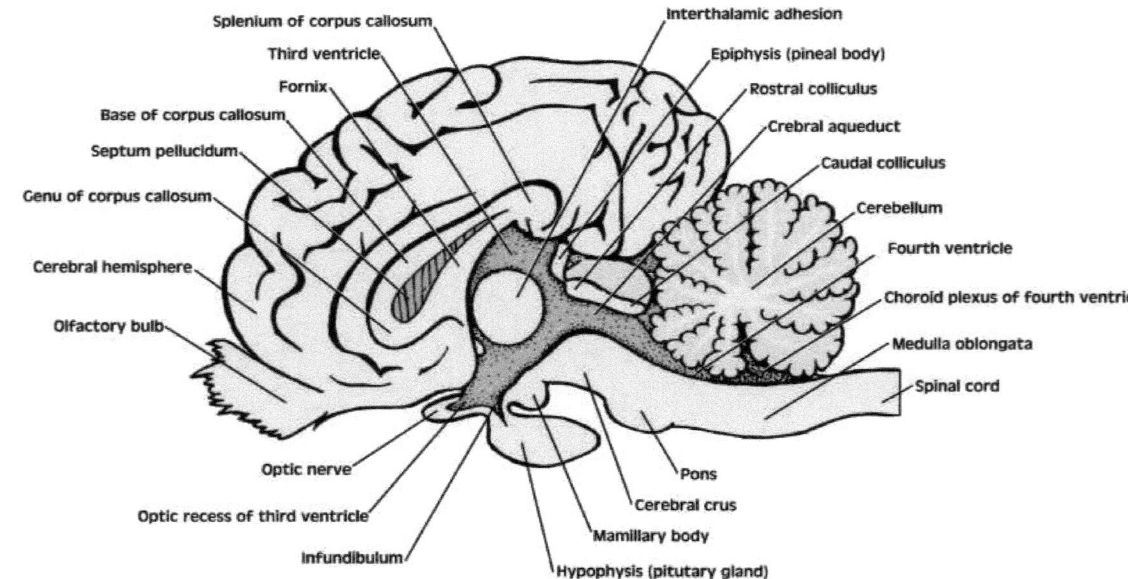

Fig. 45. Midsagittal section of brain

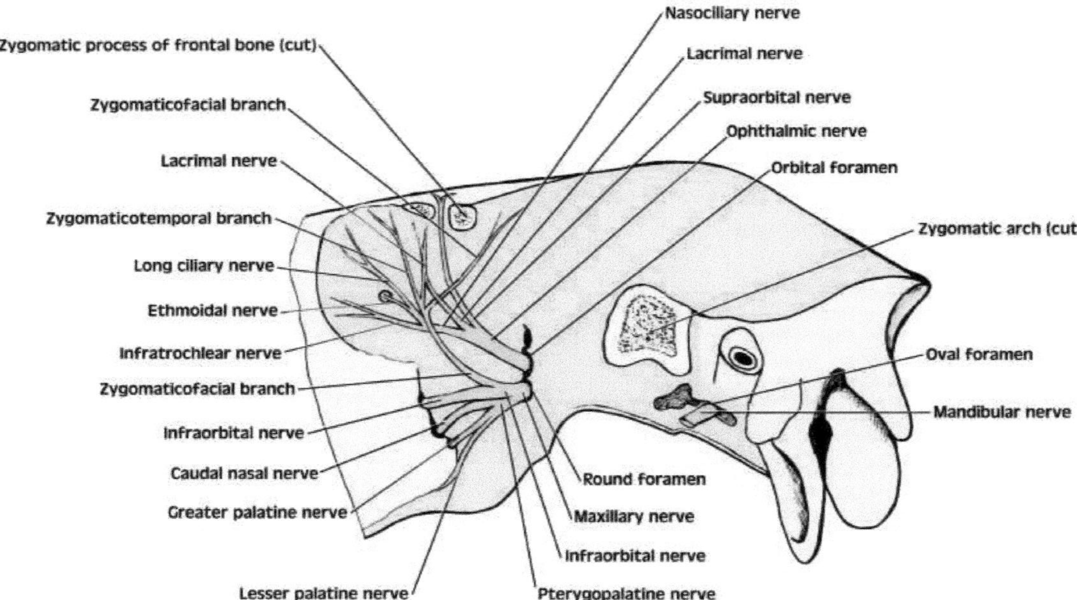

Fig.46. Trigeminal nerve (ophthalmic and maxillary nerves)

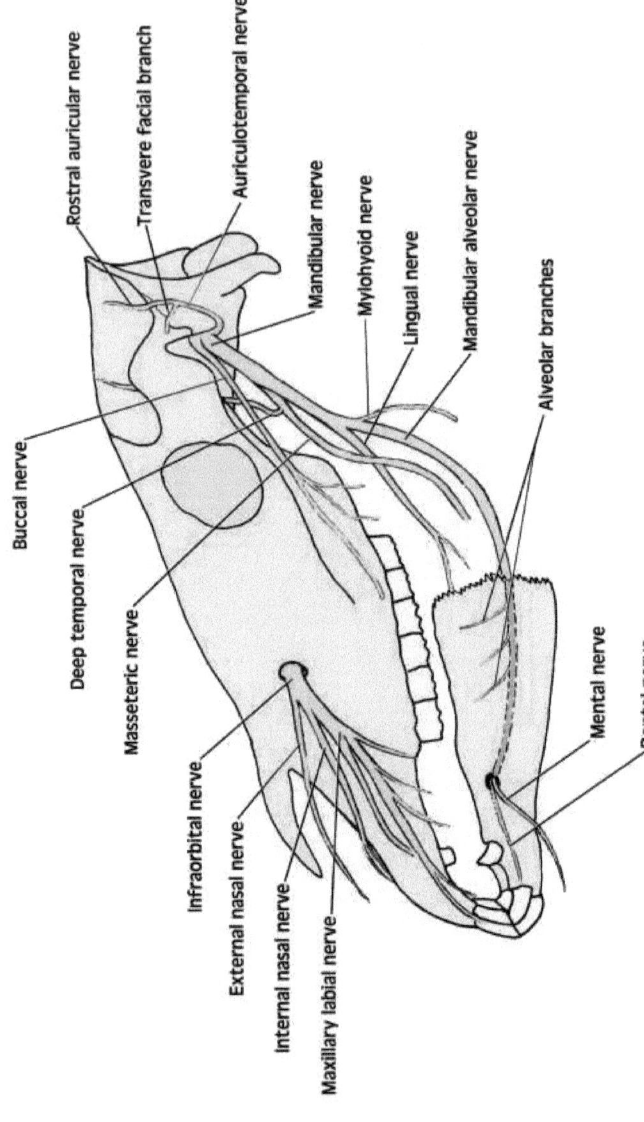

Fig.47. Mandibular and infraorbital nerves

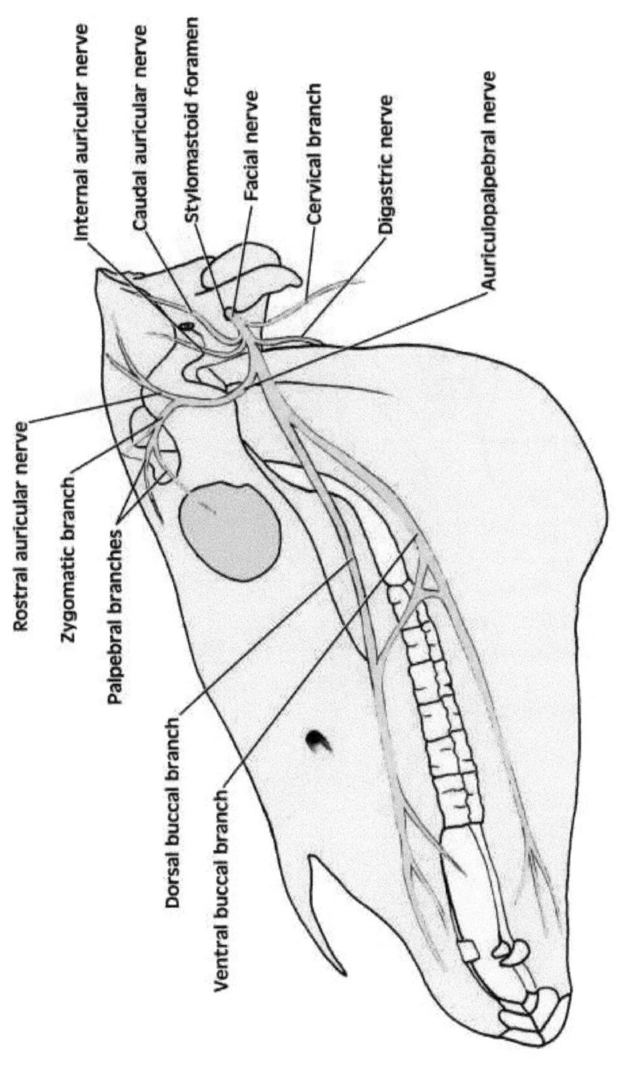

Fig.48. Facial nerve (extracanalicular part)

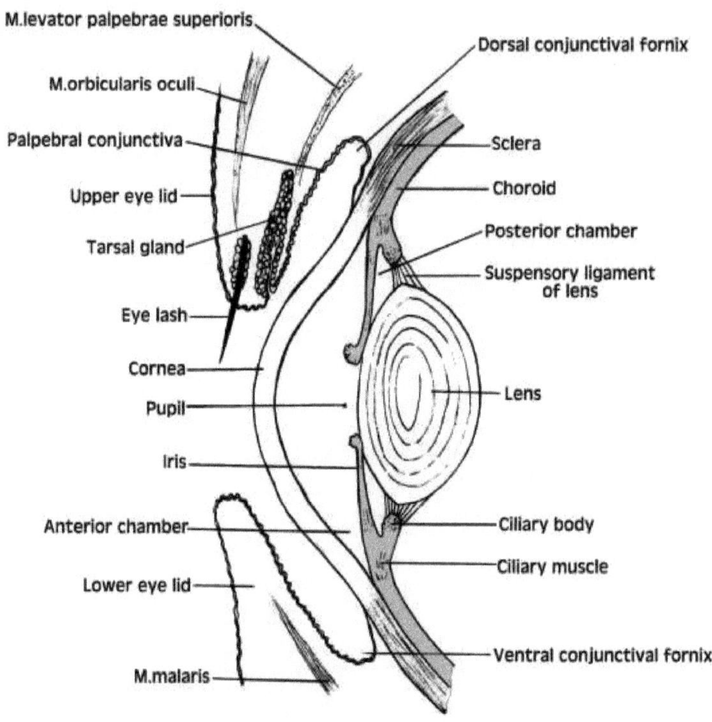

Fig.49. Eye lids and anterior part of eye ball

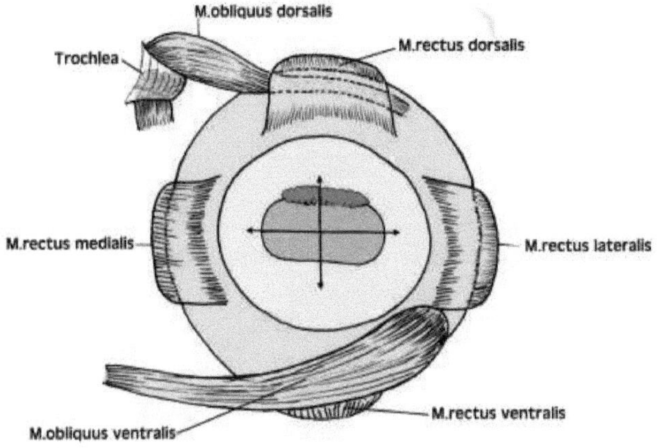

Cranial view

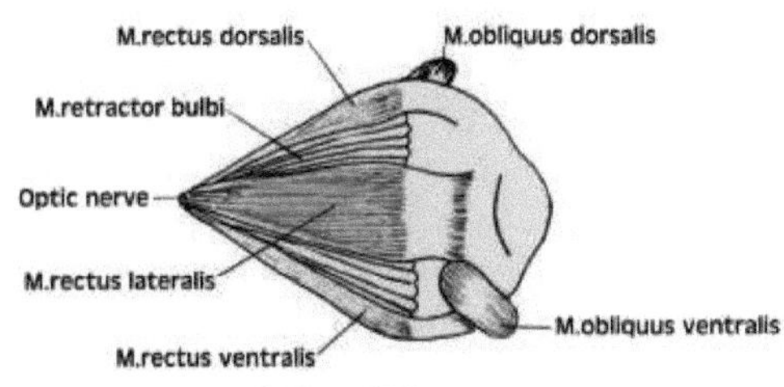

Lateral view

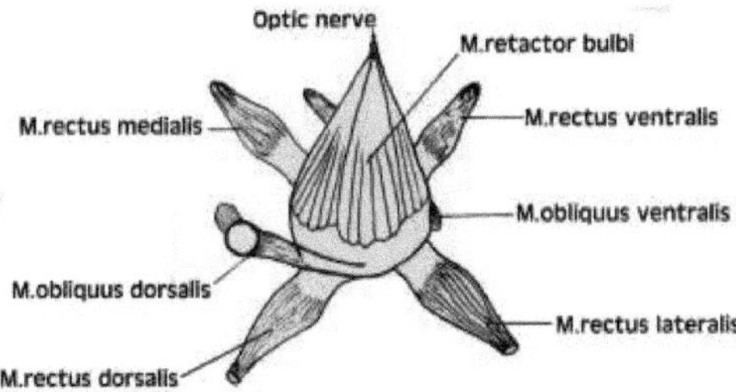

Caudodorsal view

Fig.50. Muscles of the eye ball

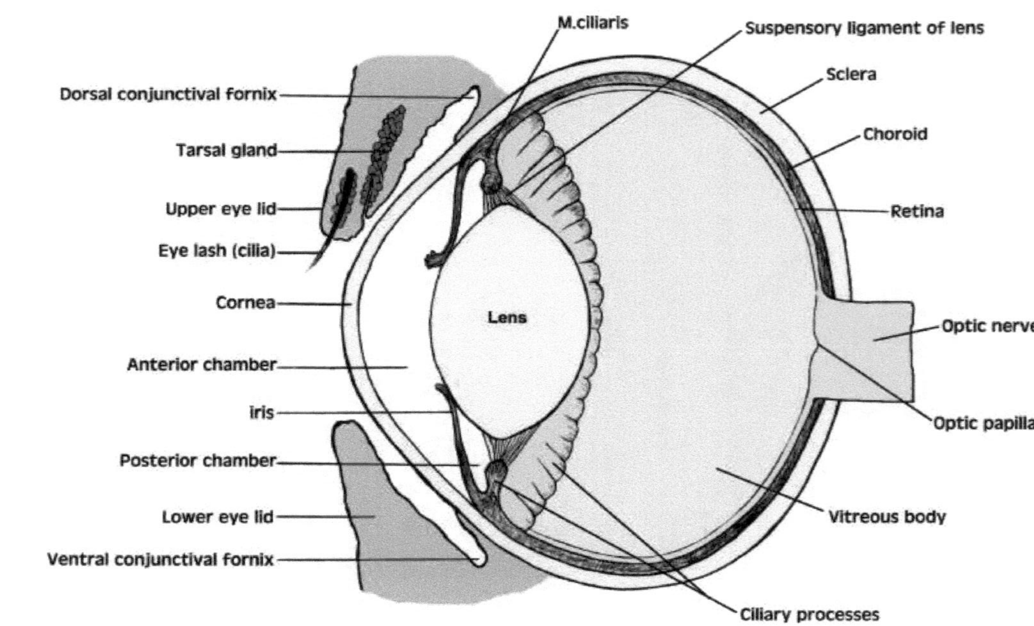

Fig.51. Sagittal section in the eye ; diagrammatic

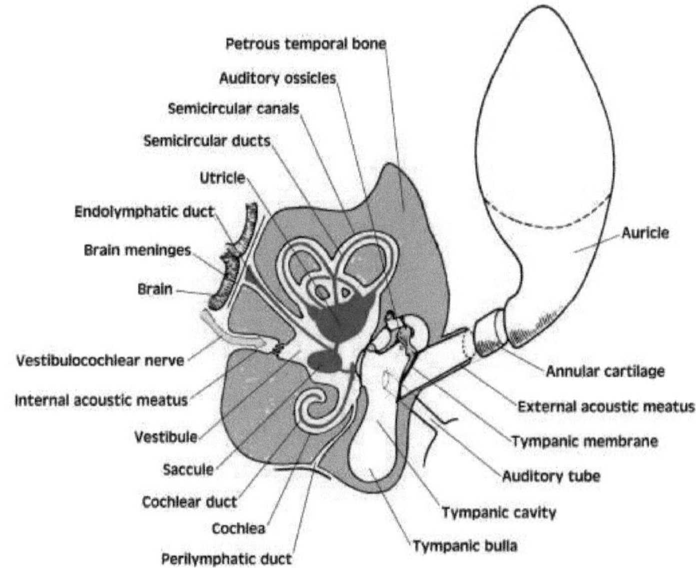

Fig.52. Right ear , caudal view ; diagrammatic

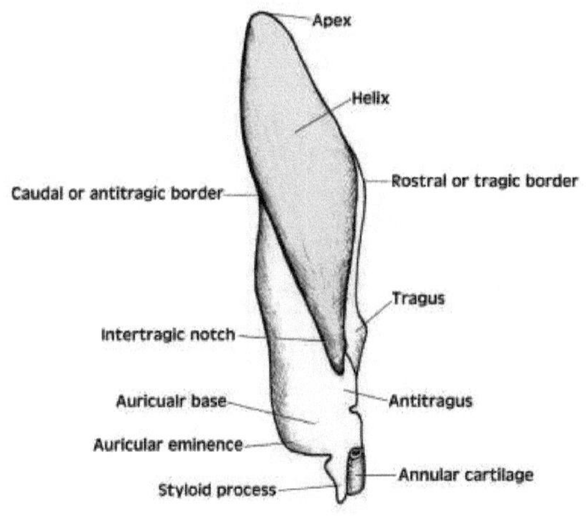

Fig.53. Right auricular cartilage

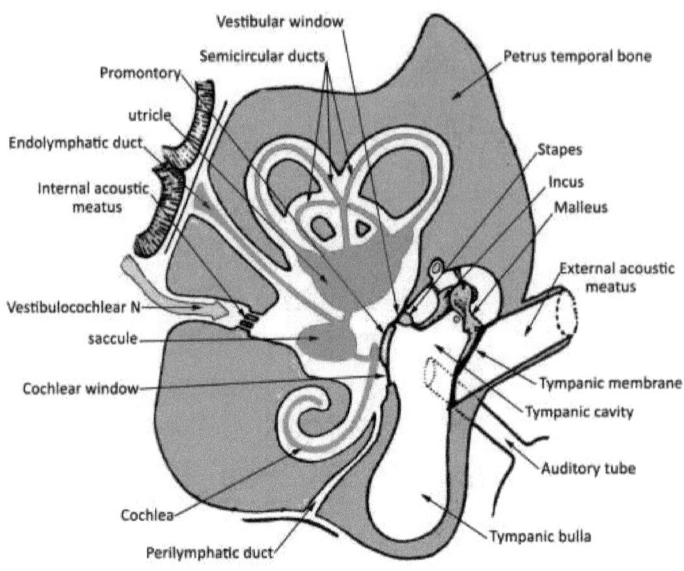

Fig.54. Osseous and membranous labyrinthes of internal ear

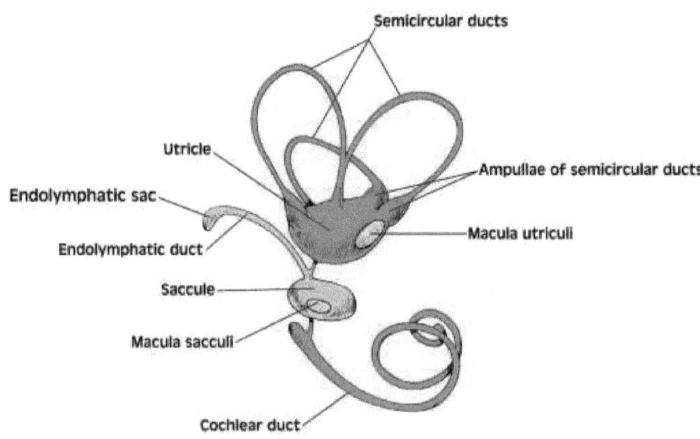

Fig.55. Membranous labyrinth of internal ear

64

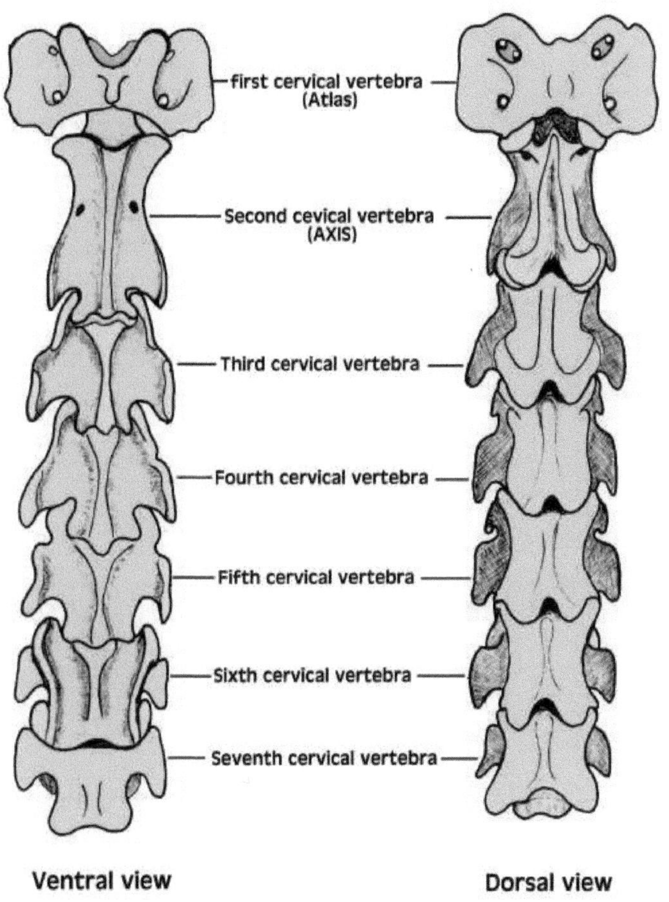

Fig.56. Cervical vertebrae

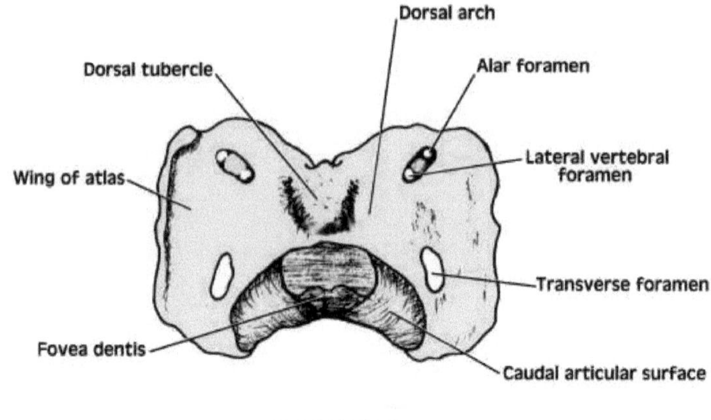

Dorsal view

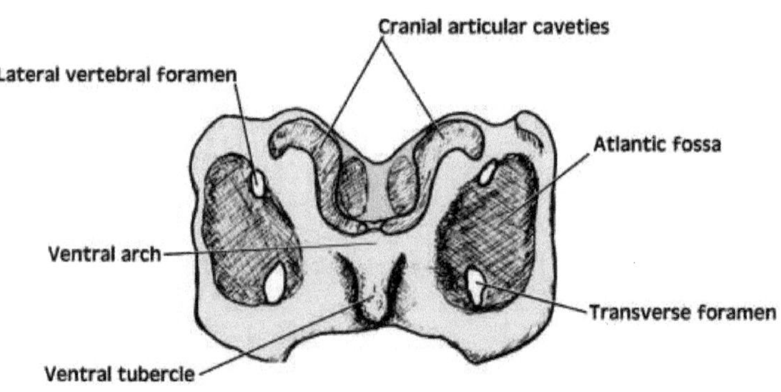

Ventral view

Fig.57.Atlas (first cervical vertebra)

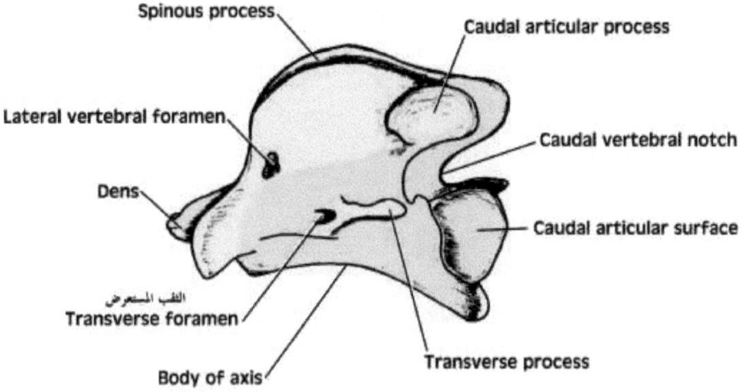

Caudo-lateral view

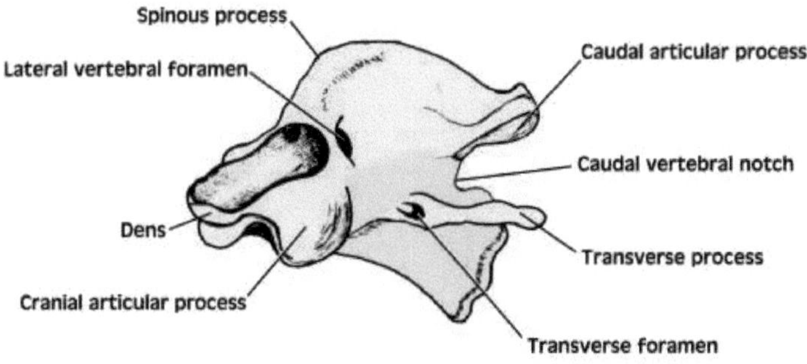

Cranio-lateral view

Fig.58. Axis (second cevical vertebra)

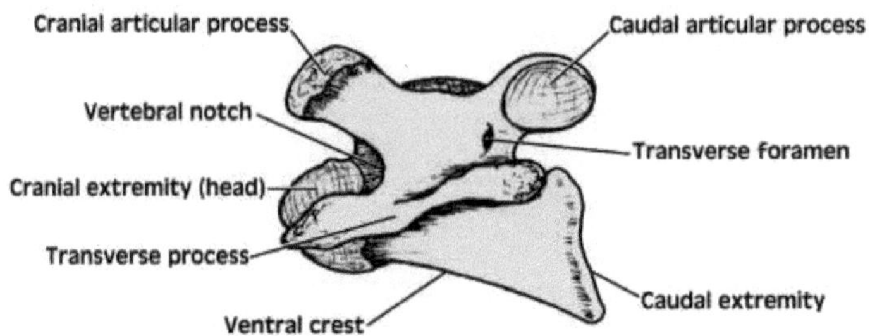

Fig.59. Third cervical vertebra, left view

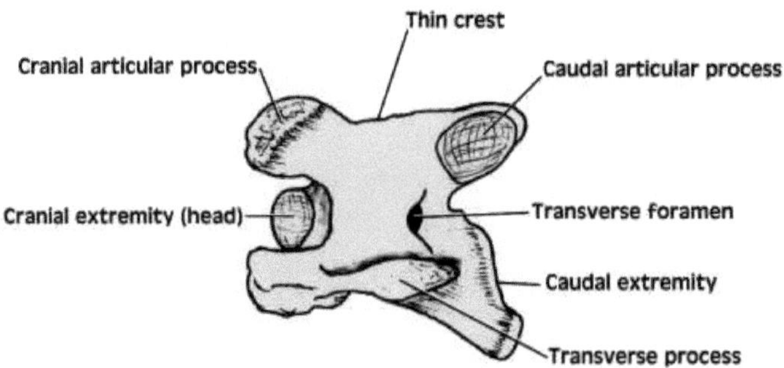

Fig.60. Fourth or fifth cervical vertebra , left view

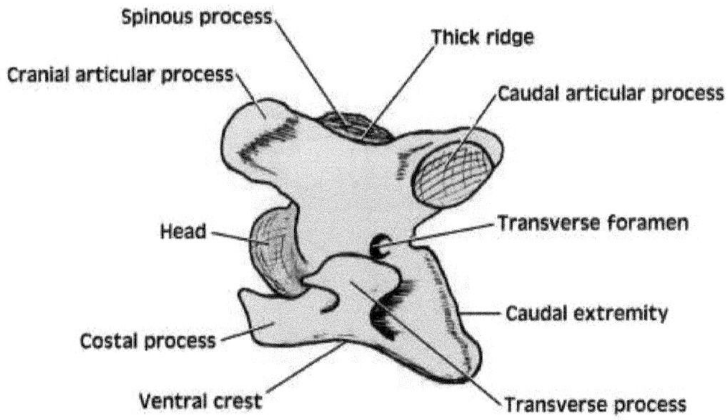

Fig.61. Sixth cervical vertebra, left lateral view

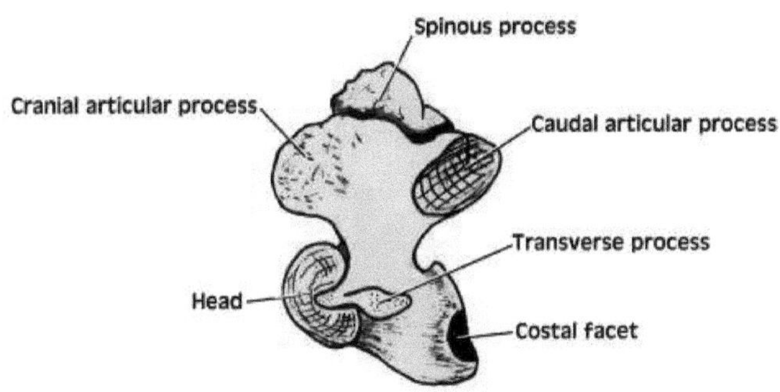

Fig.62. Seventh cervical vertebra, left lateral view

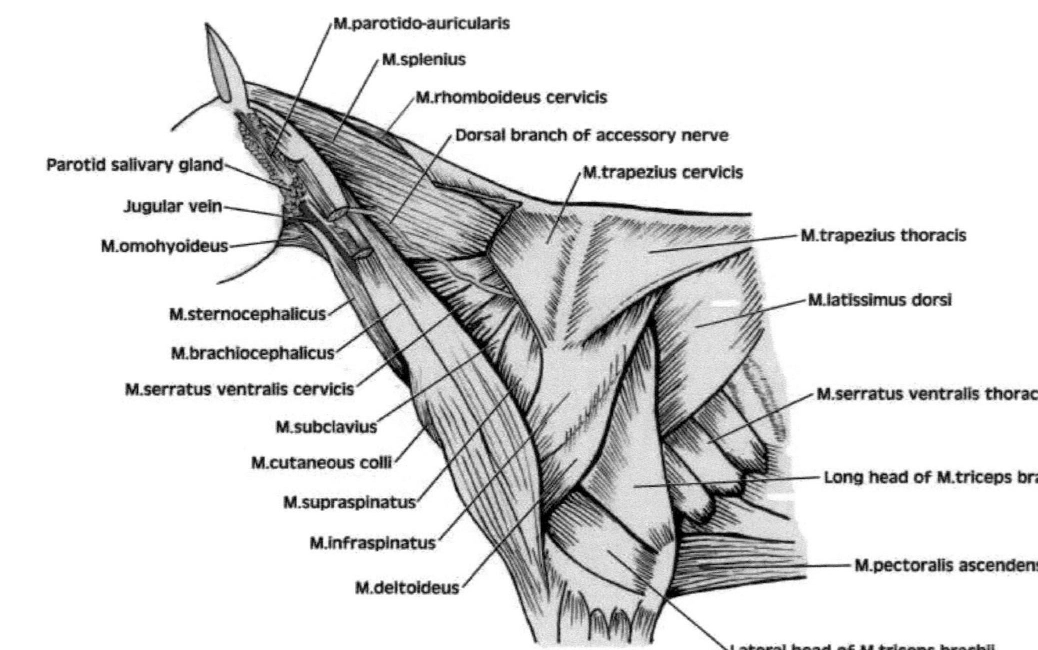

Fig.63. Dissection of the neck, superficial layer ; left lateral view

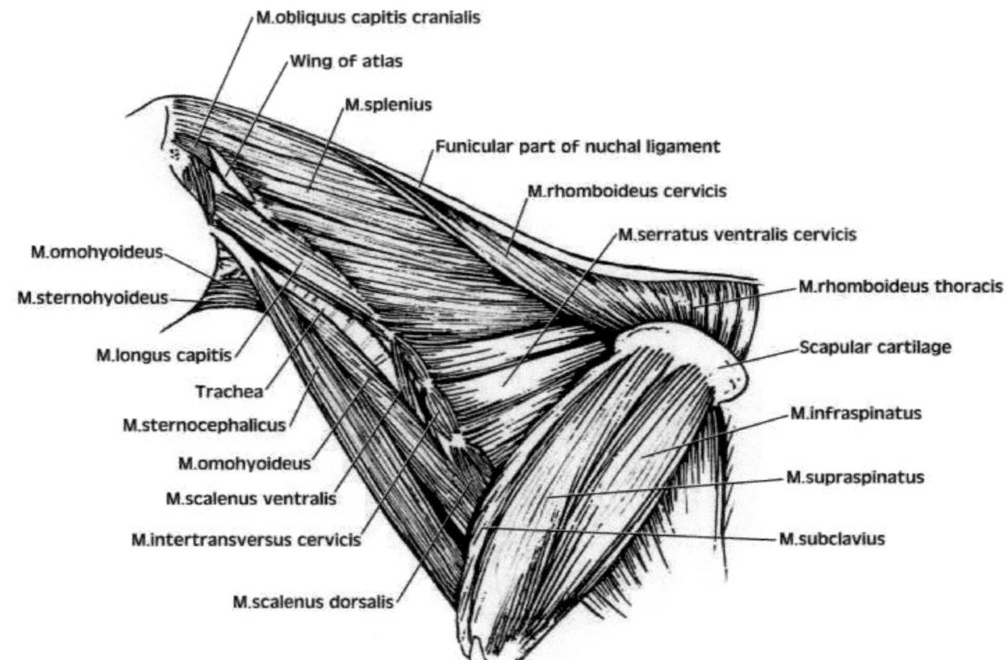

Fig.64. Dissection of neck, second layer ; lateral view

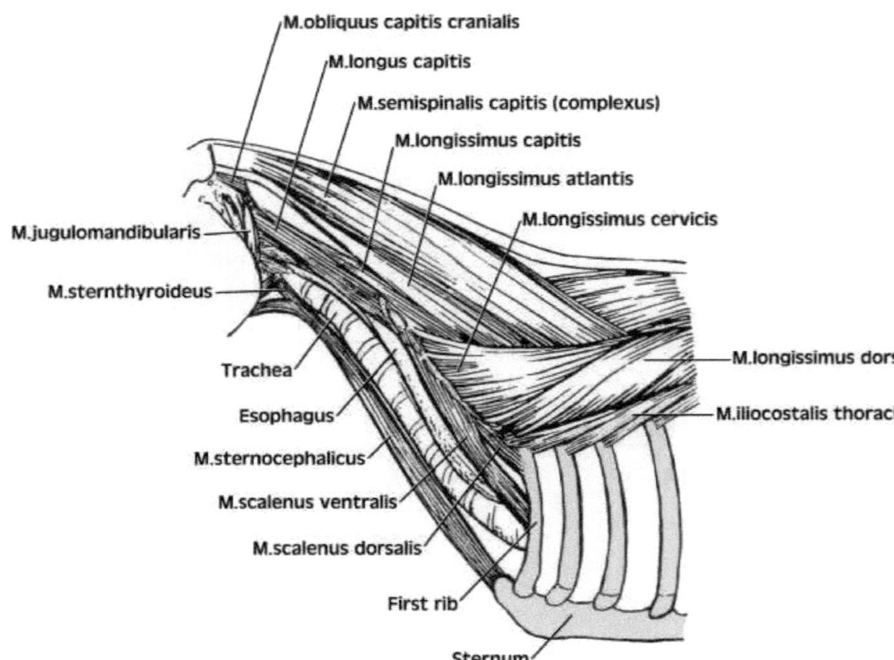

Fig.65. Dissection of neck, third layer ; lateral view

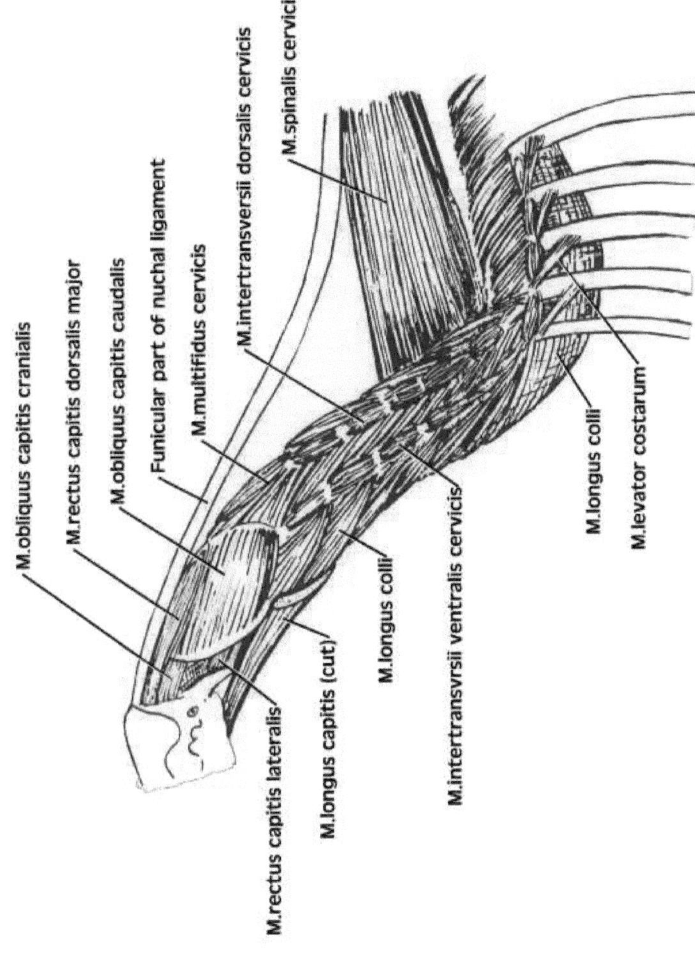

Fig.66. Dissection of neck, the deepest layer

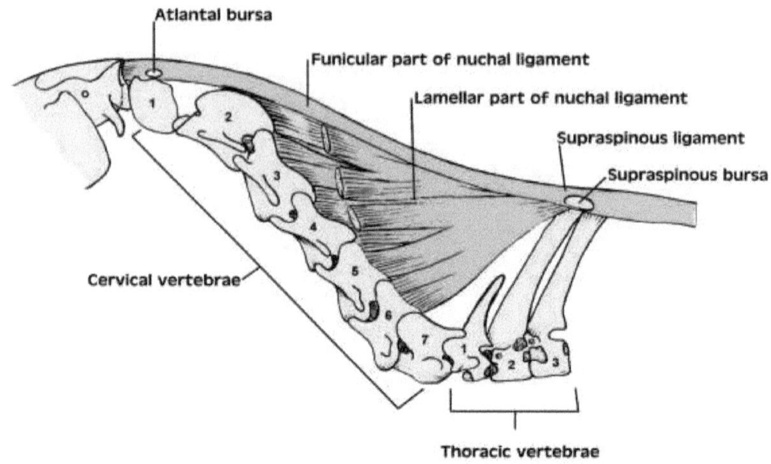

Fig.67. Nuchal ligament

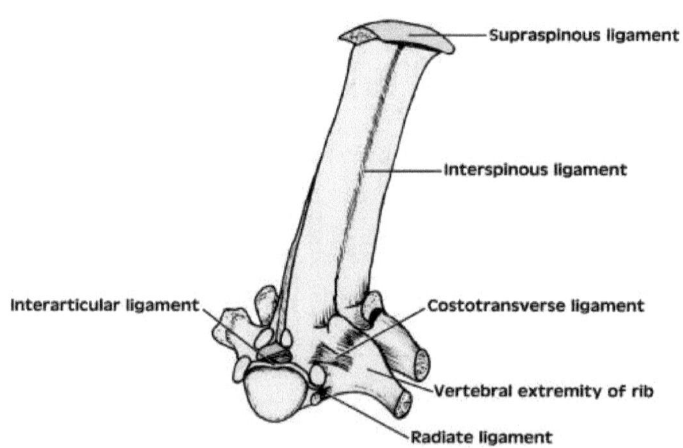

Fig.68. Costovertebral articulation

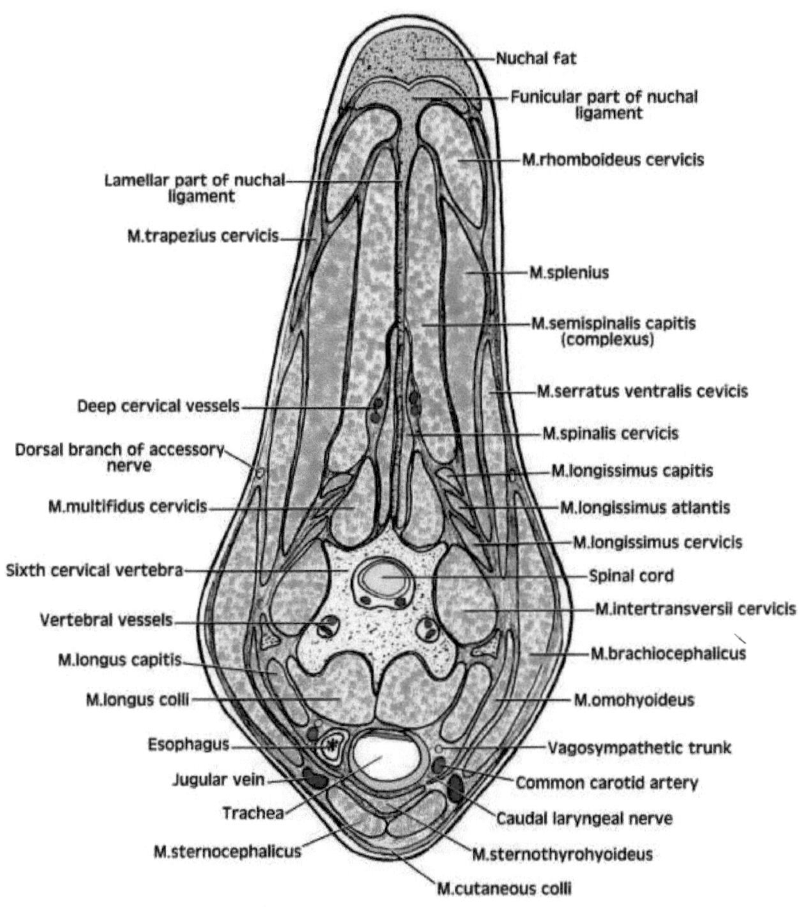

Fig.69. Cross section of neck passing through the sixth cervical vertebra

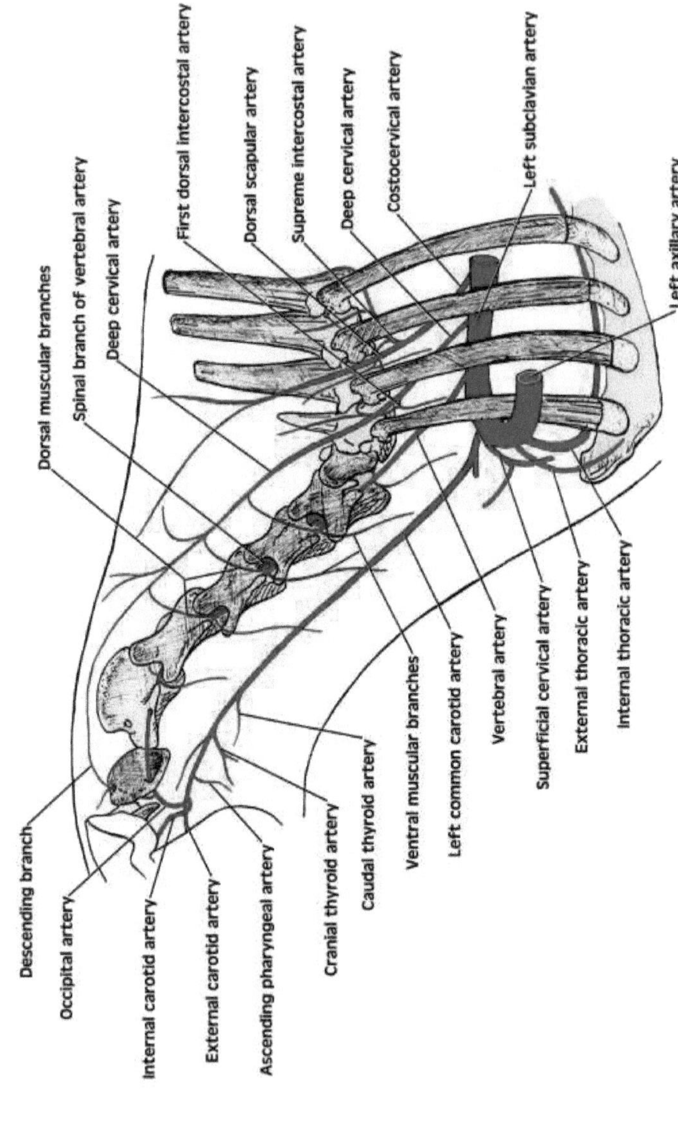

Fig.70. Arteries of neck and cranial part of thoracic wall

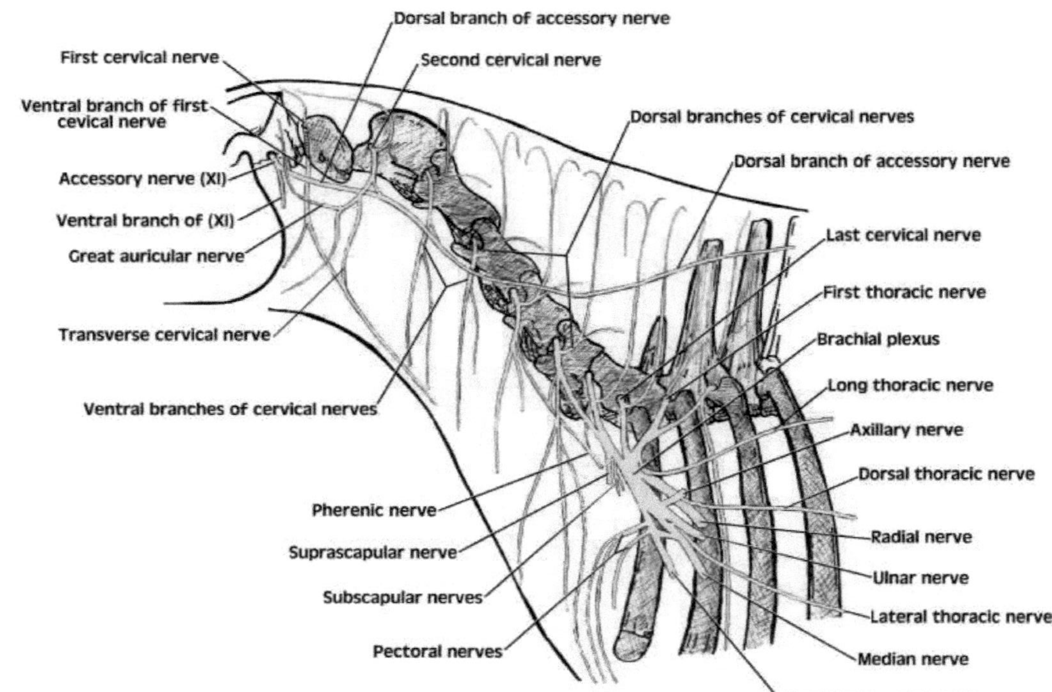

Fig.71. Cervical nerves and brachial plexus, diagrammatic

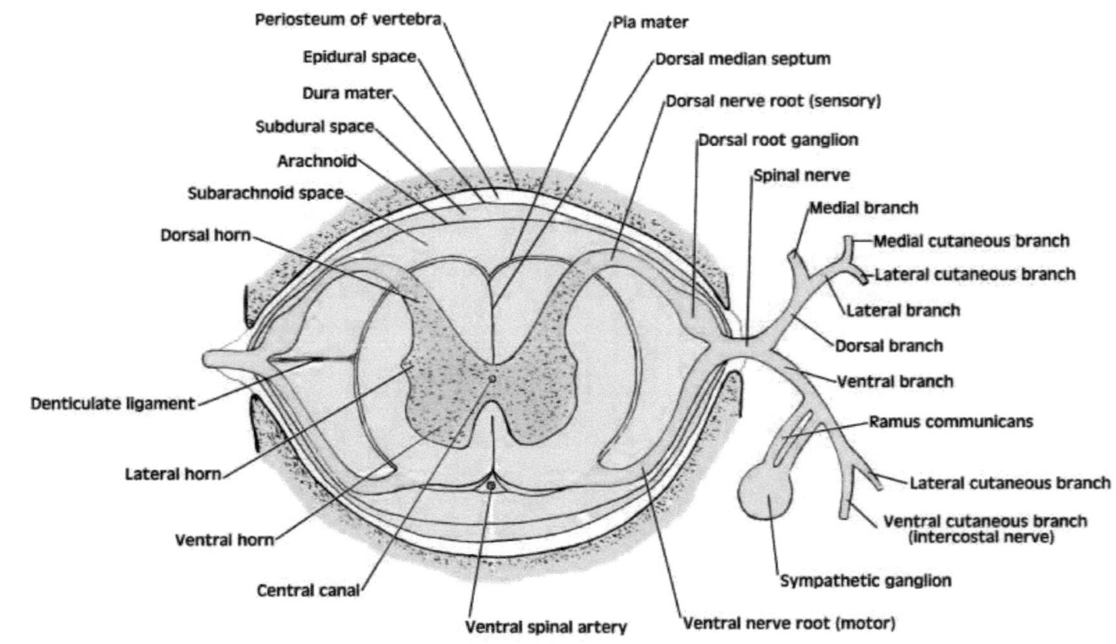

Fig.71 : .Spinal cord and spinal meninges, diagrammatic

Chapter 3
Thorax, Abdomen and Pelvis

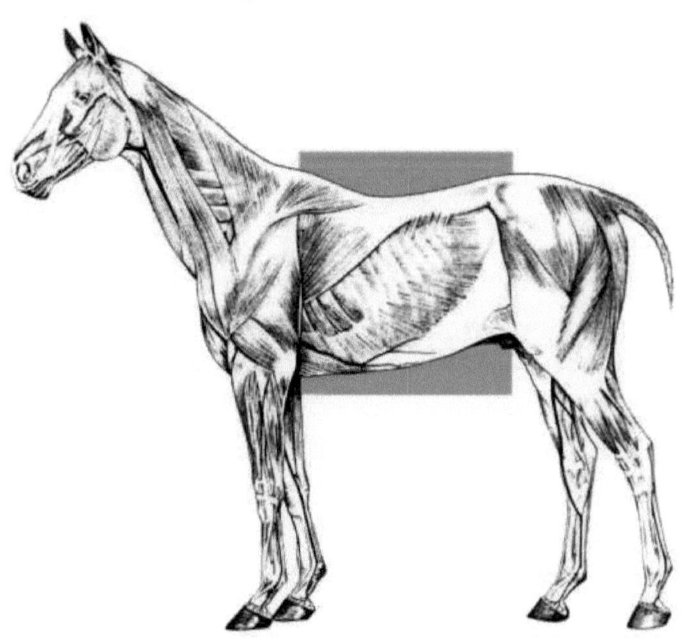

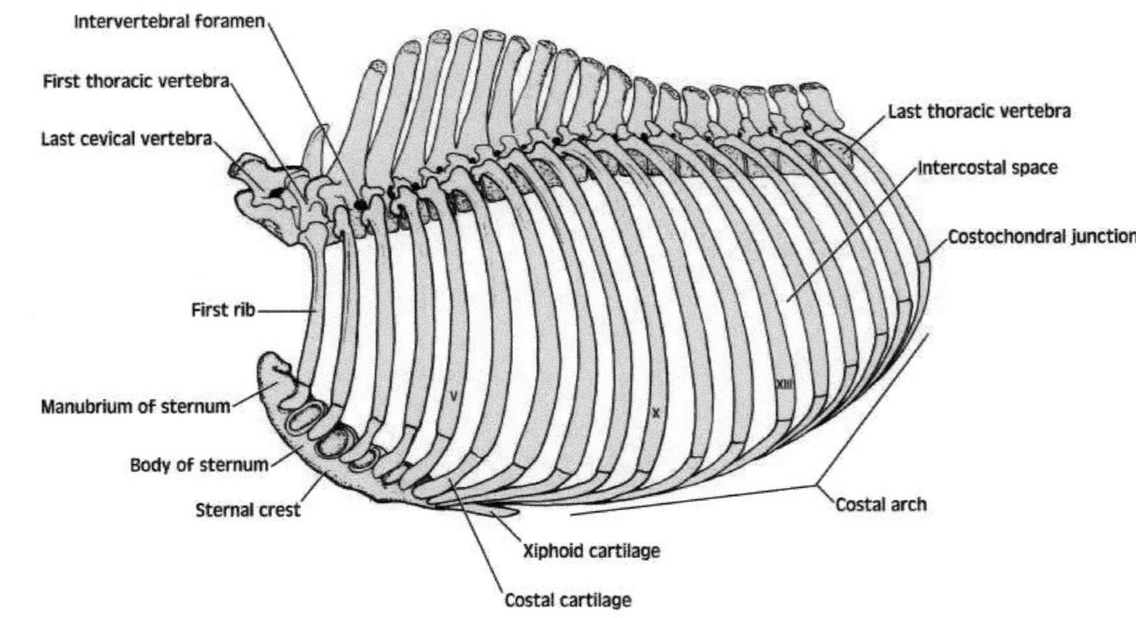

Fig.72. Bony thorax, left lateral view

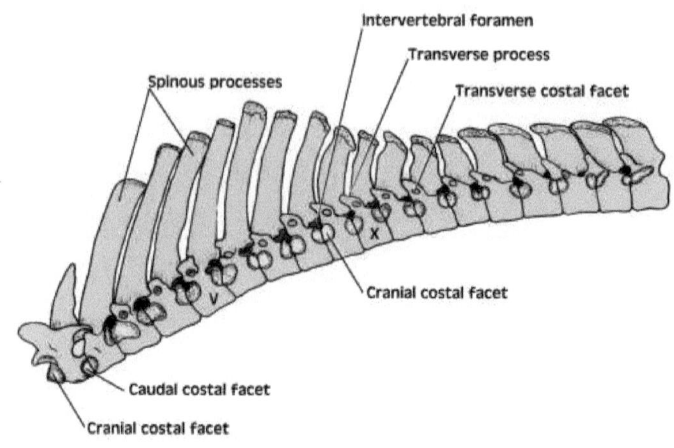

Thoracic vertebrae , lateral view

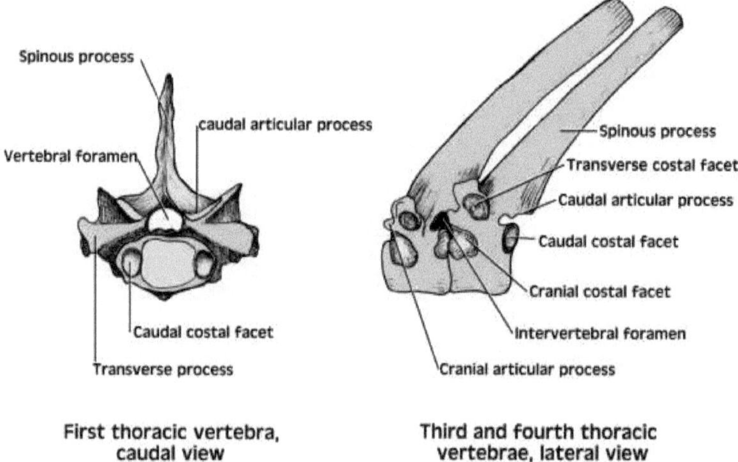

First thoracic vertebra,
caudal view

Third and fourth thoracic
vertebrae, lateral view

Fig.73. Thoracic vertebrae

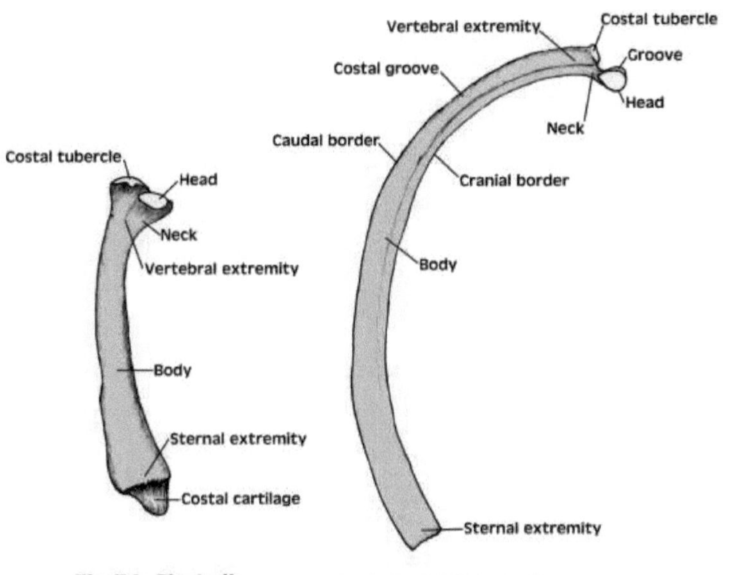

Fig.74. First rib,
medial view

Fig.75. Right seventh rib,
medial view

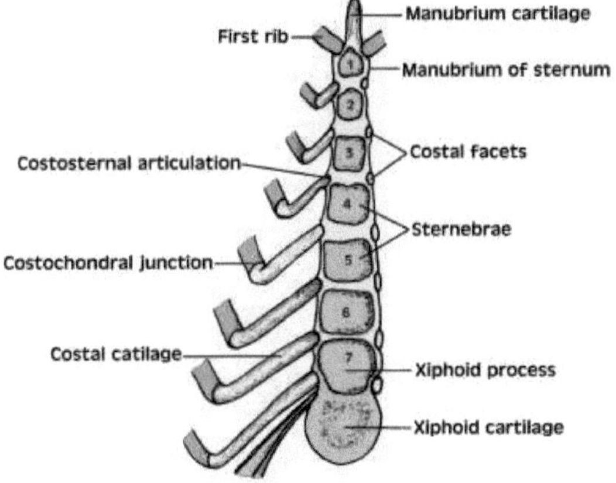

Fig.76. Sternum and costal catilages , dorsal view

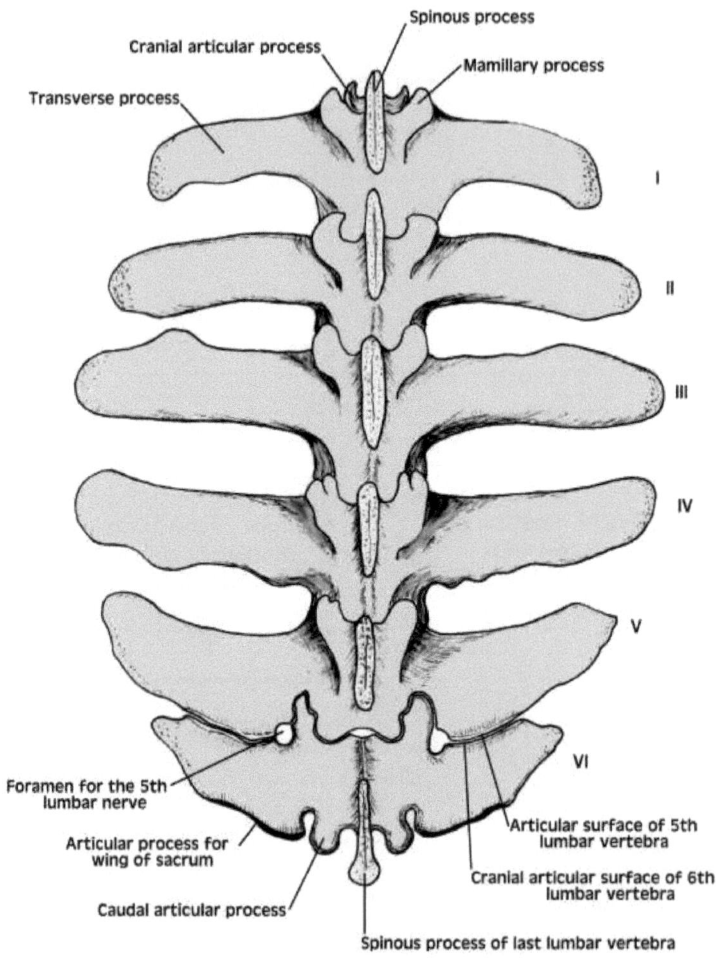

Fig.77. Lumbar vertebrae, dorsal view

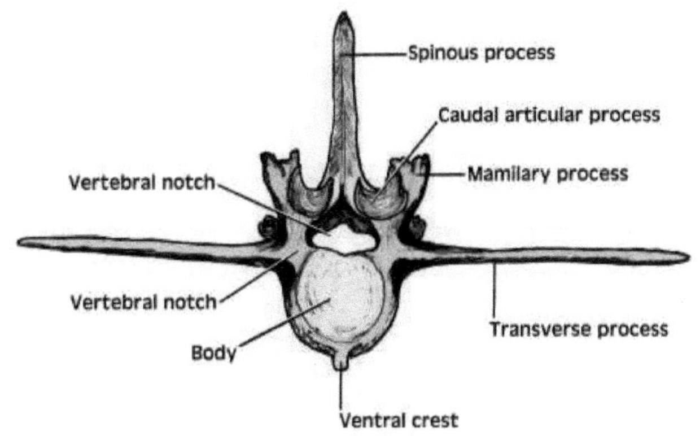

Second lumbar vertebra , caudal view

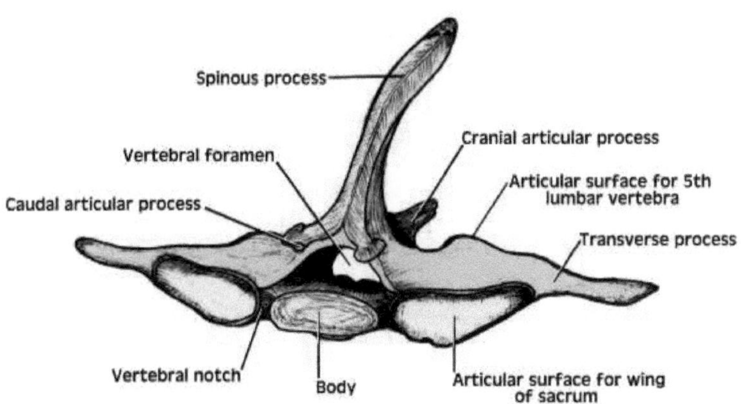

Last lumbar vertebra , caudal view

Fig.78. Lumbar vertebrae

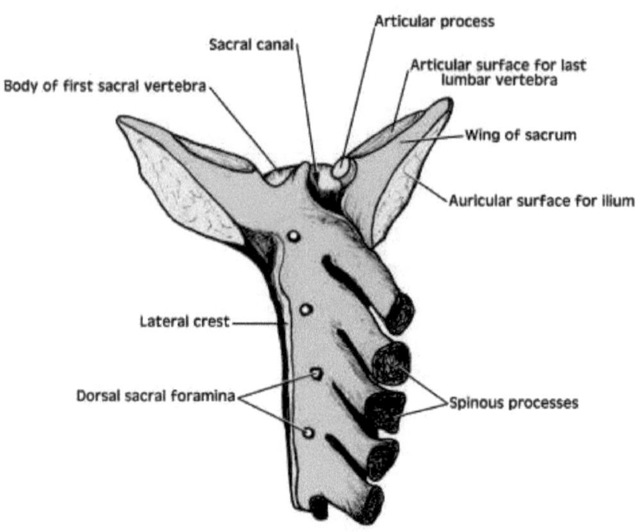

Sacrum , dorsolateral view

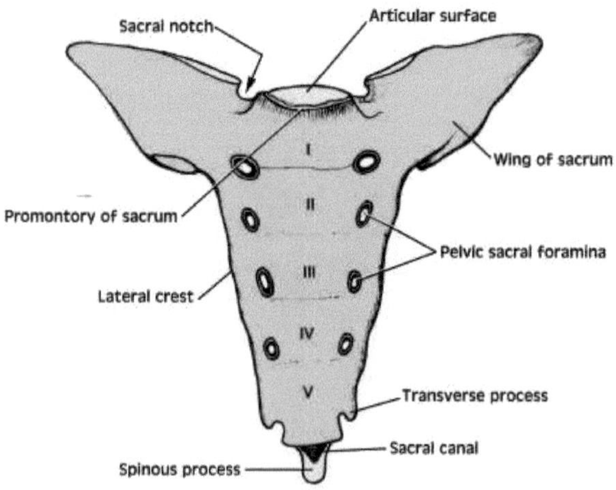

Sacrum , ventral view

Fig.79. Sacrum

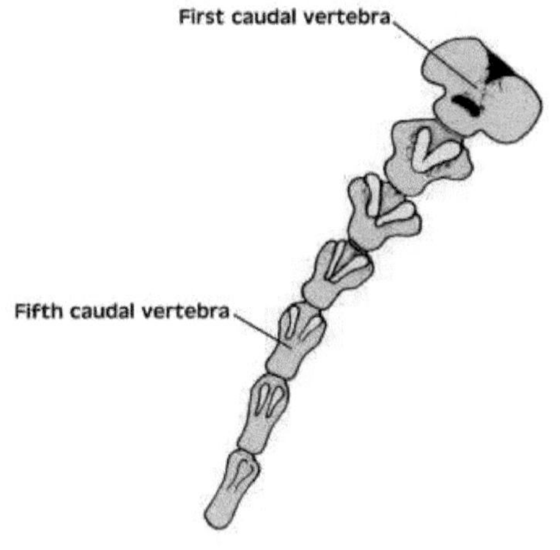

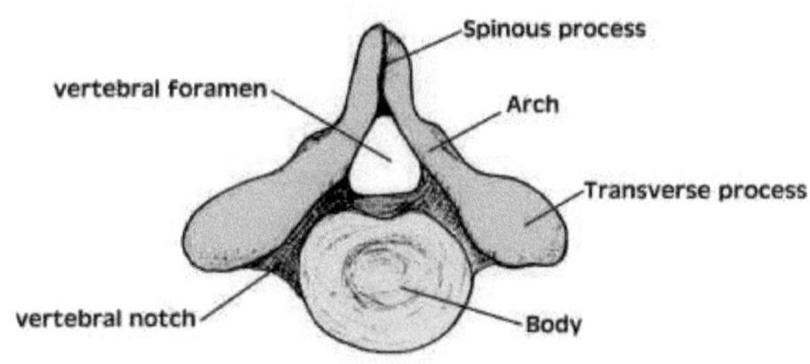

First caudal vertebra, caudal view

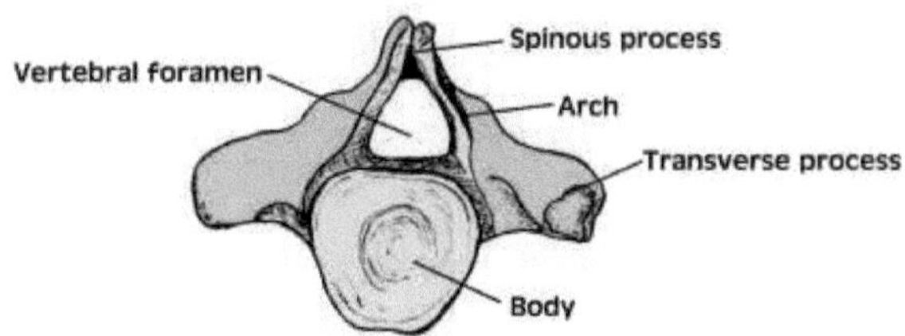

Second caudal vertebra, caudal view

Fig.80. Caudal vertebrae

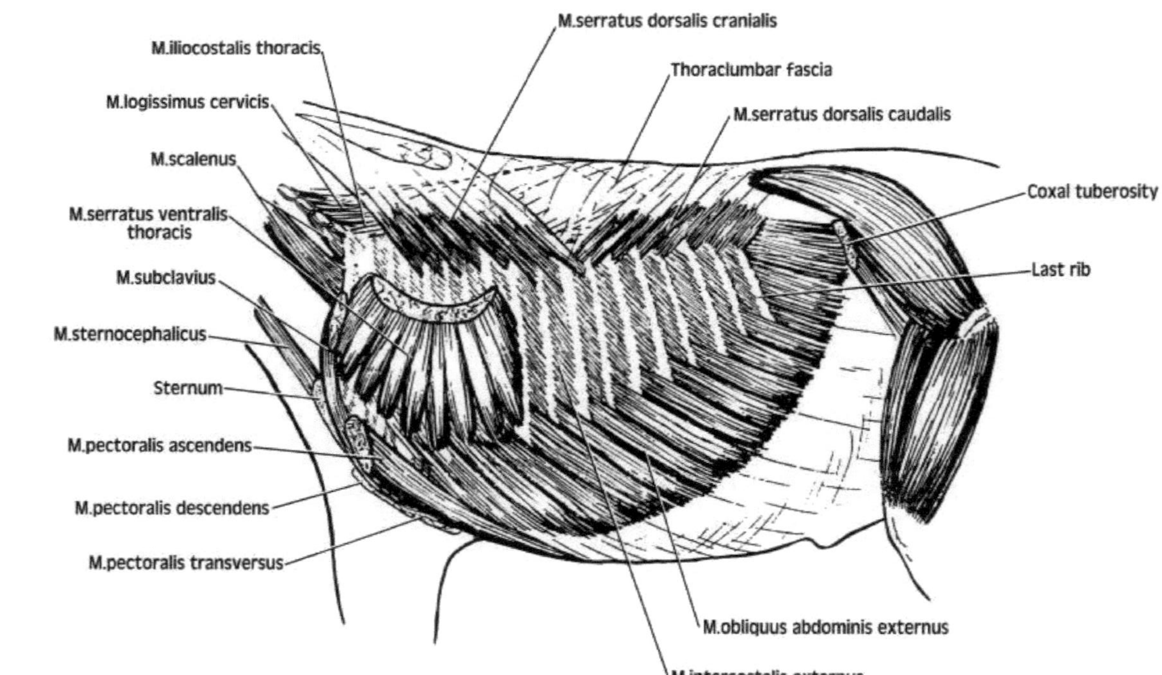

Fig.81.Superficial dissection of thoracic and abdominal walls
(after removal of thoracic limb)

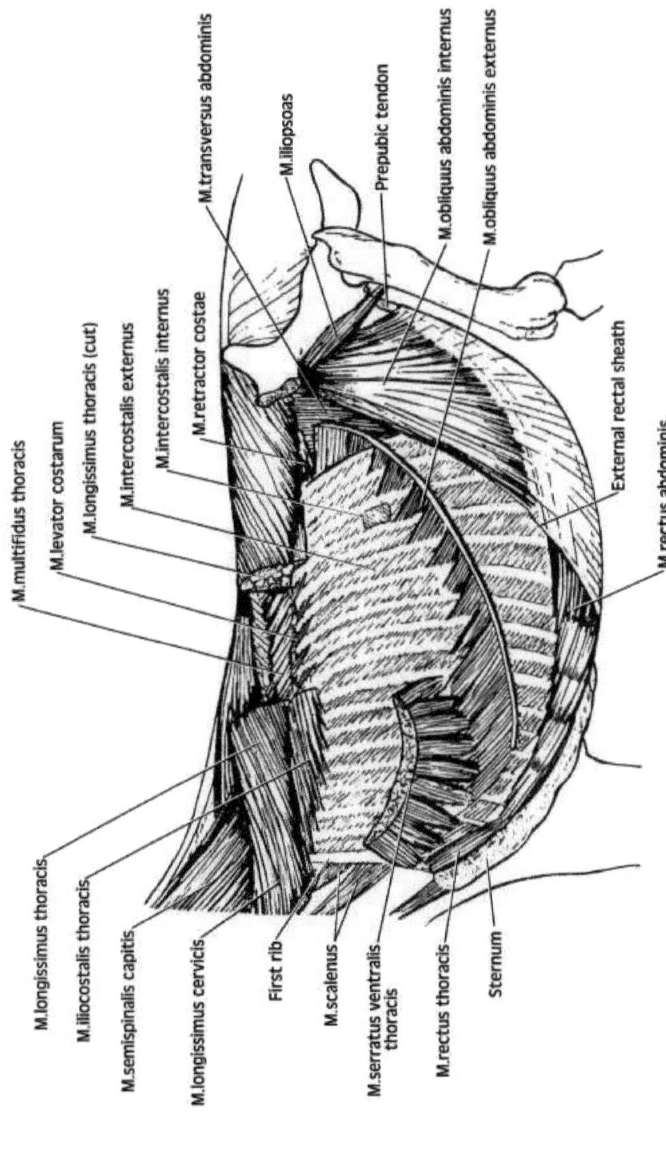

Fig.82. Deep dissection of thoracic and abdominal walls

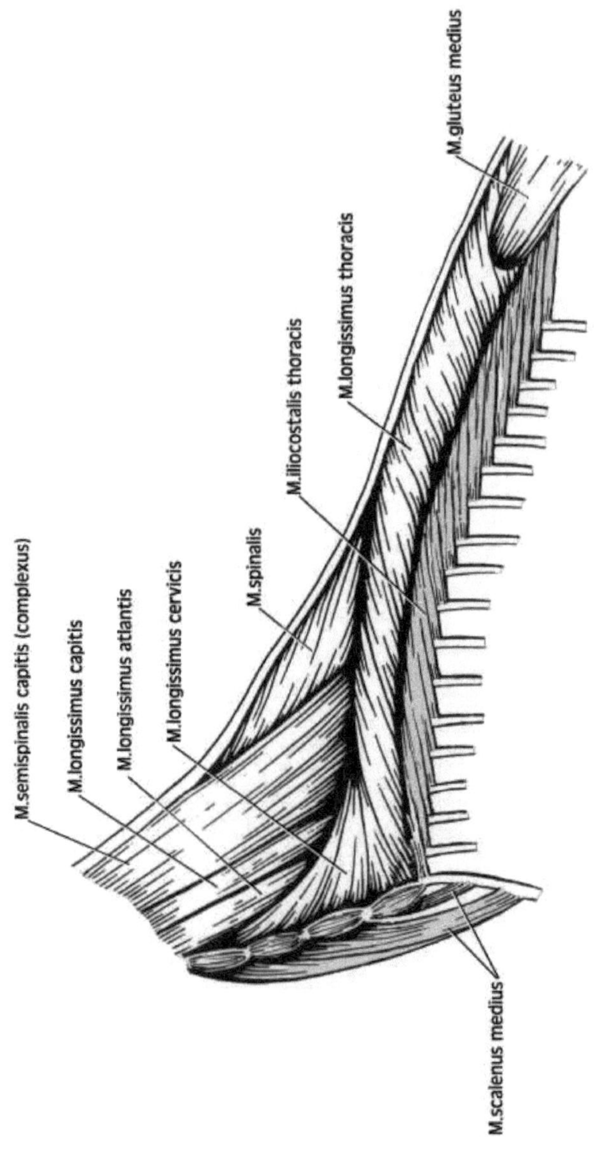

Fig.83. Muscles of back and loins , left lateral view

90

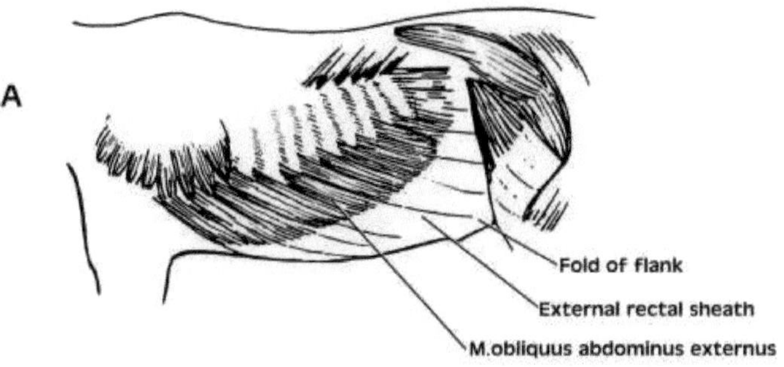

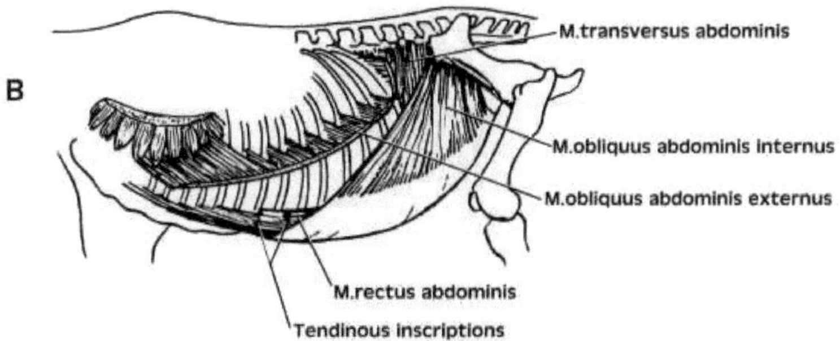

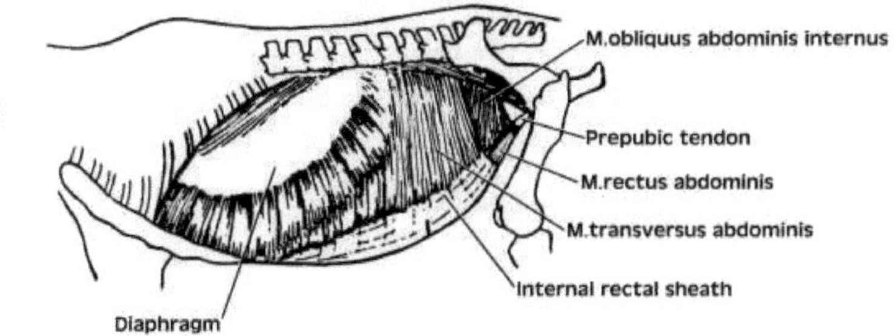

Fig.84. Abdominal muscles

91

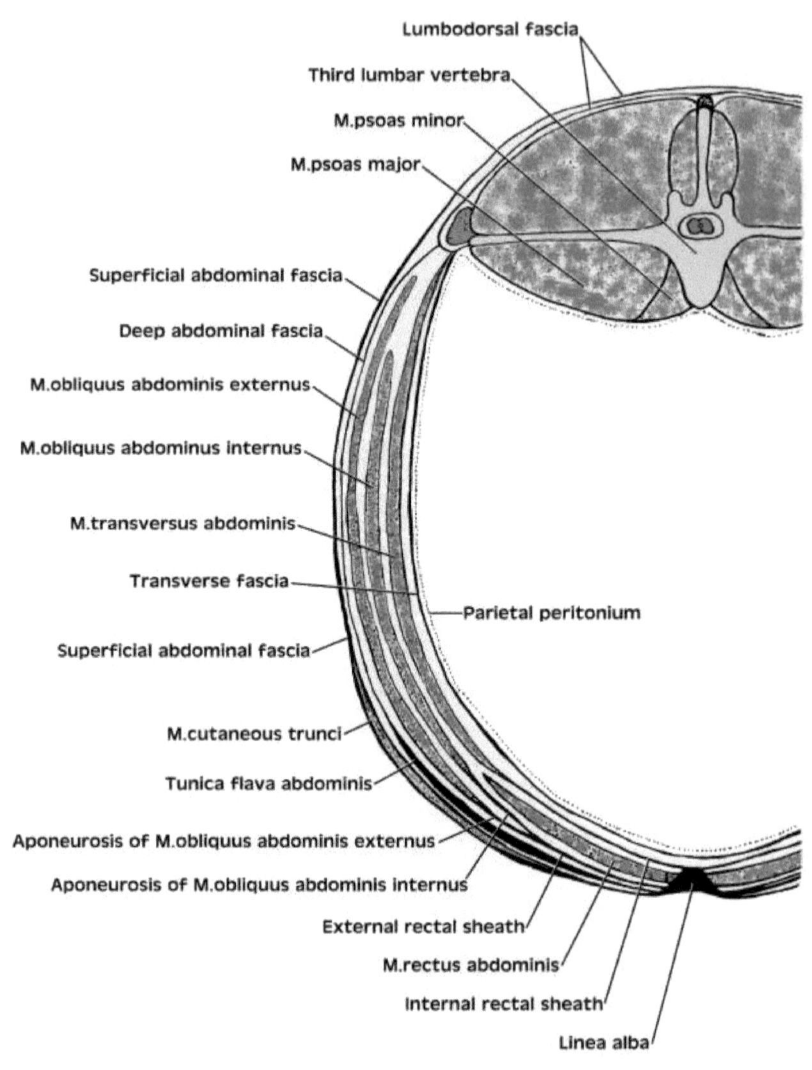

Fig.85. Cross section in the abdomenal wall

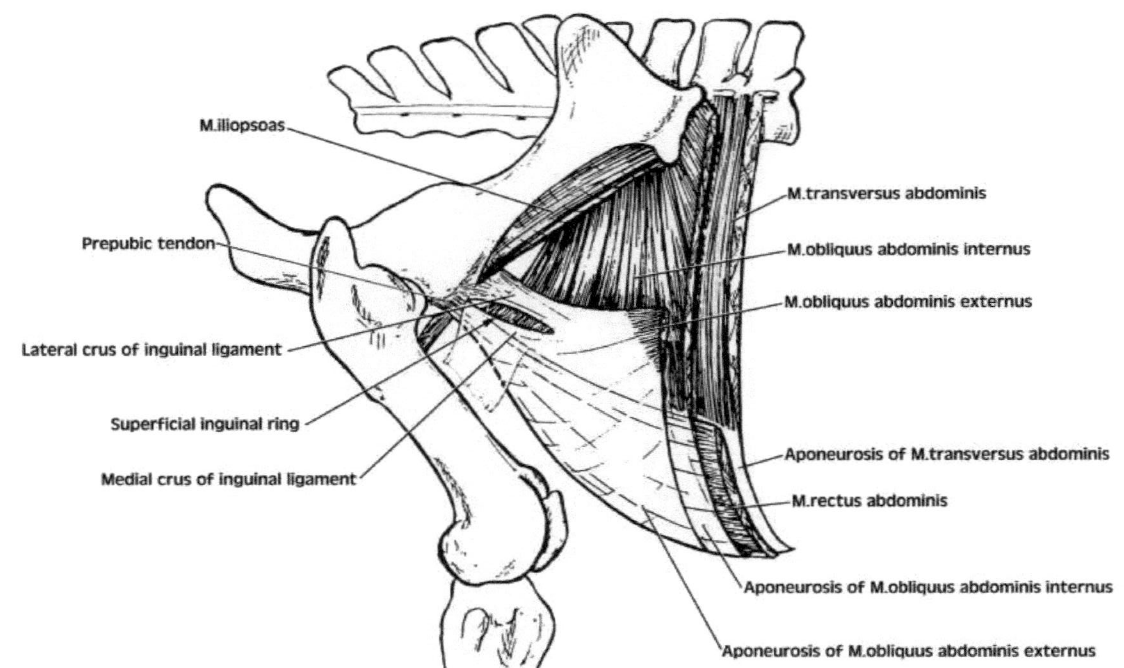

Fig.86. Muscles of the inguinal region , right lateral view

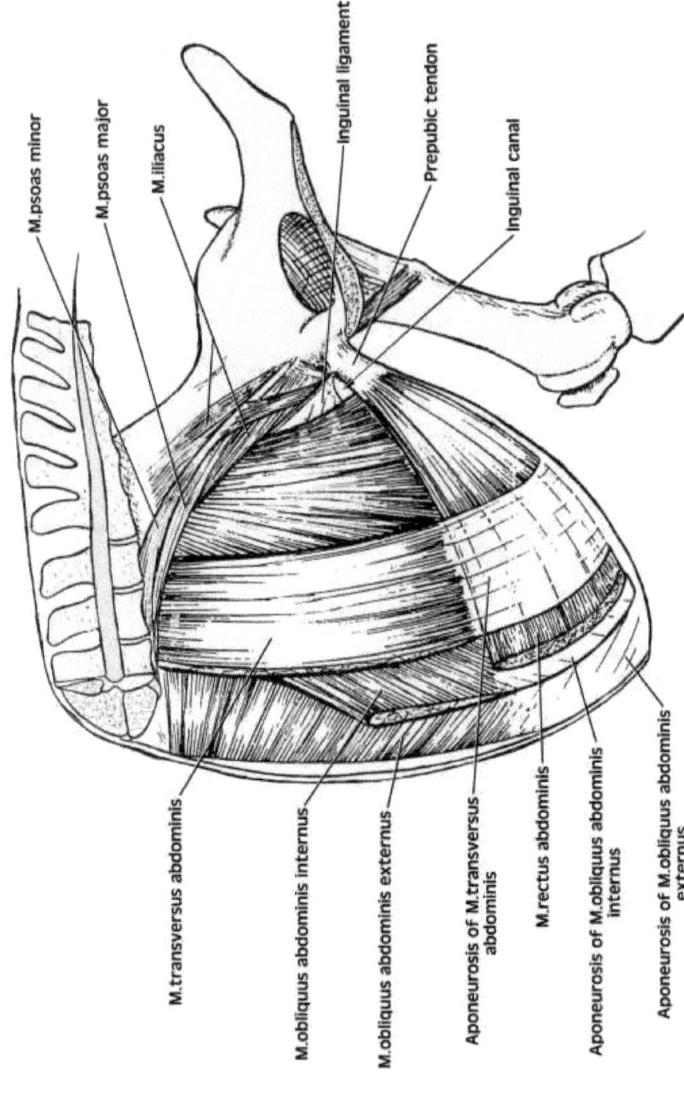

Fig.87. Muscles of inguinal region , right medial view

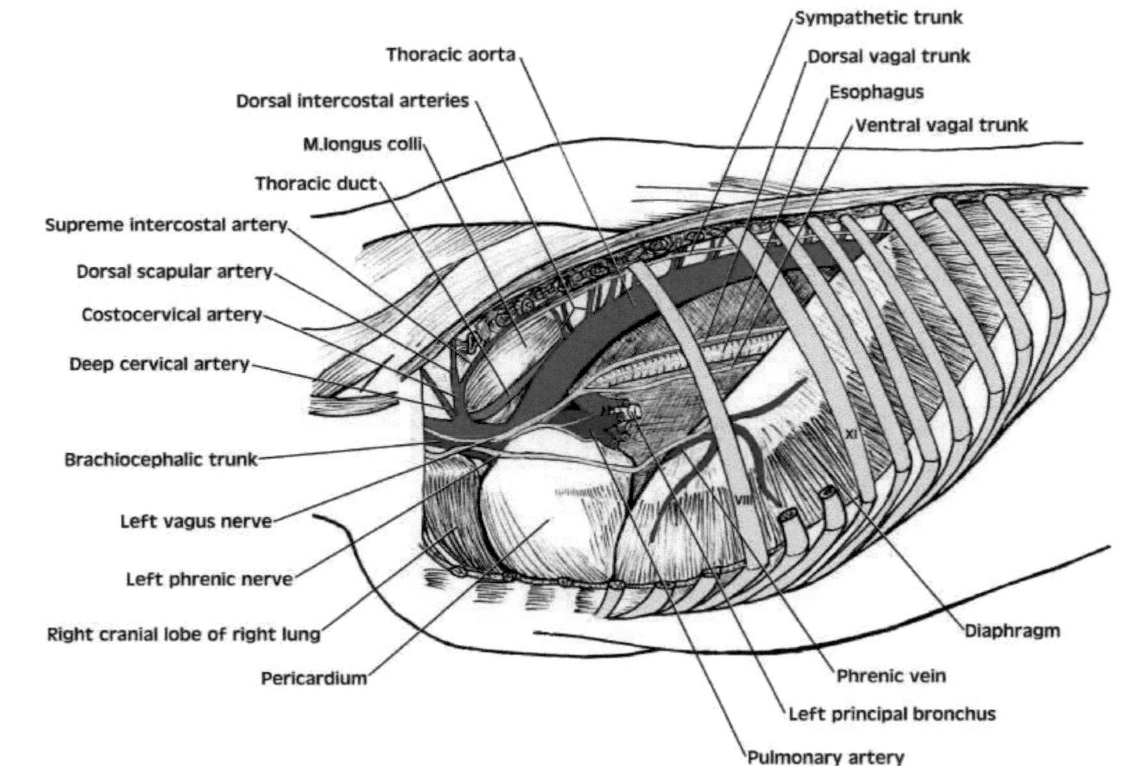

Fig.88. Thoracic contents after removal of left lung , left view

95

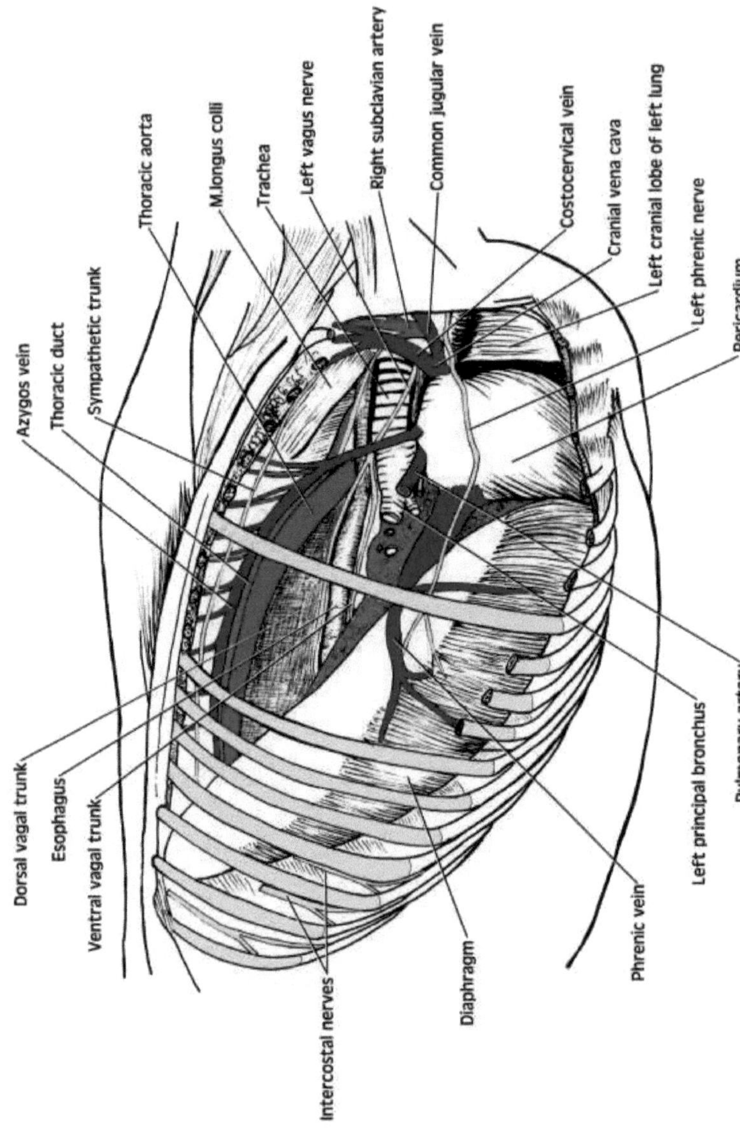

Fig.89. Thoracic contents after removal of right lung, right view

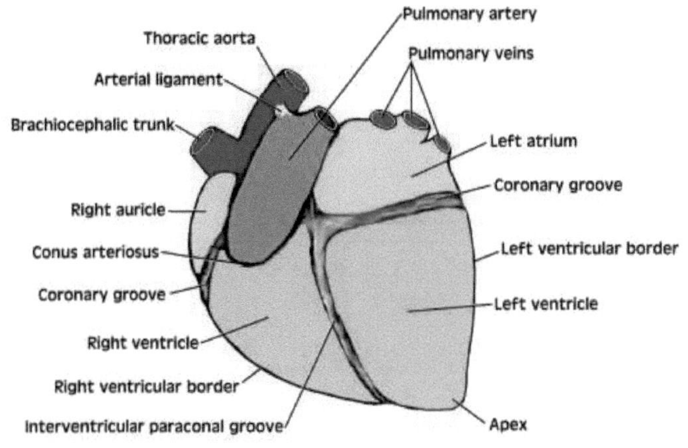

Fig.90. Heart , left surface

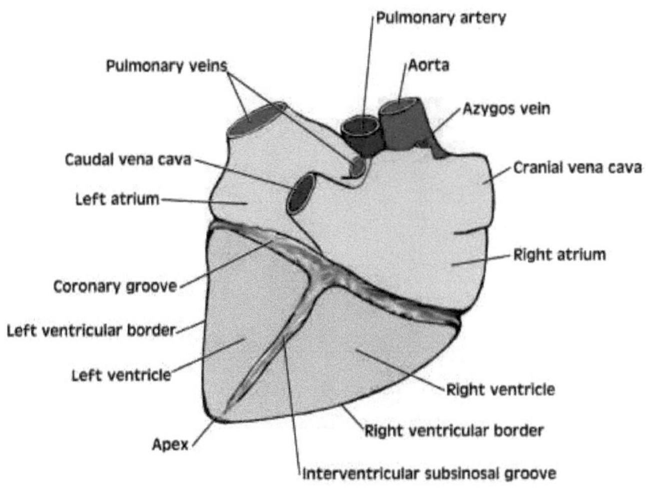

Fig.91. Heart , right surface

97

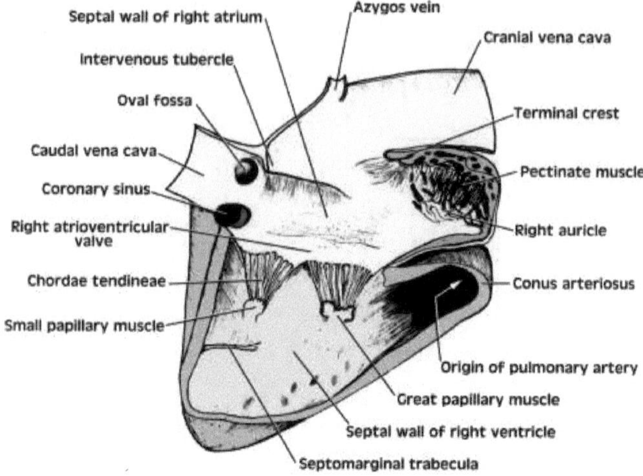

Fig.92. Right atrium and ventricle

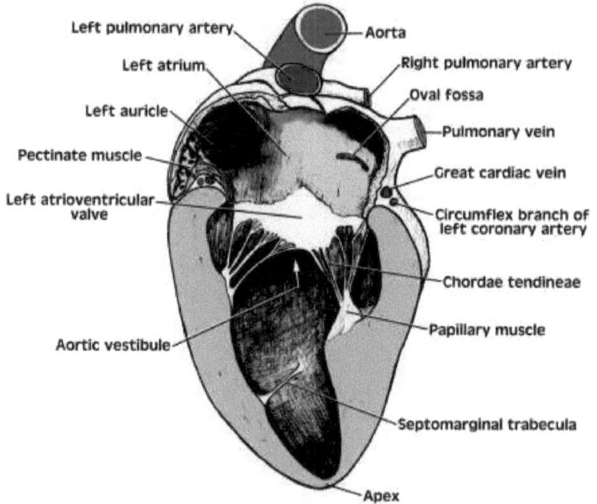

Fig.93. Left atrium and ventricle

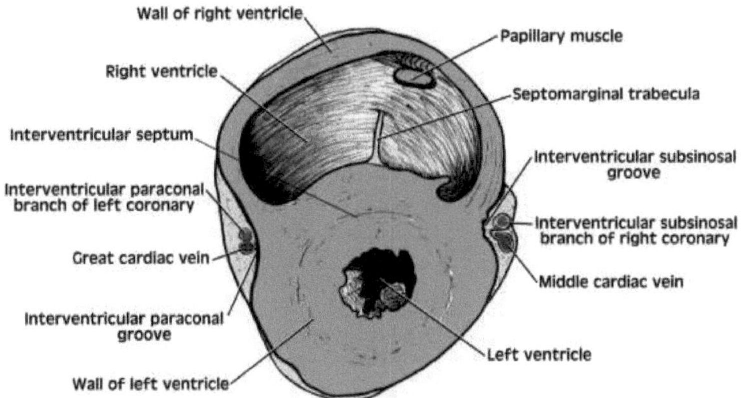

Fig.94.Cross section of ventricular mass

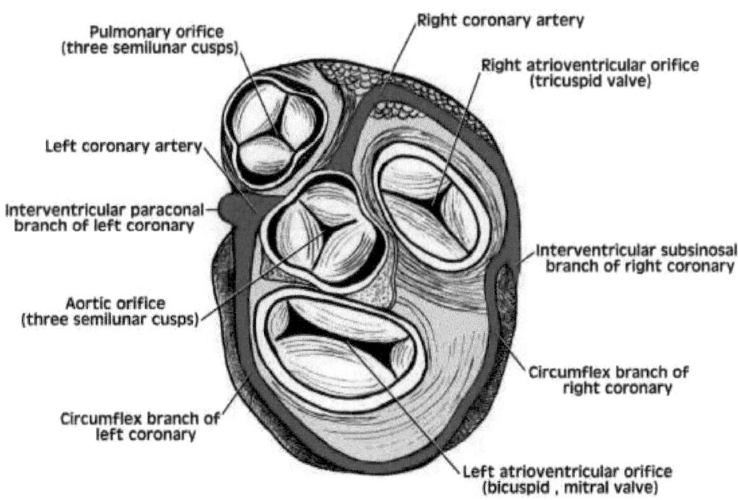

Fig.95. Ventricular base of heart

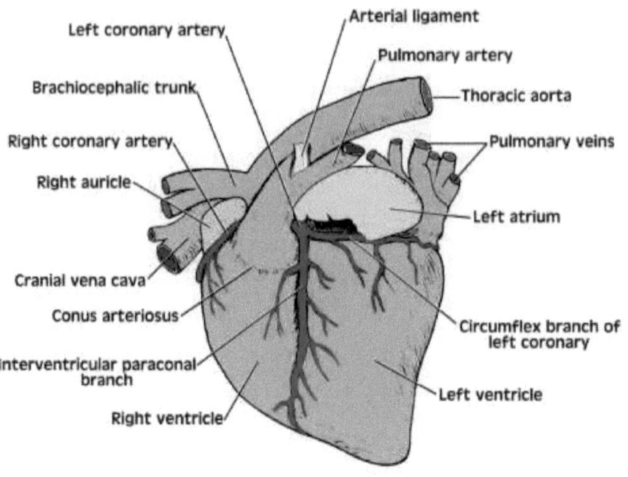

Left coronary artery

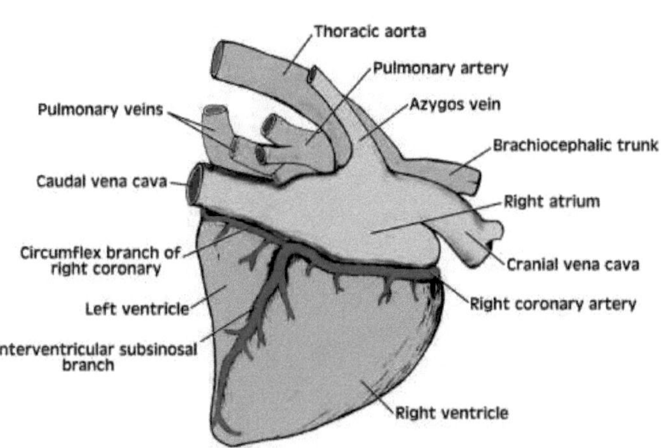

Right coronary artery

Fig.96. Arteries of heart

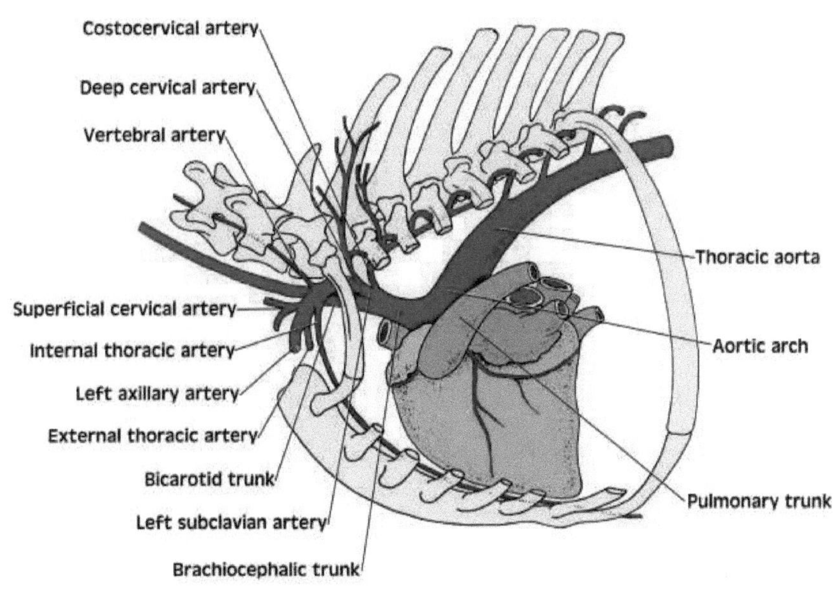

Fig.97. Origin and branching of brachiocephalic trunk

101

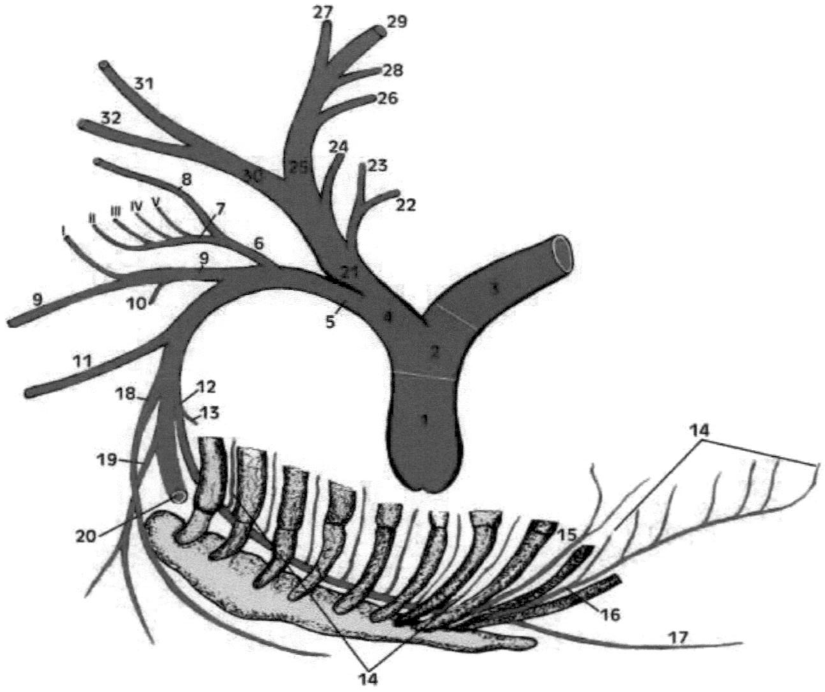

Fig.98. Pattern of distribution of brachiocephalic trunk, diagrammatic

Fig.98. Pattern of distribution of brachiocephalic trunk, diagrammatic

1. Ascending aorta
2. Aortic arch
3. Descending aorta (thoracic aorta)
4. Brachiocephalic trunk
5. Left subclavian artery
6. Left costocervical artery
7. Supreme intercostal artery
8. Dorsal scapular artery
9. Left deep cervical artery
10. Mediastinal branch
11. Left vertebral artery
12. Left internal thoracic artery
13. Thymic branch
14. Ventral intercostal arteries
15. Pericardiophrenic artery
16. Musculophrenic artery
17. Cranial epigastric artery
18. Left superficial cervical artery
19. Left external thoracic artery
20. Left axillary artery
21. Brachiocephalic artery
22. Right costocervical artery
23. Right deep cervical artery
24. Right vertebral artery
25. Right subclavian artery
26. Right internal thoracic artery
27. Right superficial cervical artery
28. Right external thoracic artery
29. Right axillary artery
30. Bicarotid trunk
31. Right common carotid artery
32. Left common carotid artery

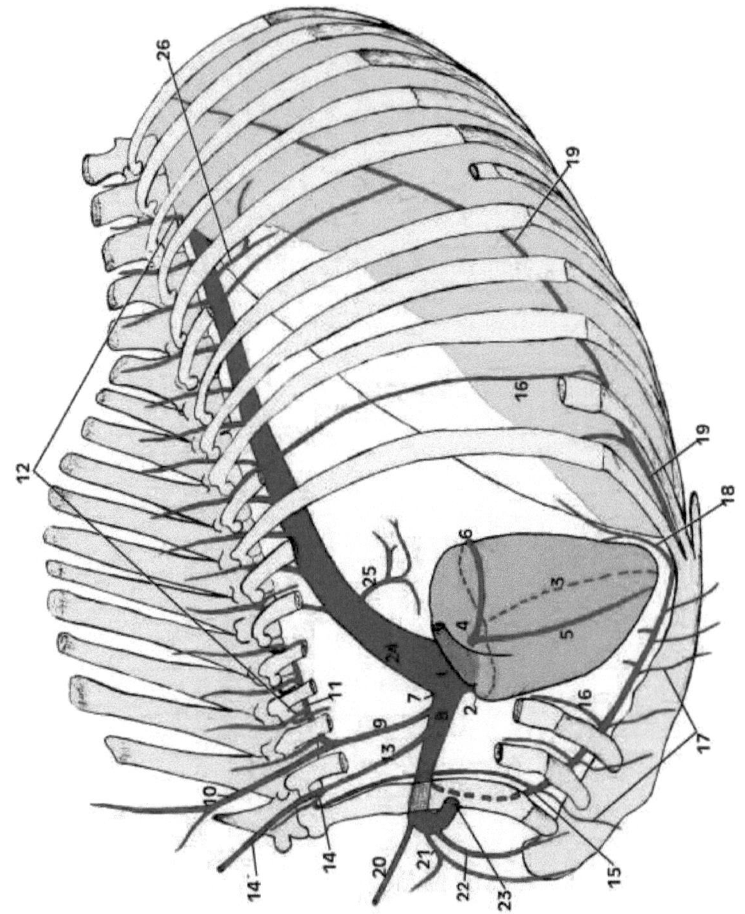

Fig.99. Arterial blood supply of thorax , left view ; diagrammatic

Fig. 99. Arterial blood supply of thorax, left view; diagrammatic

1. Aortic arch
2. Right coronary artery
3. Interventricular subsinosal branch
4. Left coronary artery
5. Interventricular paraconal branch
6. Right and left circumflex branches
7. Brachiocephalic trunk
8. Left subclavian artery
9. Costocervical artery
10. Dorsal scapular artery
11. Supreme intercostals artery
12. Dorsal intercostal arteries
13. Deep cervical artery
14. First dorsal intercostal artery
15. Internal thoracic artery
16. Ventral intercostal arteries
17. Perforating branches
18. Pericardiophrenic artery
19. Musculophrenic artery
20. Vertebral artery
21. Superficial cervical artery
22. External thoracic artery
23. Left axillary artery
24. Thoracic aorta
25. Bronchesophageal artery
26. Cranial phrenic artery

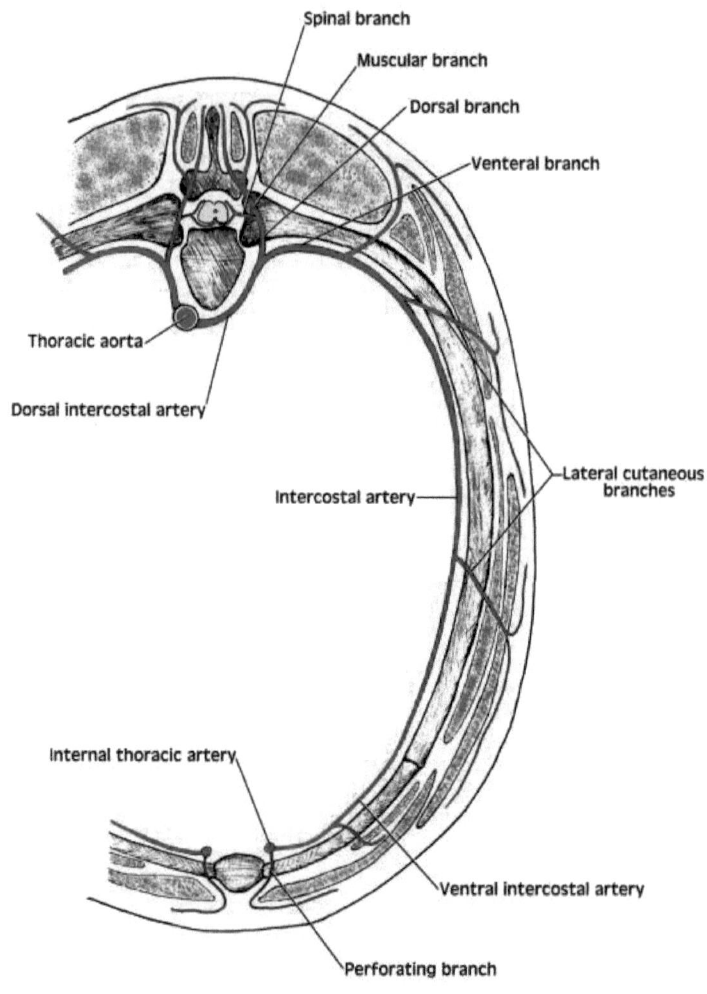

Fig.100. Arteries of thoracic wall, cross section diagrammatic

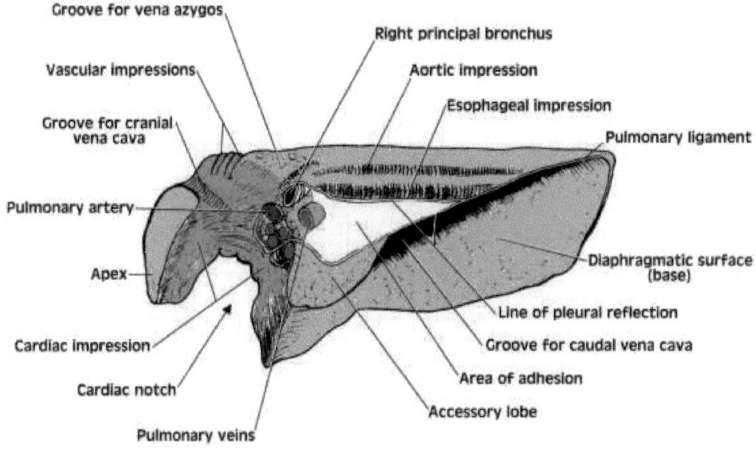

Right lung

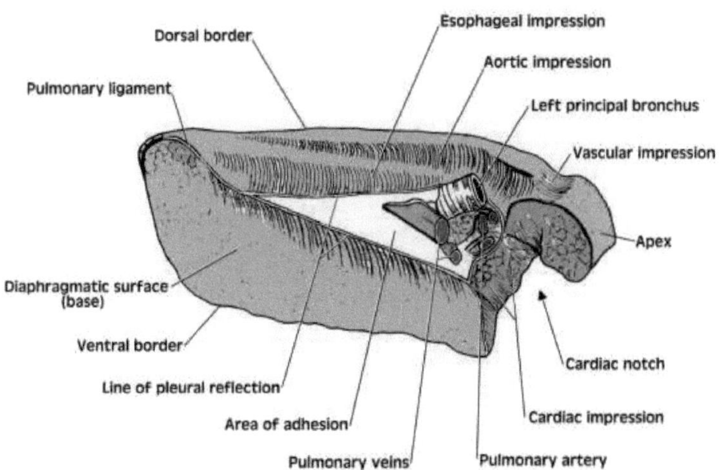

Left lung

Fig.101. Mediastinal and diaphragmatic surfaces of the lung

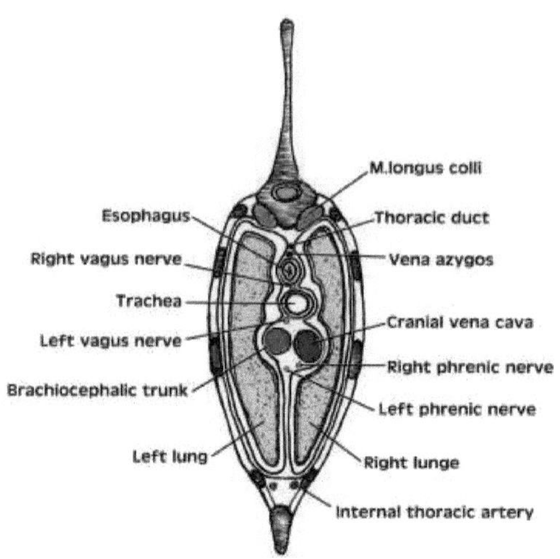

Fig.102. Transverse section in cranial mediastinum

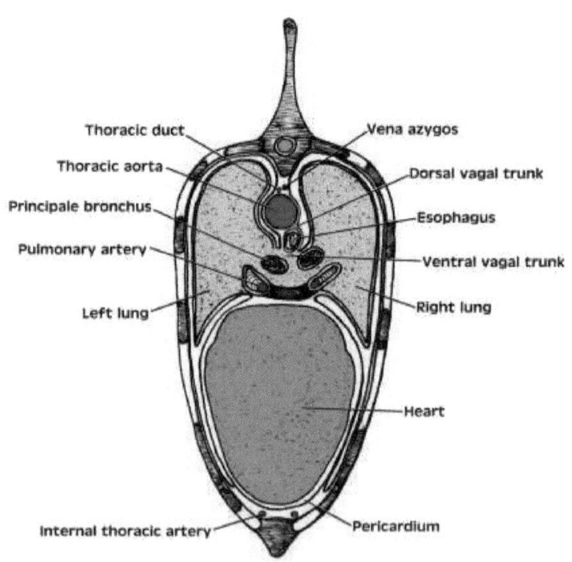

Fig.103. Transverse section in cardiac mediastinum

108

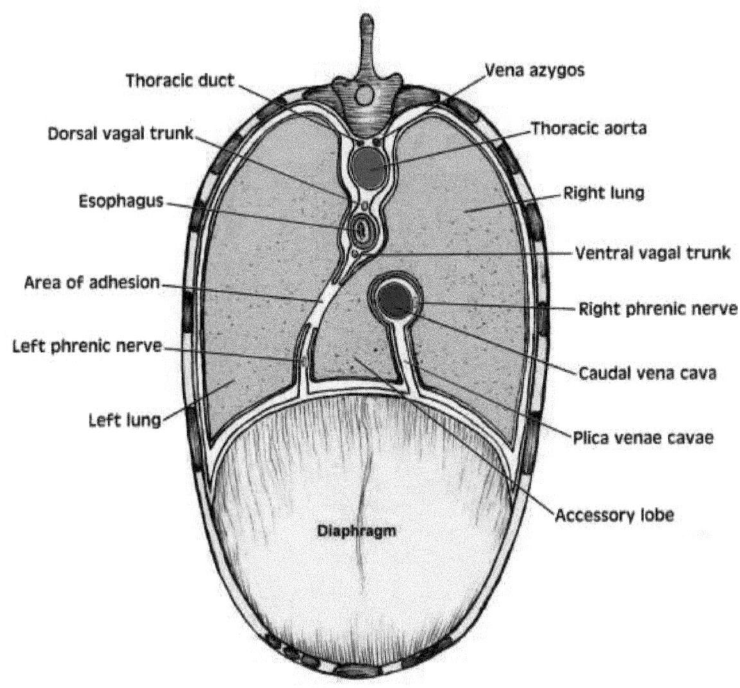

Fig 104. Transverse section in caudal mediastinum

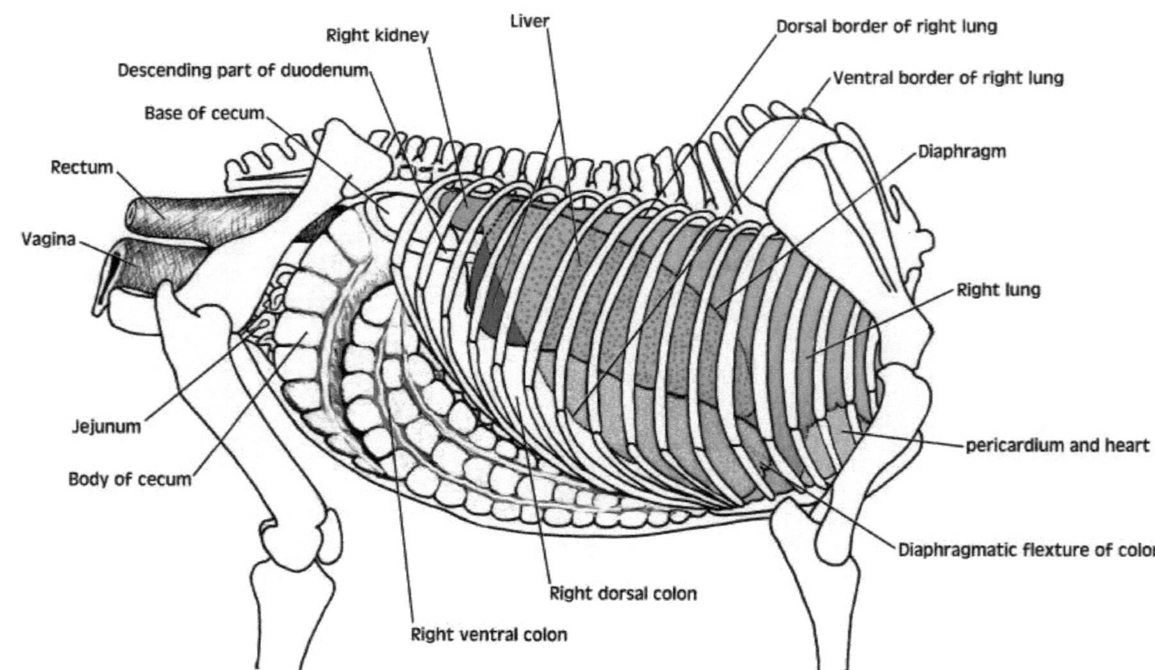

Fig 105. Topography of the viscera in mare , right view

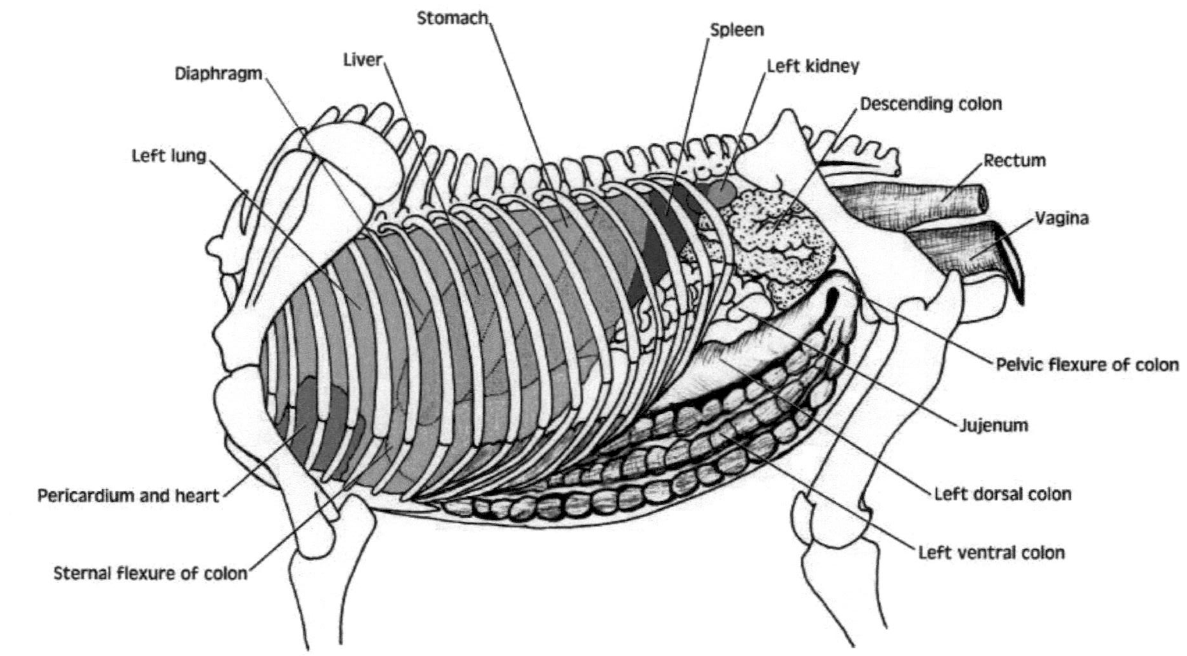

Fig.106. Topography of the viscera in mare , left view

111

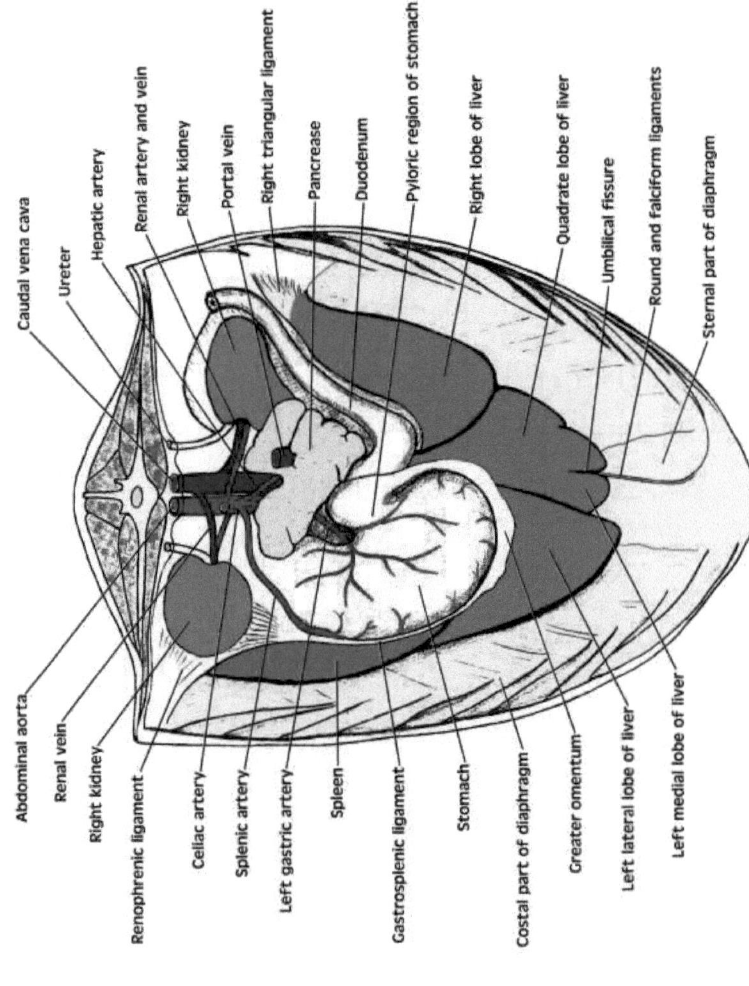

Fig.107. Contents of the cranial part of abdominal cavity , organs in situ

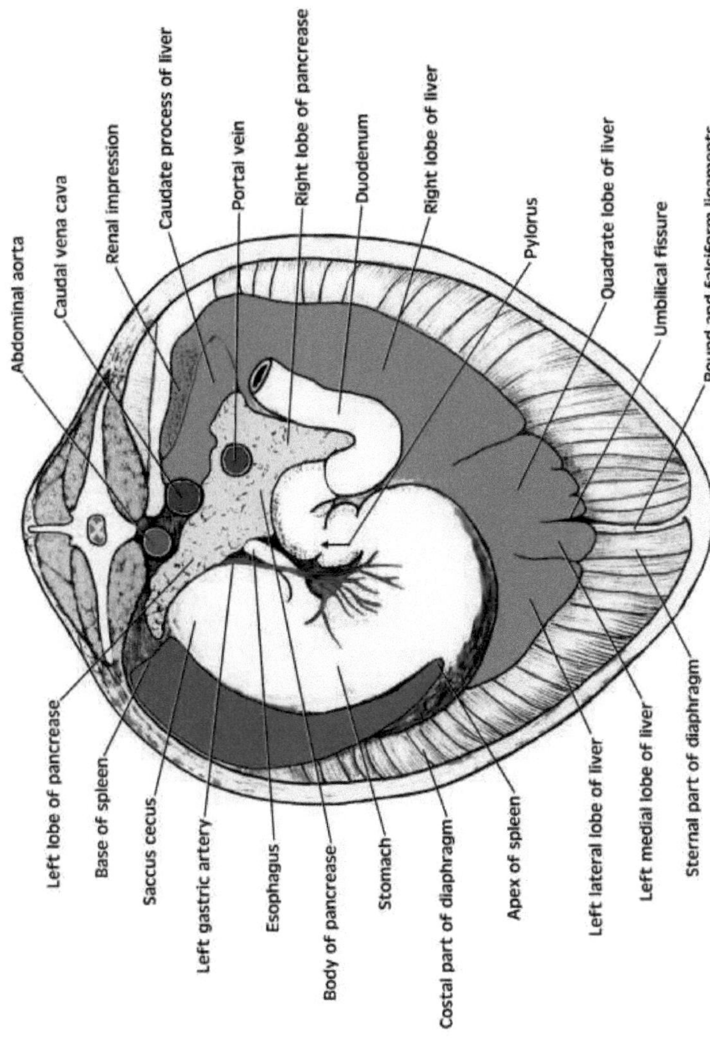

Fig.108. Contents of the cranial part of abdominal cavity after removal of kidneys

113

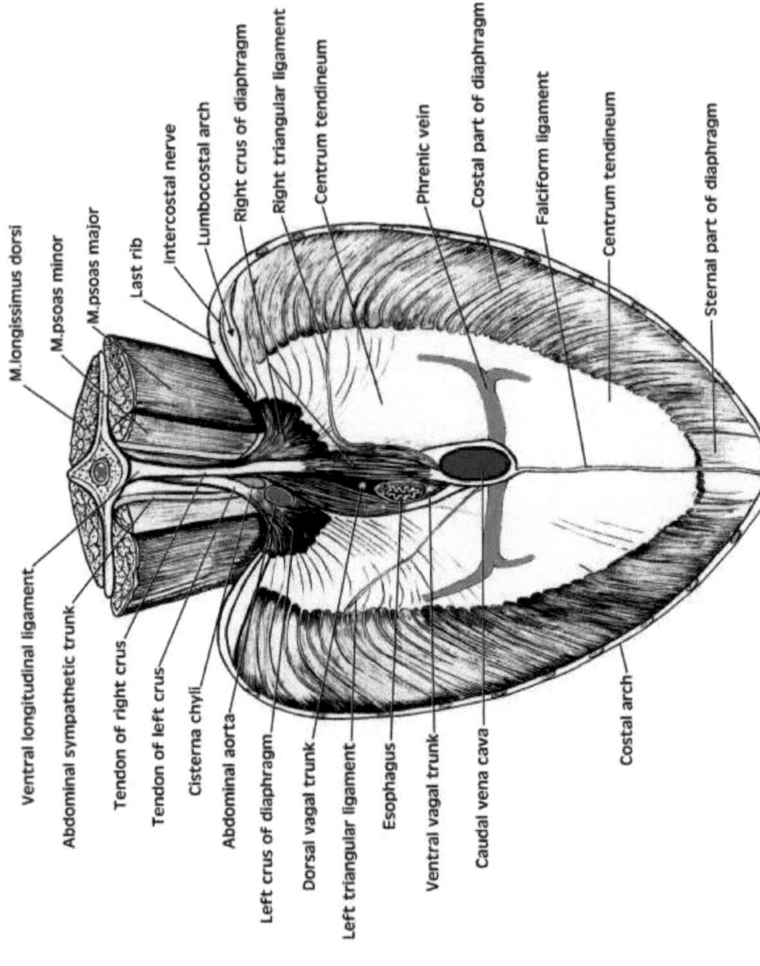

Fig.109. Diaphragm , abdominal surface

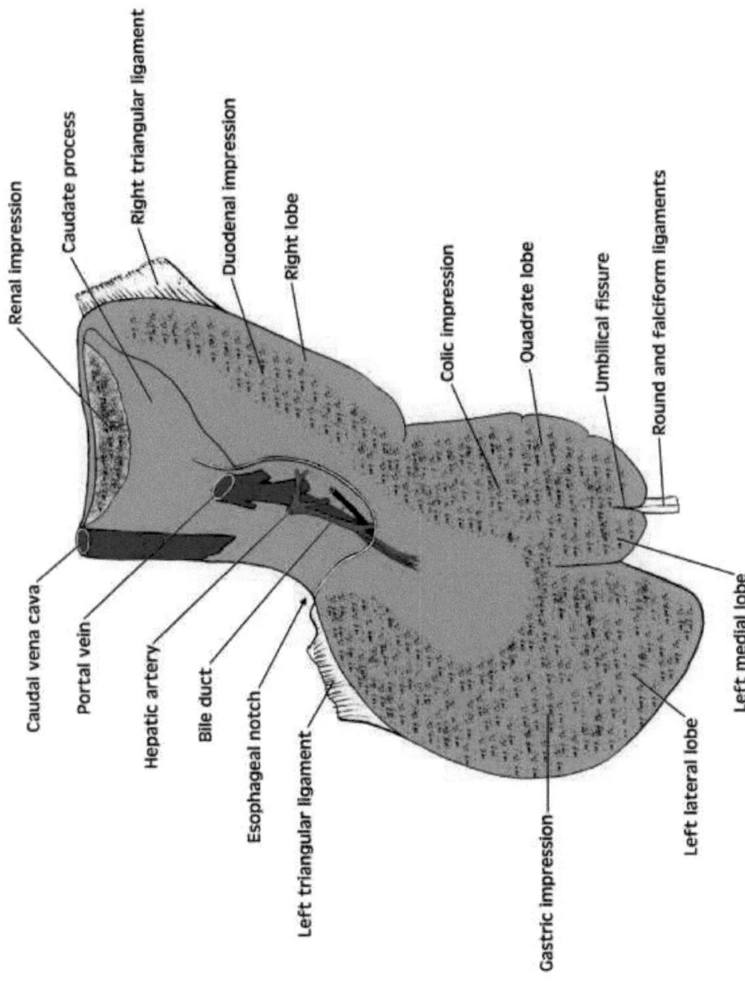

Fig.110. Liver , visceral surface

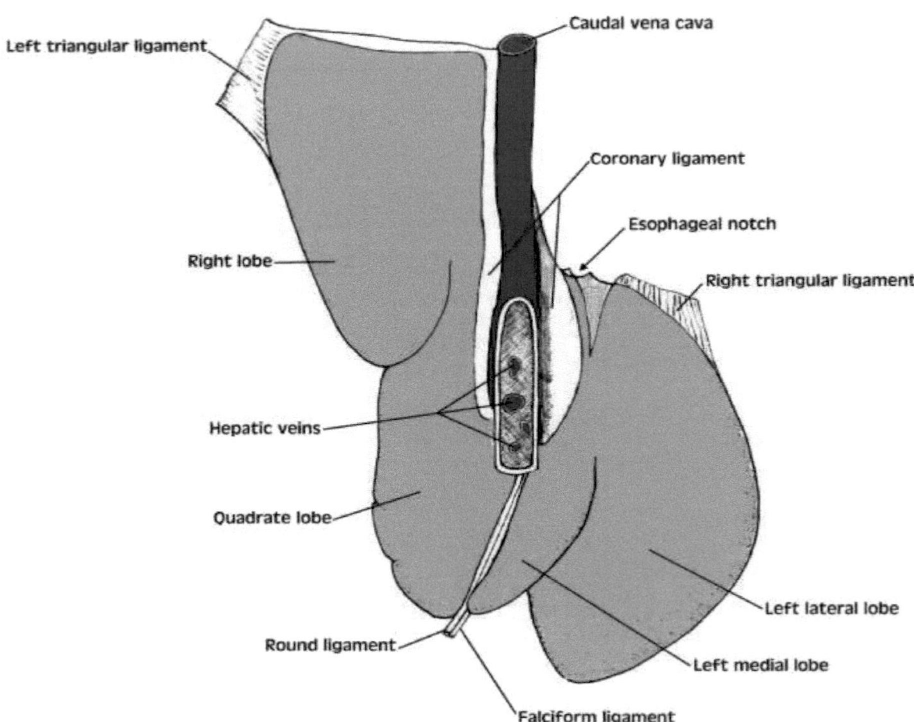

Fig.111. Liver , diaphragmatic surface

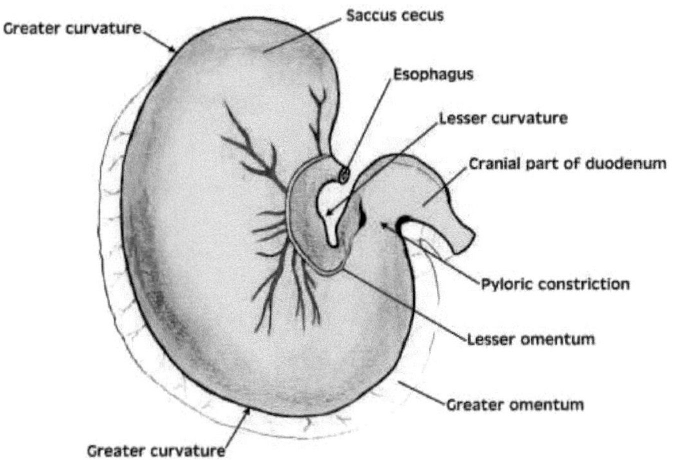

Stomach , visceral surface

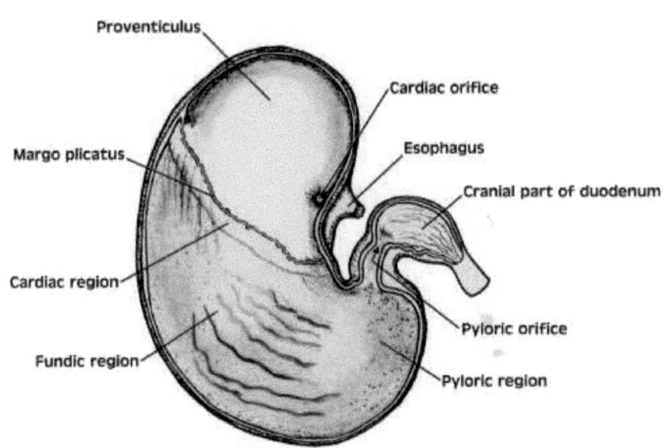

Interior of the stomach

Fig.112. Stomach

117

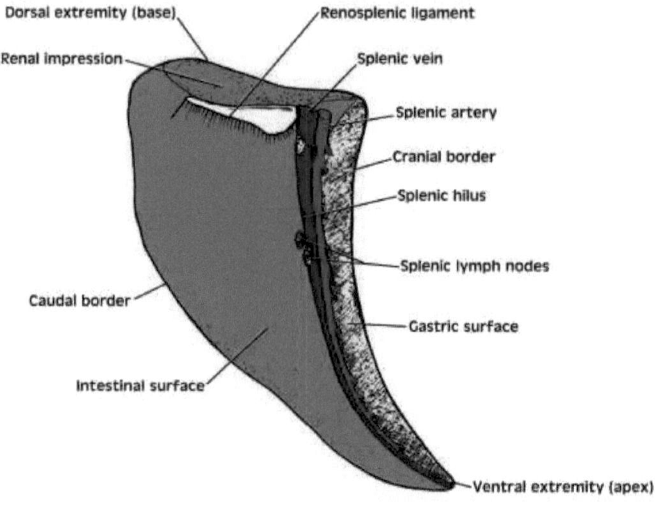

Visceral surface of the spleen

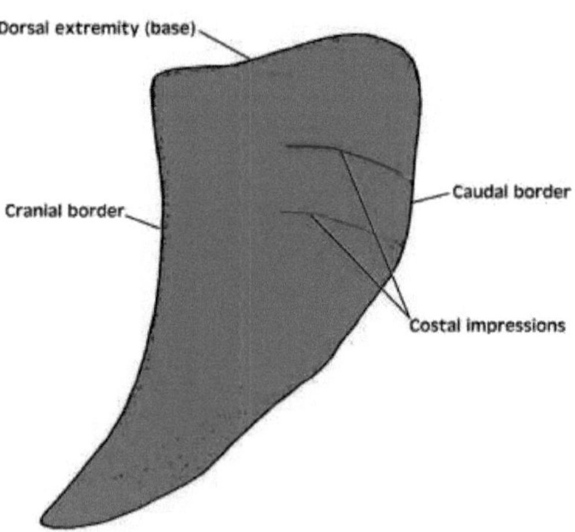

Parietal surface of the spleen

Fig.113. spleen

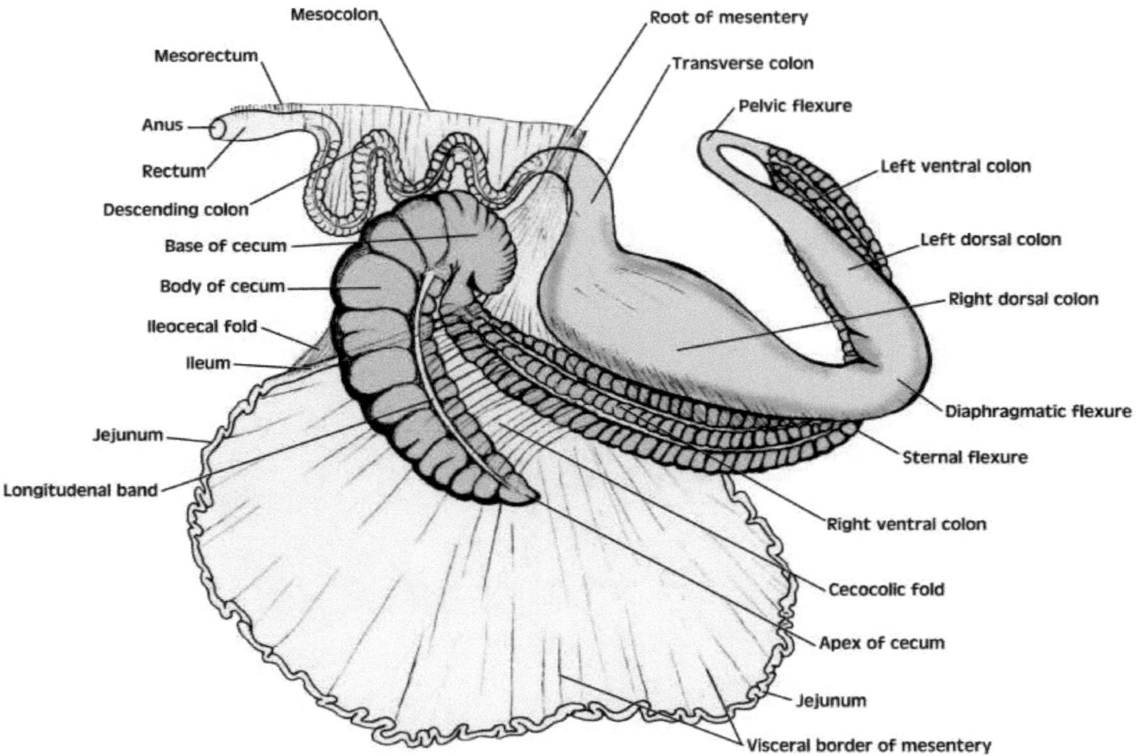

Fig.114. Intestine , right view

119

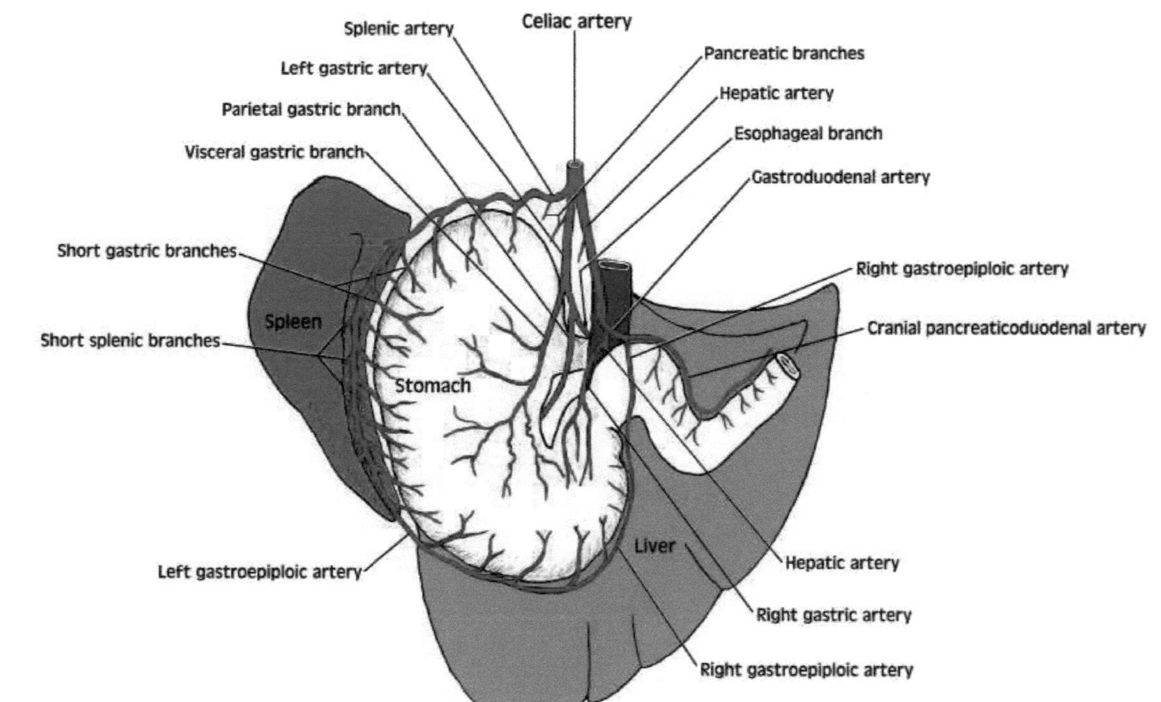

Fig.115. Distibution of the celiac artery , diagrammatic

120

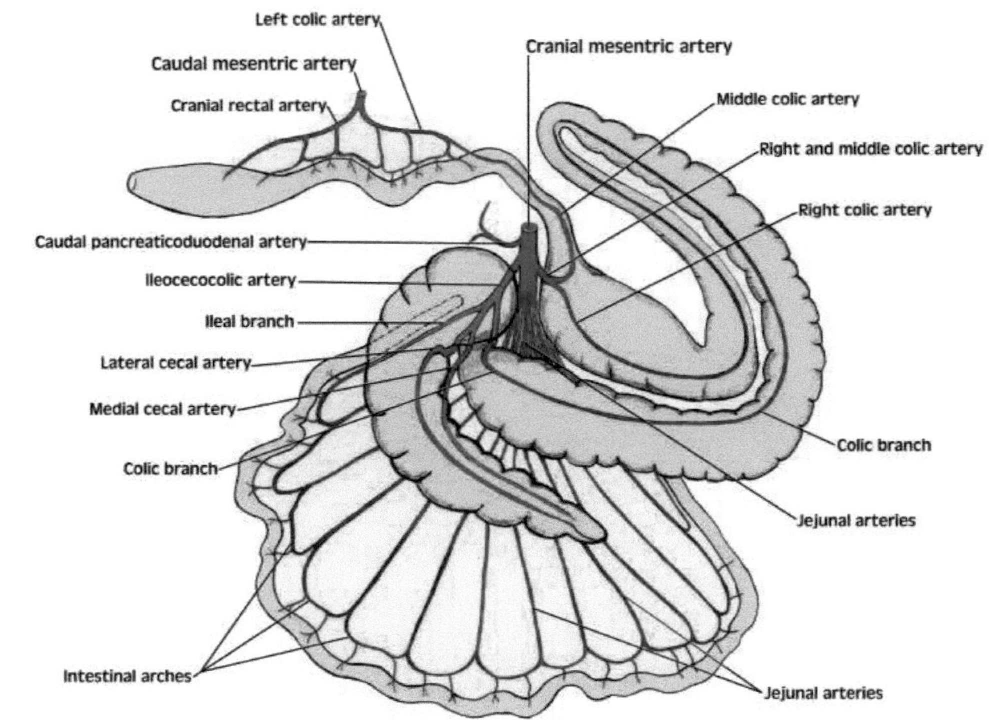

Fig.116. Distribution of the cranial and caudal mesentric arteries , diagrammatic

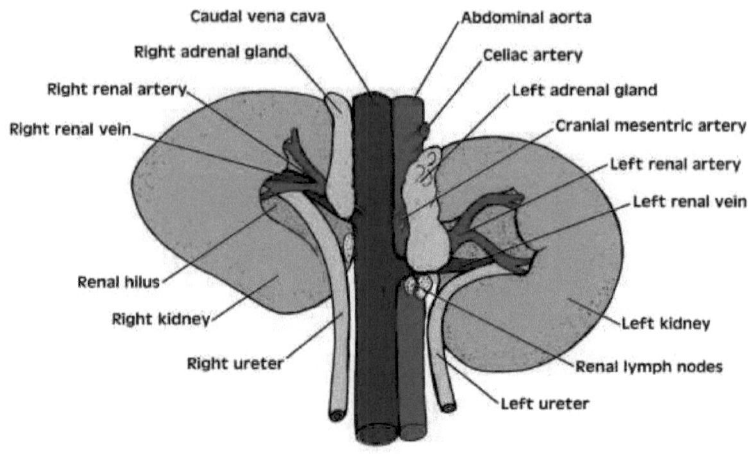

Kidneys and adrenal glands , ventral view

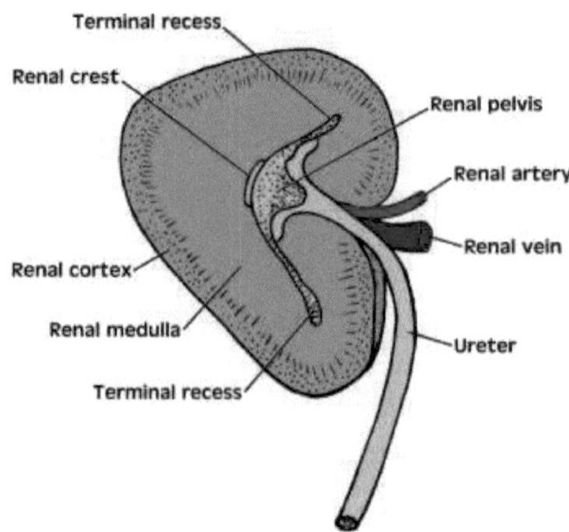

Horizontal section in the right kidney

Fig.117. kidneys

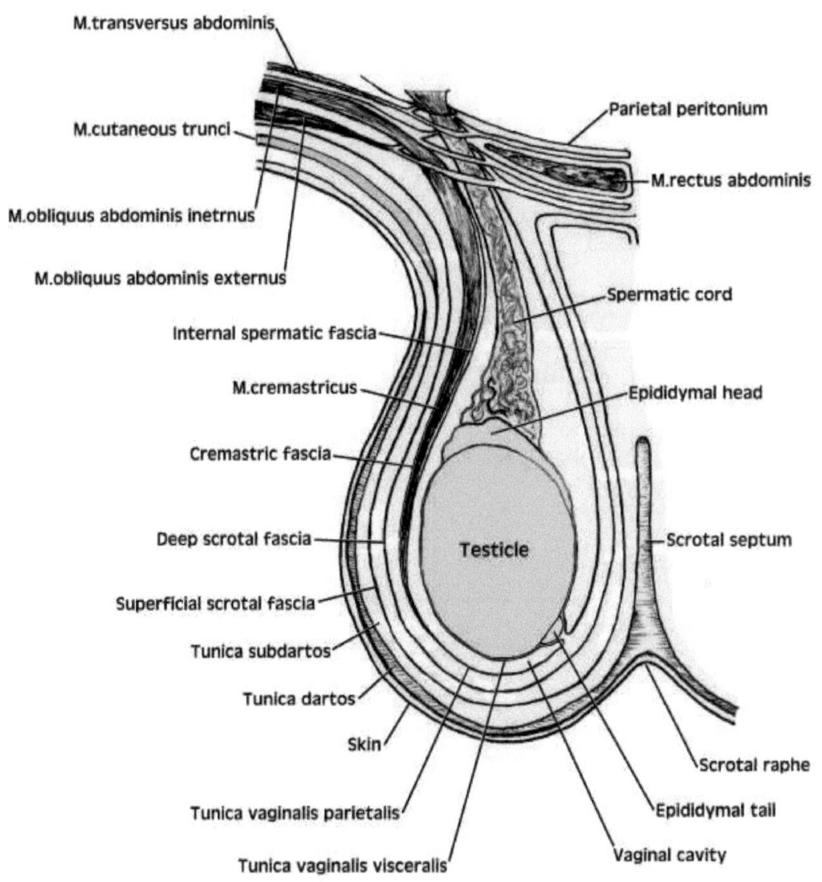

Fig.118. Scrotum and testicle , diagrammatic

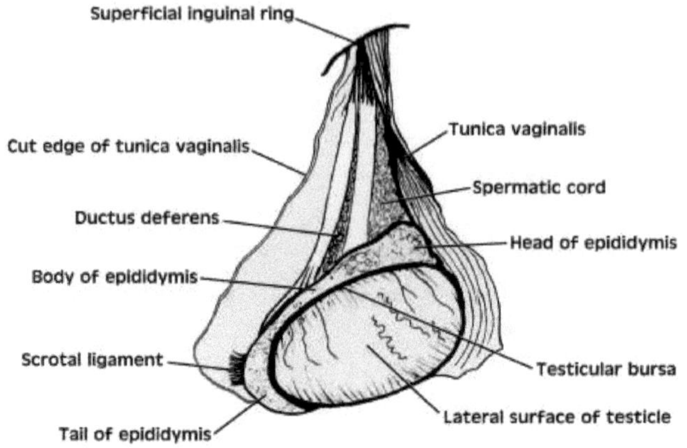

Fig.119. Right testicle and epididymis , lateral view

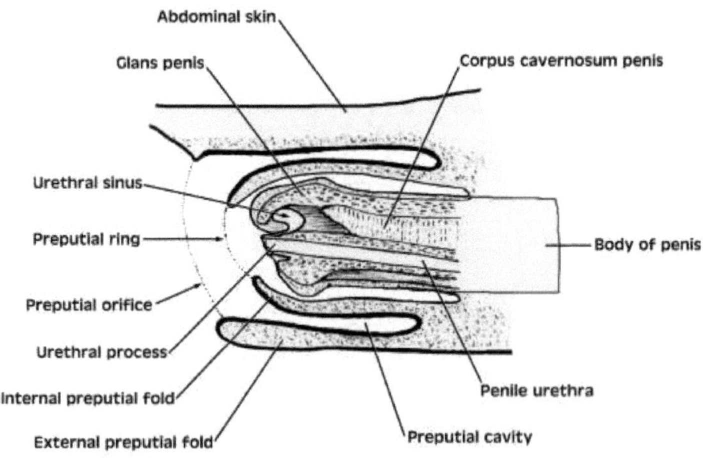

**Fig.120. Prepuce and cranial part of penis ,
sagittal section**

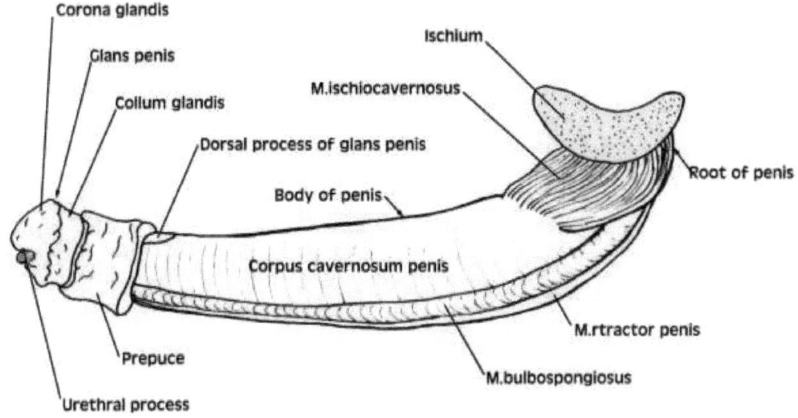

Penis , lateral view

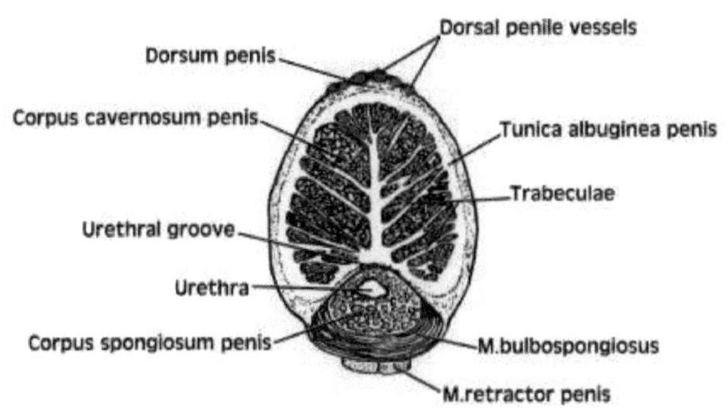

Cross section in the body of penis

Fig.121. penis

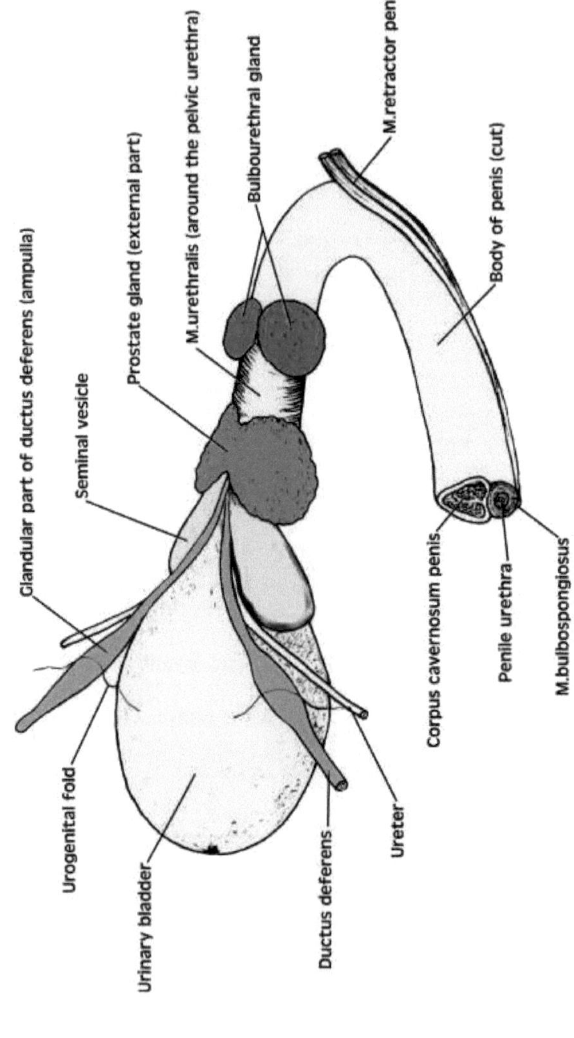

Fig.122. Accessory genital glands ,dorsolateral view ; diagrammatic

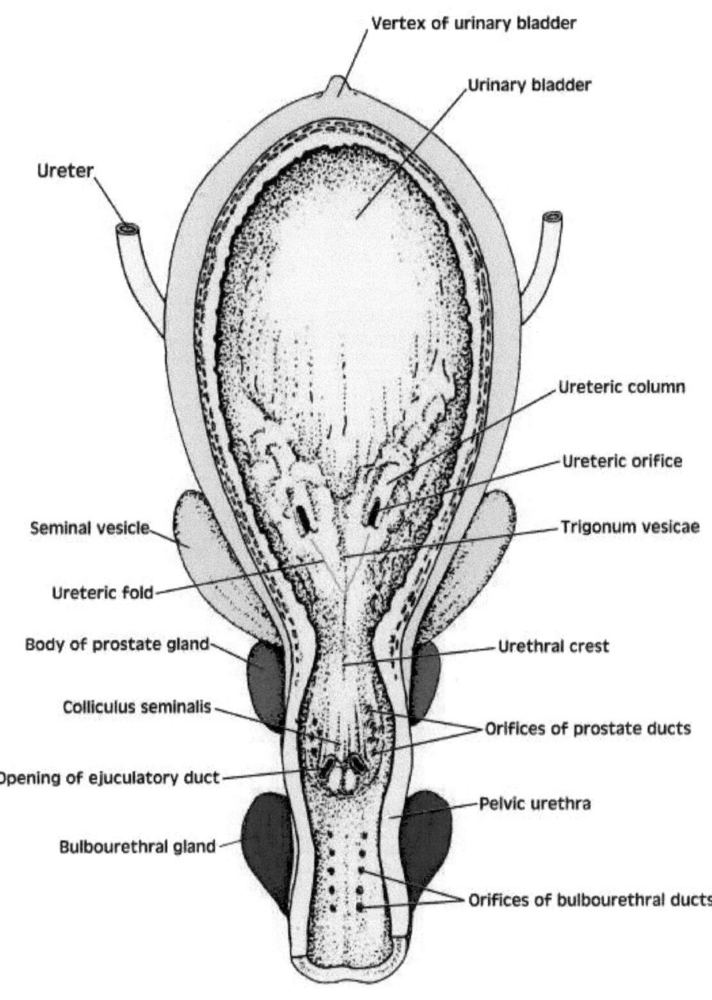

Fig.123. Opened urinary bladder and pelvic urethra of stallion , ventral view

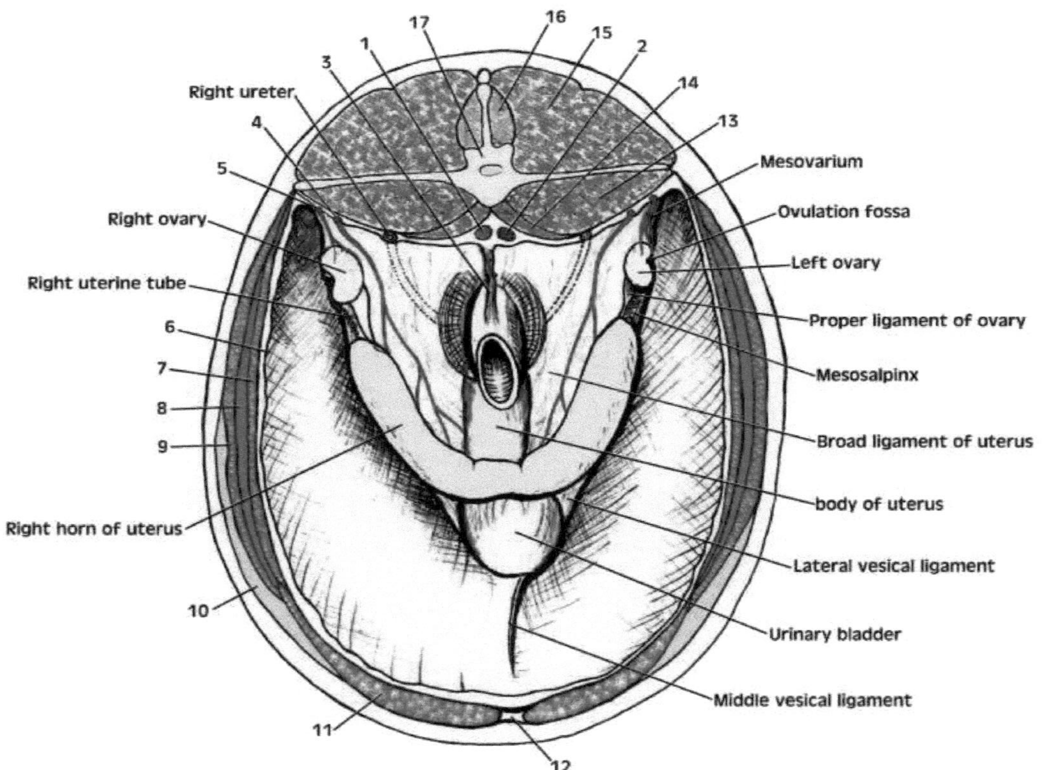

Fig.124. Female genital organs in situ , cranial view

Fig. 124. Female genital organs in situ, cranial view

1. Abdominal aorta
2. Caudal vena cava
3. Mesorectum
4. Uterine artery
5. Ovarian artery
6. Parietal peritoneum
7. M. transversus abdominis
8. M. obliquus abdominis internus
9. M. obliquus abdominis externus
10. M. cutaneous trunci
11. M. rectus abdominis
12. Linea alba
13. M. psoas major
14. M. psoas minor
15. M. longissimus dorsi
16. M. multifidus dorsi
17. Third lumbar vertebra

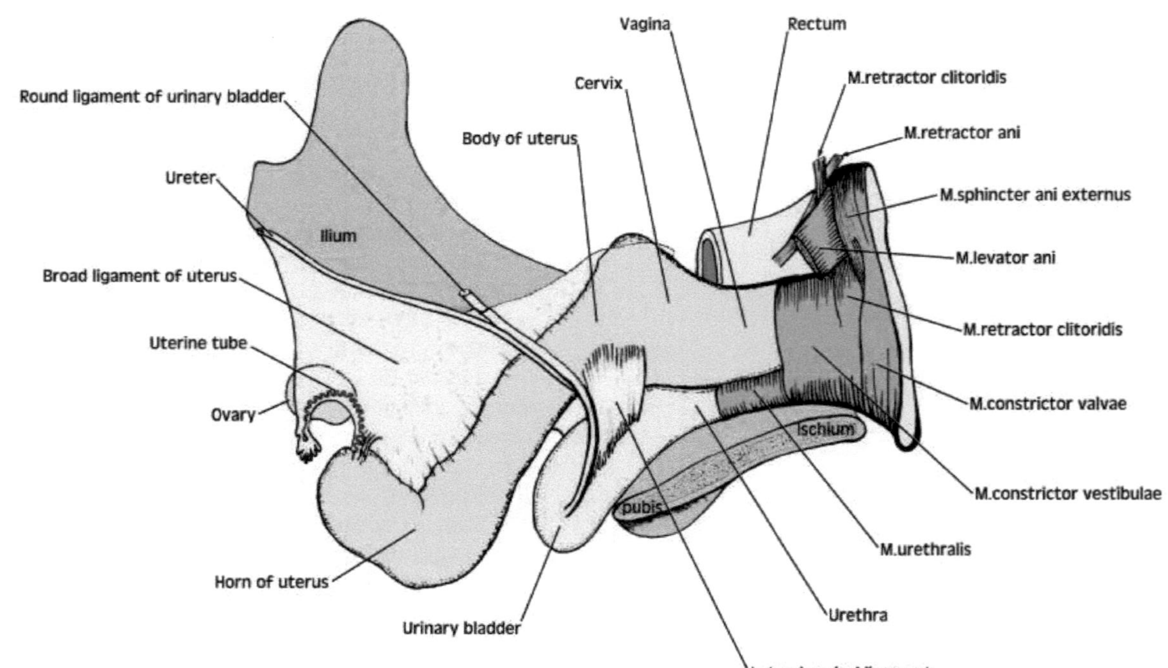

Fig.125. Female genital organs , lateral view ; diagrammatic

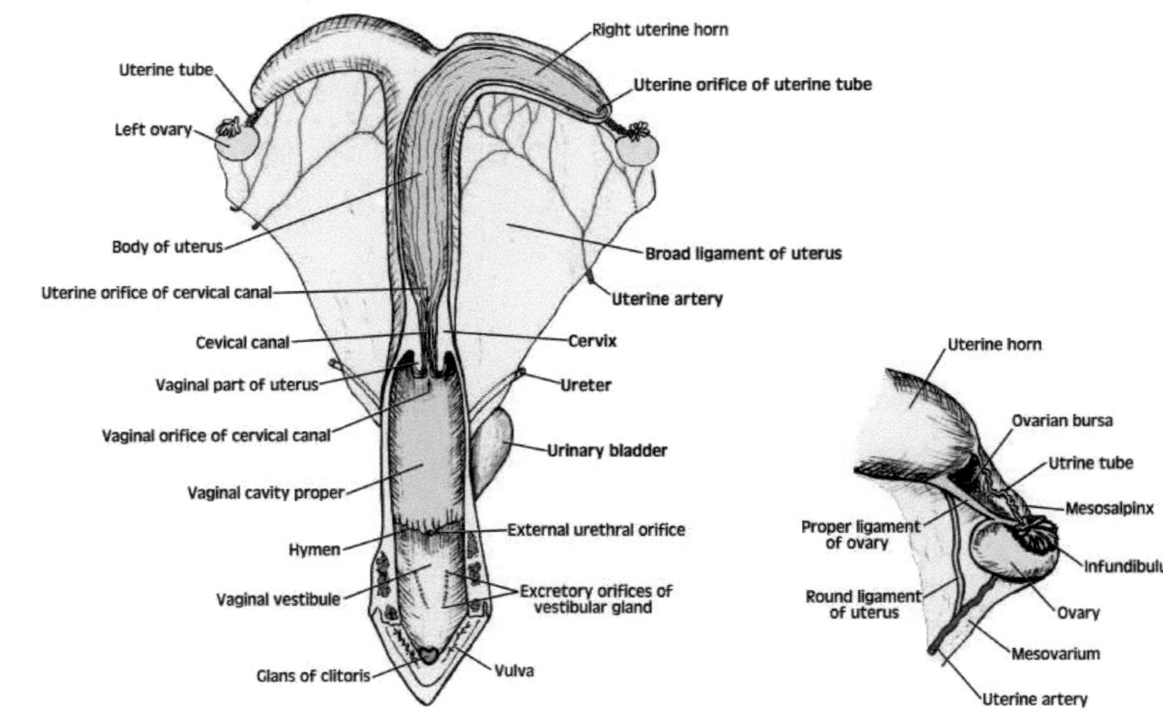

Opened female genital organs , dorsal view

Right ovary and uterine tube

Fig.126. Genital organs in mare

131

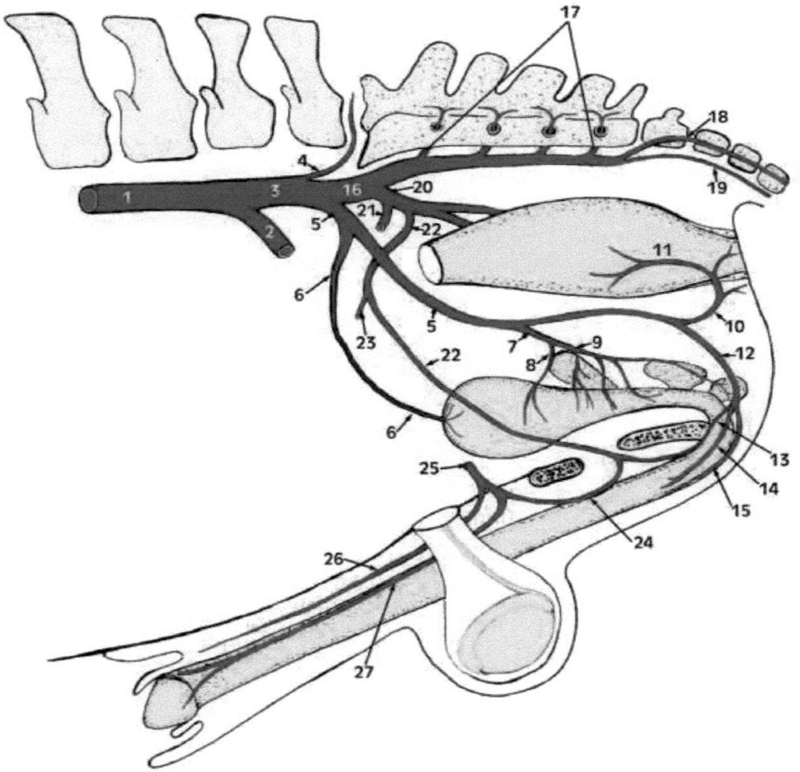

Fig.127. Distribution of internal iliac artery in stallion , diagrammatic

Fig. 127. Distribution of internal iliac artery in stallion, diagrammatic

1. Abdominal aorta
2. External iliac artery
3. Internal iliac artery
4. Last lumbar artery
5. Internal pudendal artery
6. Umbilical artery (round ligament of urinary bladder)
7. Urogenital artery (prostatic artery)
8. Caudal vesical artery
9. Ramus ductus deferens
10. Ventral perineal artery
11. Caudal rectal artery
12. Artery of the penis
13. Dorsal artery of the penis
14. Deep artery of the penis
15. Artery of the bulb
16. Caudal gluteal artery
17. Sacral branches
18. Ventrolateral caudal artery
19. Median caudal artery
20. Cranial gluteal artery
21. Iliolumbar artery
22. Obturator artery
23. Iliacofemoral artery
24. Middle artery of the penis
25. External pudendal artery
26. Superficial caudal epigastric artery
27. Cranial artery of the penis

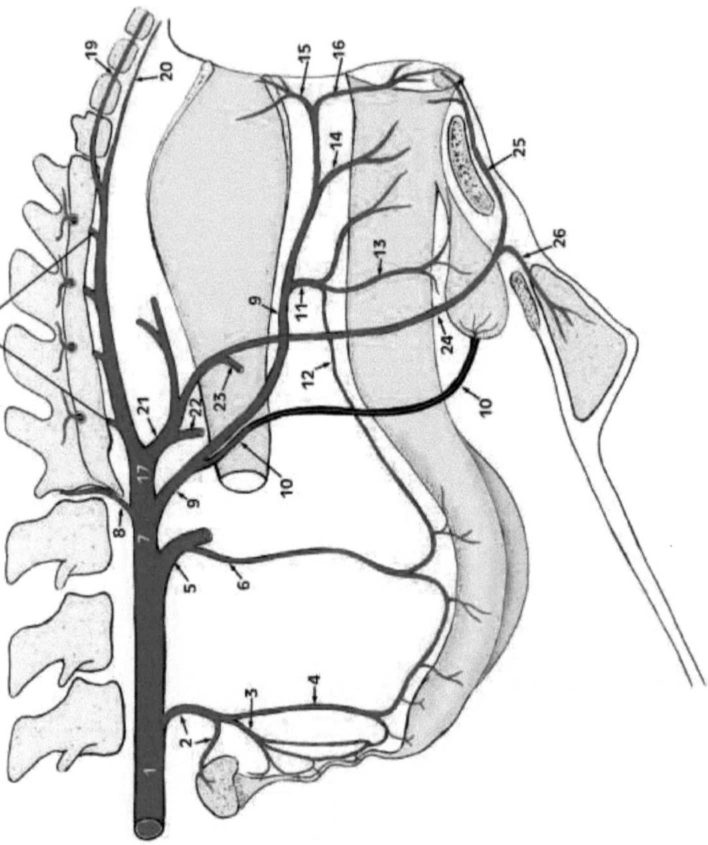

Fig.128. Arterial supply of female genital organs , diagrammatic

134

Fig.128. Arterial supply of female genital organs, diagrammatic

1. Abdominal aorta
2. Ovarian artery
3. Tubal branch of ovarian artery
4. Uterine branch (cranial uterine artery) of ovarian artery
5. External iliac artery
6. Uterine artery (middle uterine artery)
7. Internal iliac artery
8. Last lumbar artery
9. Internal pudendal artery
10. Umbilical artery (round ligament of urinary bladder)
11. Urogenital artery (vaginal artery)
12. Uterine branch (caudal uterine artery)
13. Caudal vesicular artery
14. Vestibular branch
15. Ventral perineal artery
16. Artery of the vestibular bulb
17. Caudal gluteal artery
18. Sacral branches
19. Ventrolateral caudal artery
20. Median caudal artery
21. Cranial gluteal artery
22. Iliolumbar artery
23. Iliacofemoral artery
24. Obturator artery
25. Middle artery of the clitoris
26. Caudal mammary artery

Chapter 4

Thoracic Limb

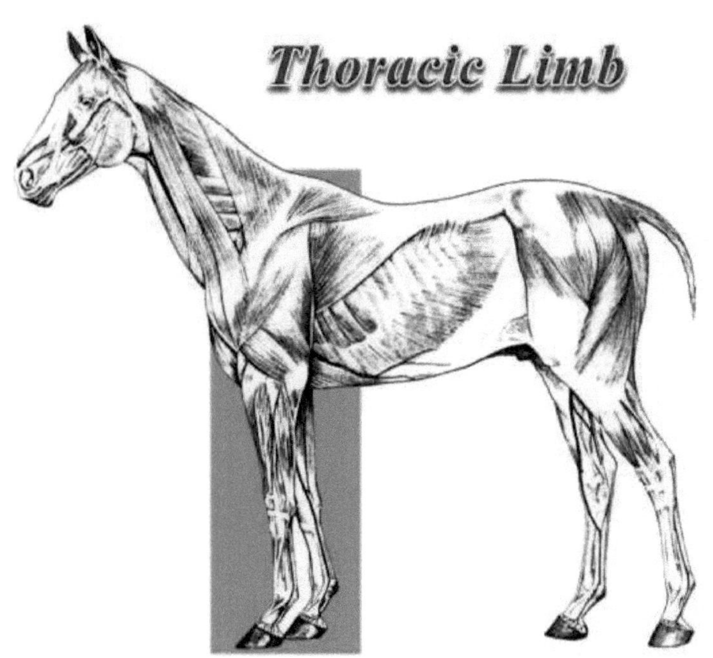

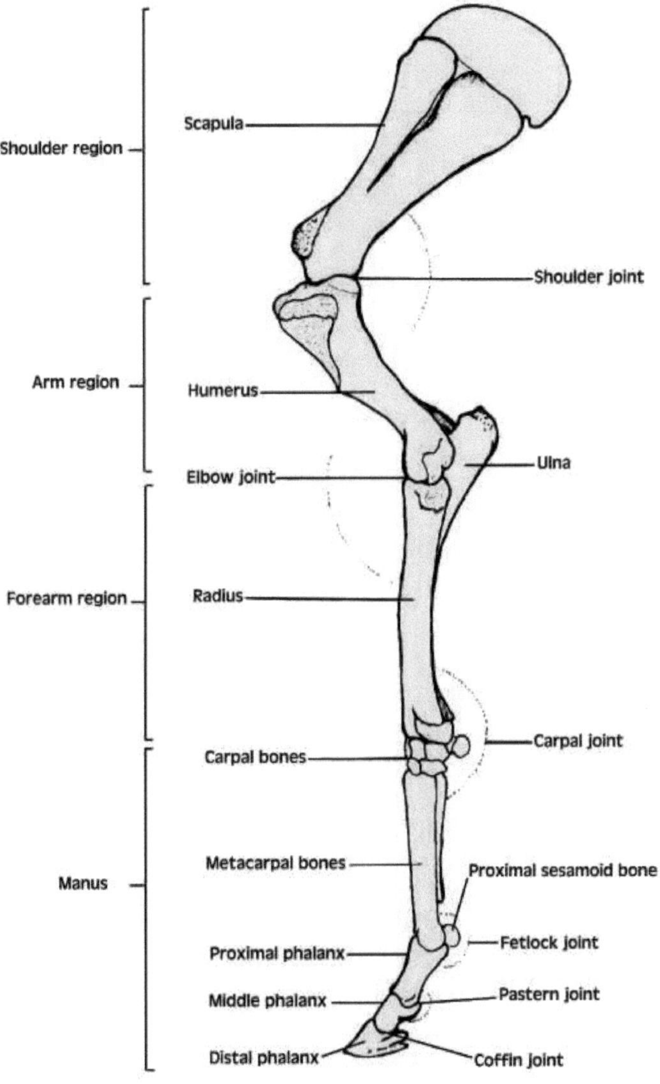

Fig 129. Bones and joints of thoracic limb, lateral view

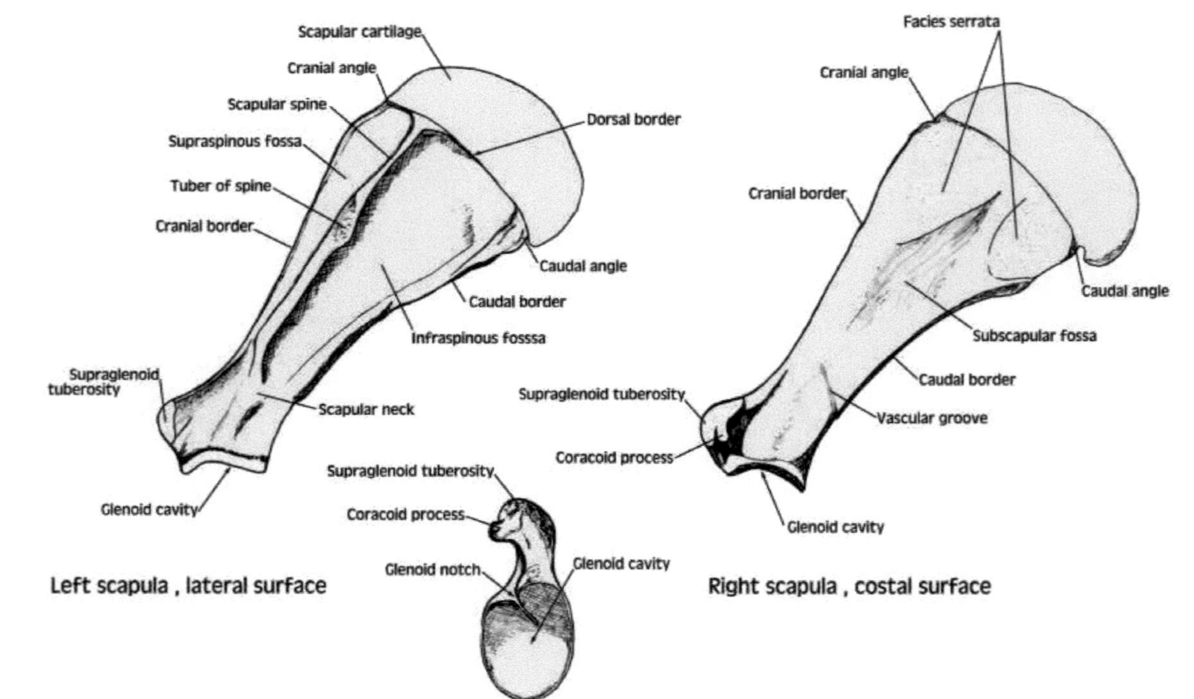

Left scapula , lateral surface

Left scapula , ventral end view

Right scapula , costal surface

Fig.130. Scapula

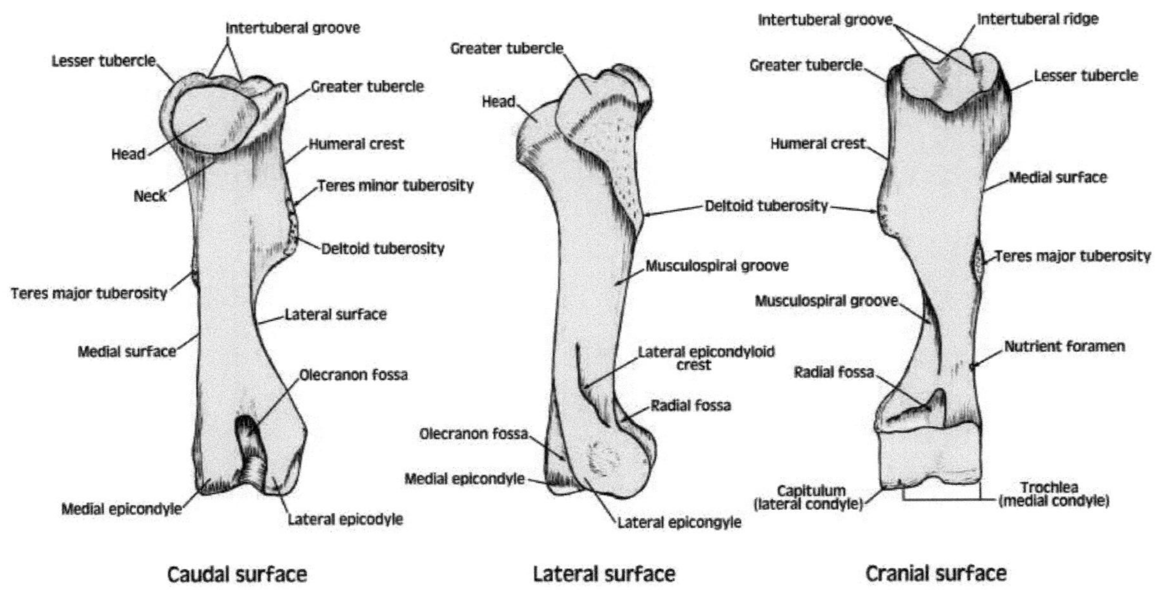

Fig.131. Right humerus

141

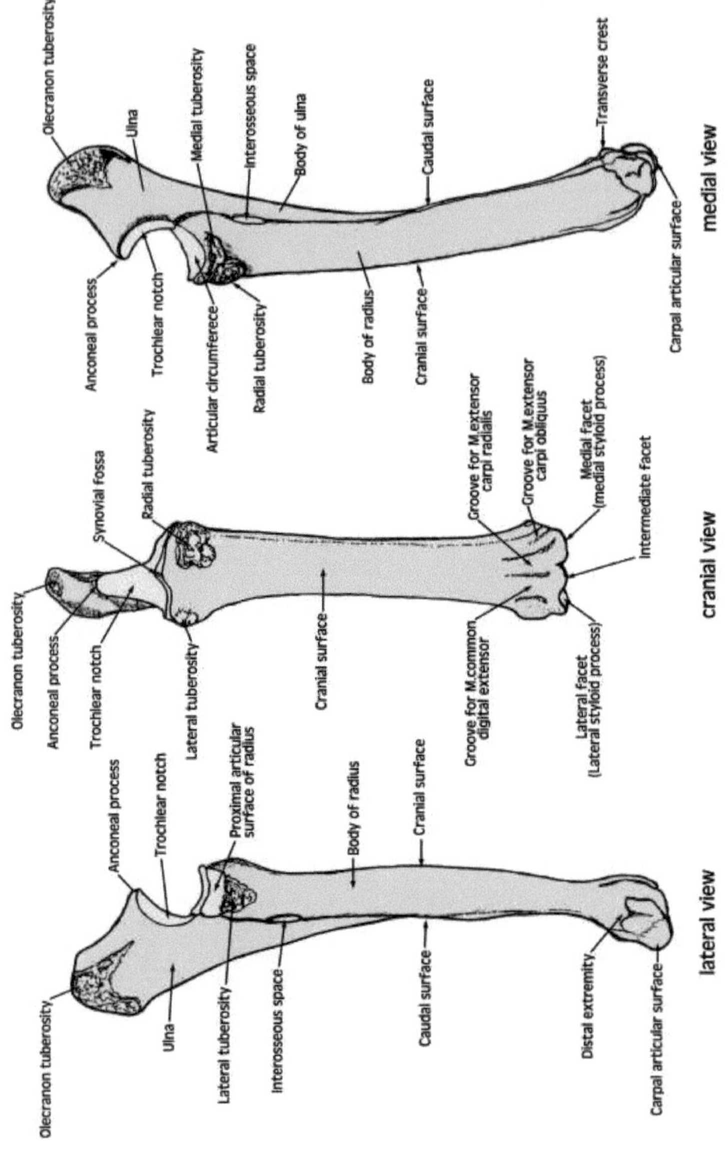

Fig.132. Right radius and ulna

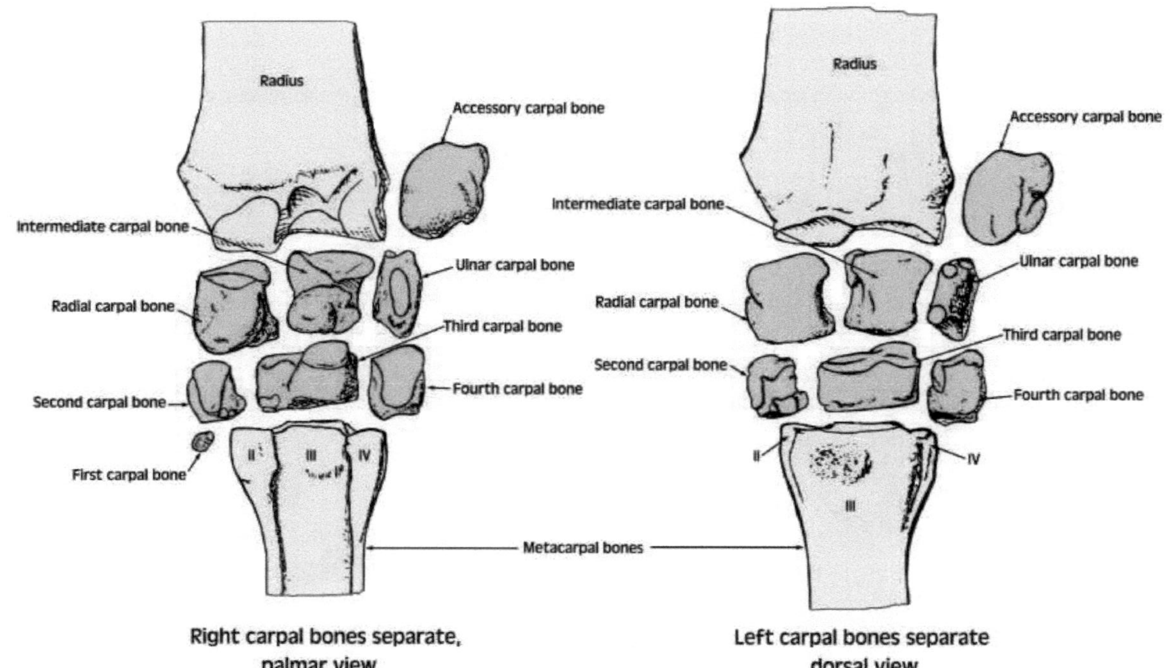

Right carpal bones separate,
palmar view

Left carpal bones separate
dorsal view

Fig.133. Carpal bones

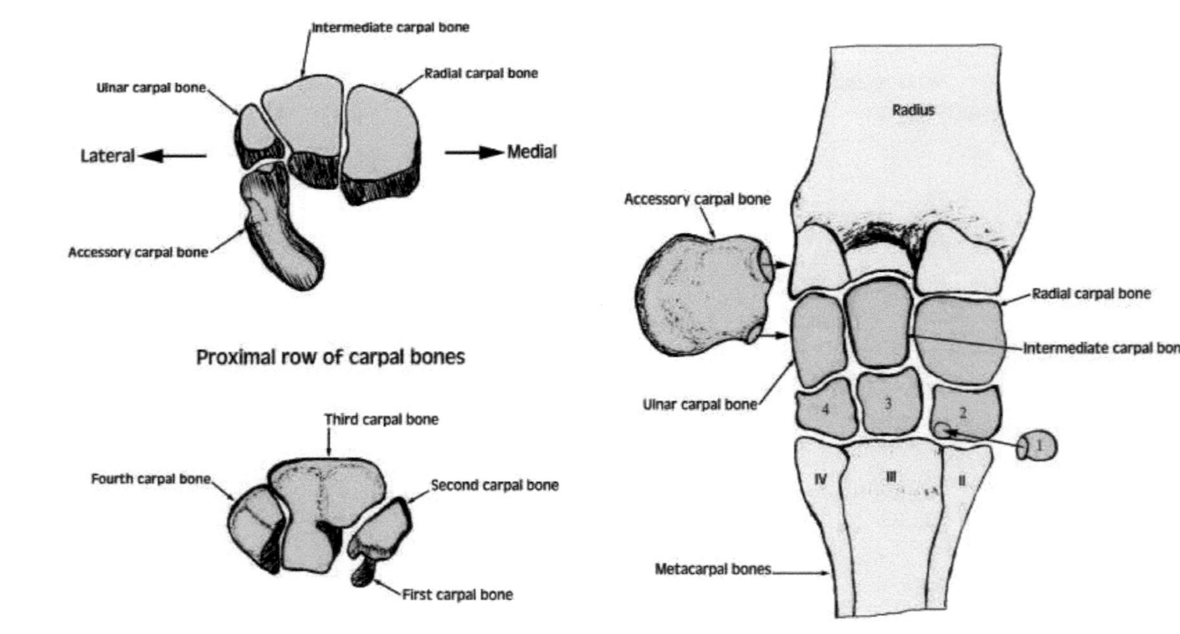

Fig.134. Carpal bones , diagrammatic

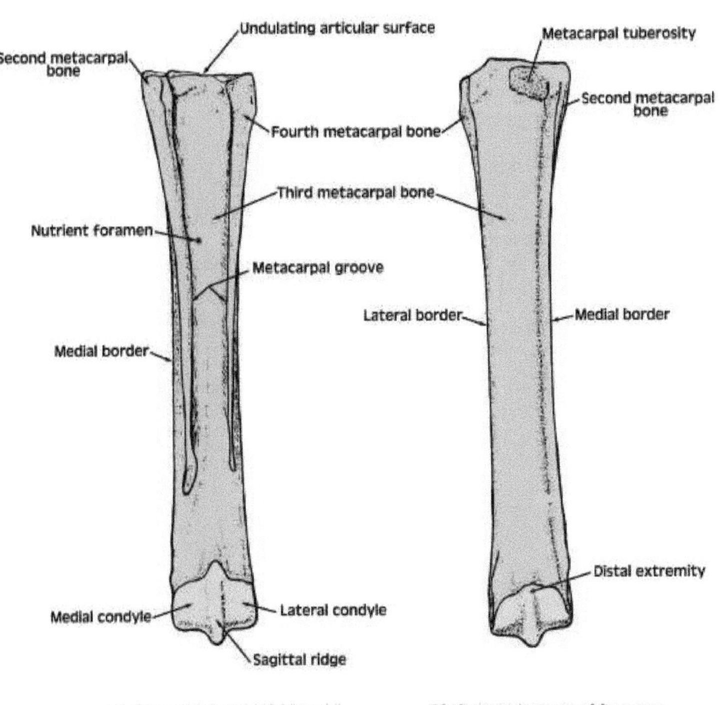

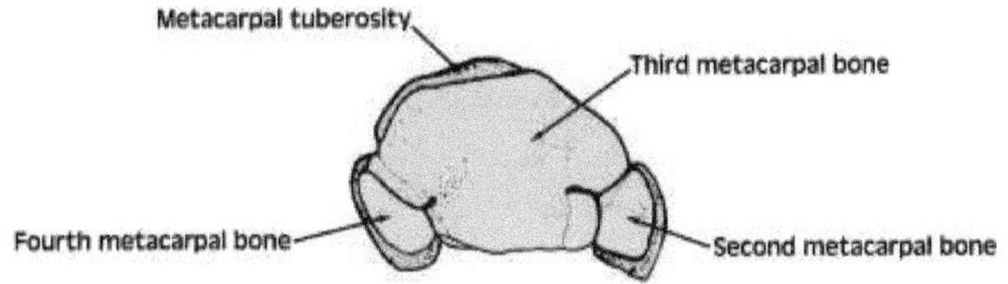

Fig.135. Metacarpal bones

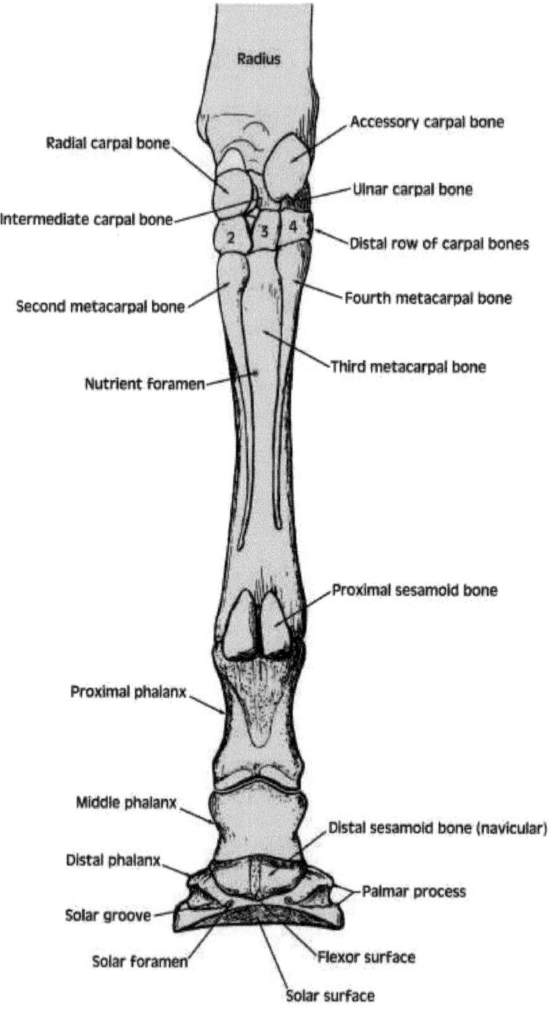

Fig.136. Right manus , palmar view

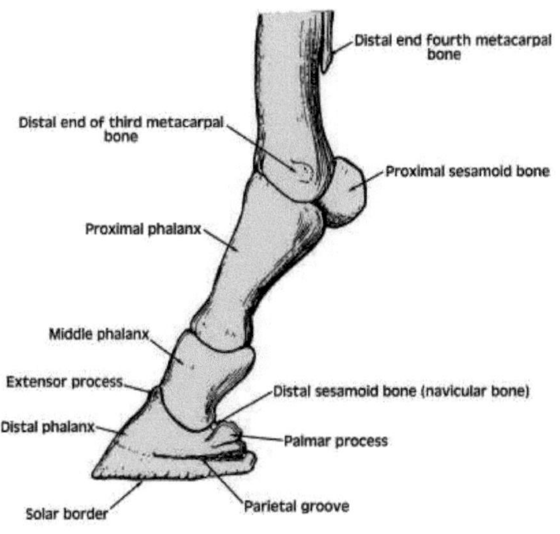

Medial surface

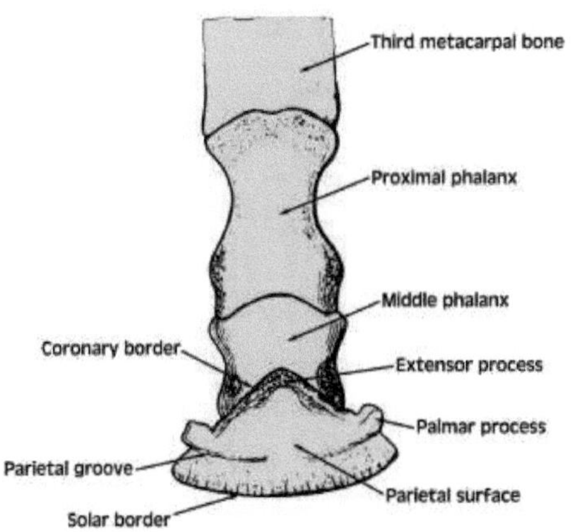

Dorsal surface

Fig 137. Left third digit

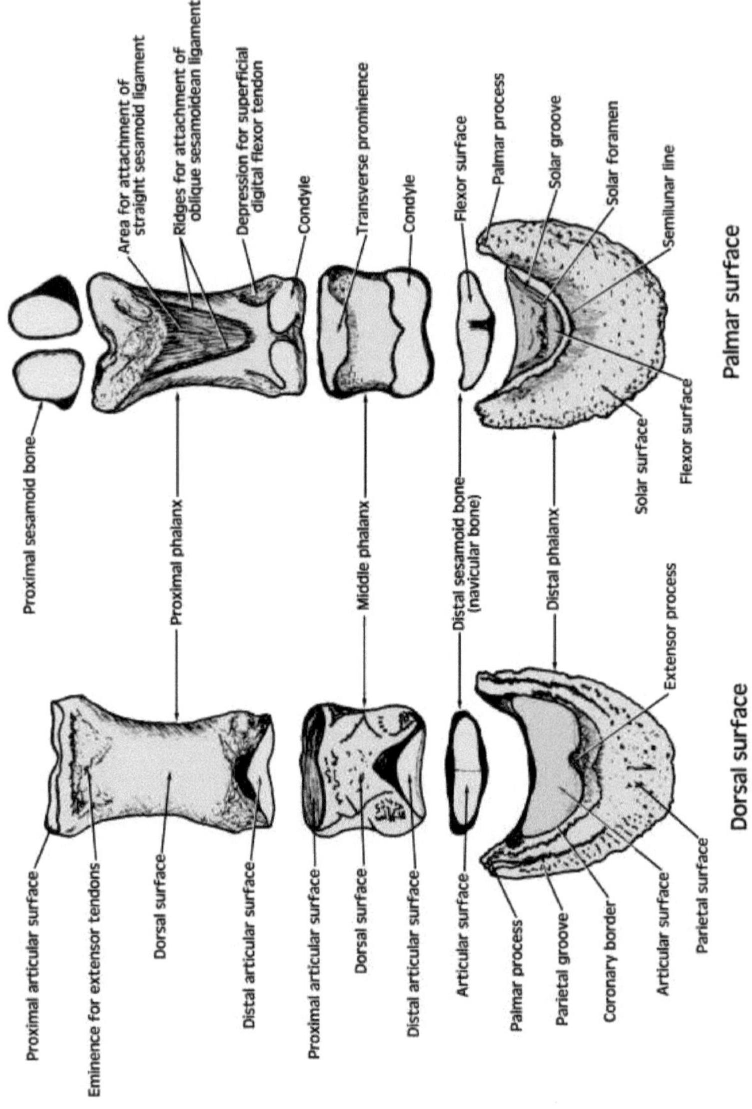

Fig.138. Phalanges of third digit and sesamoid bones

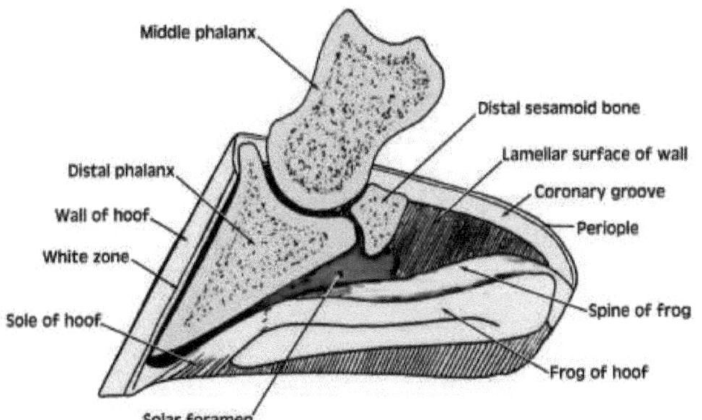

Hoof and its adjacent bones , sagittal section

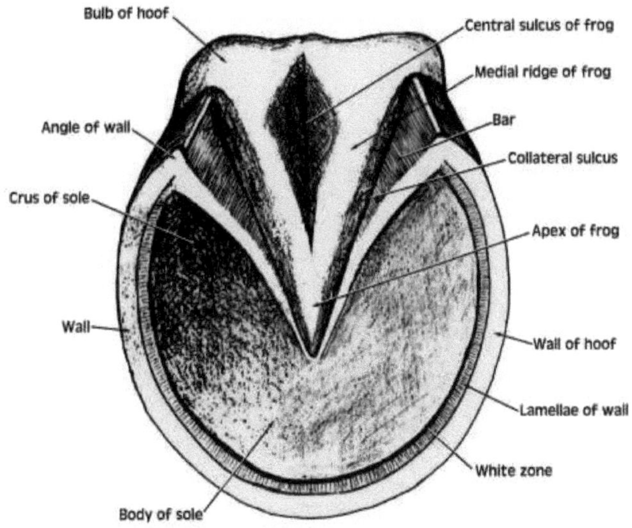

Ground surface of hoof

Fig.139. Hoof

149

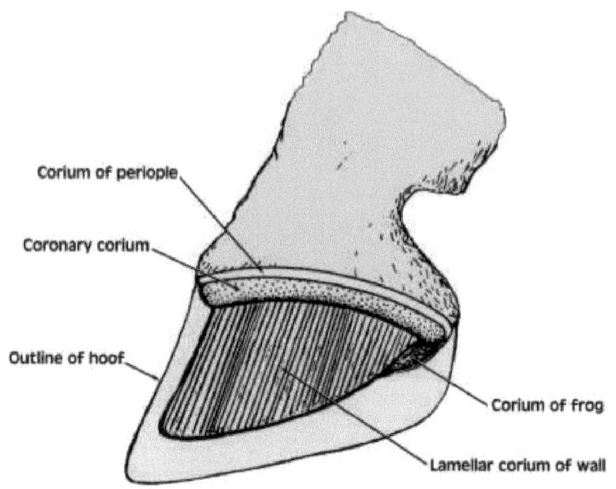

Corium of the foot , lateral view

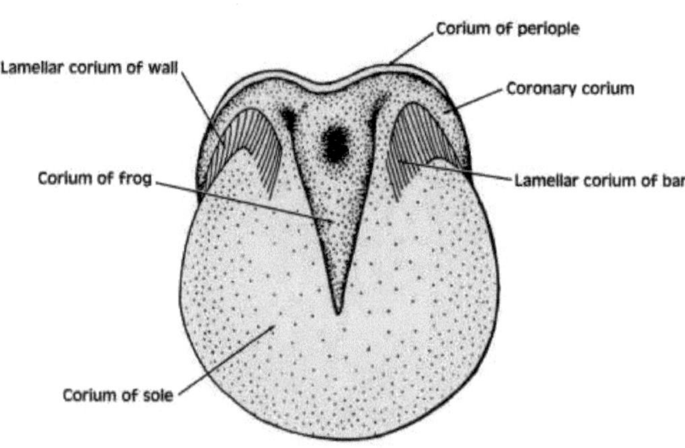

Corium of the foot , solar view

Fig.140. Corium of the foot

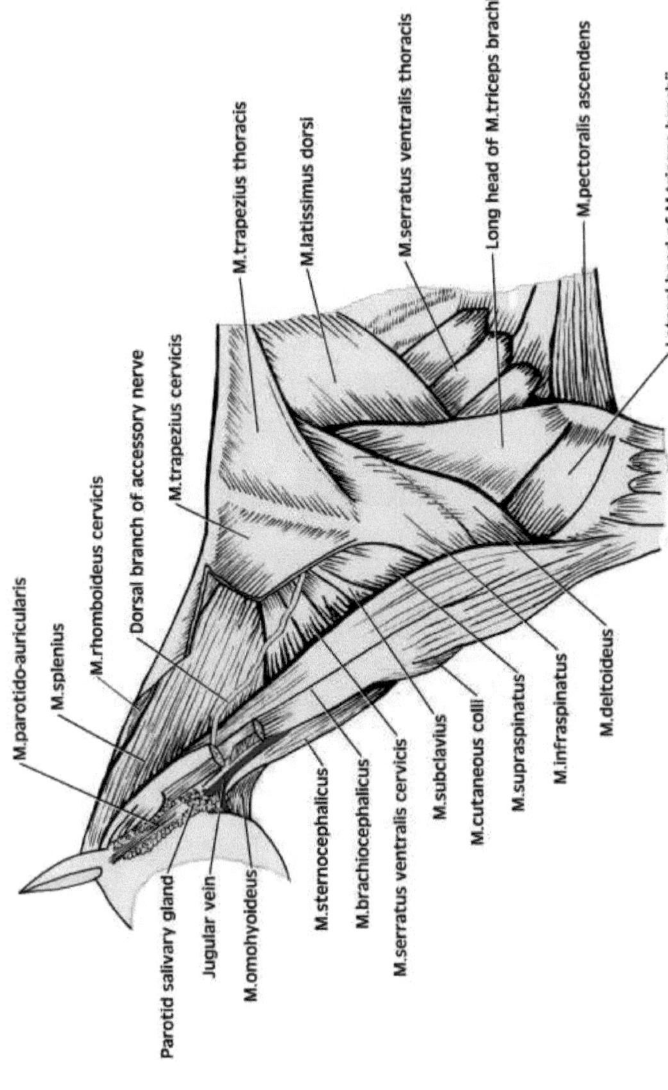

Fig.140. Dissection of the shoulder and arm regions ; left lateral view

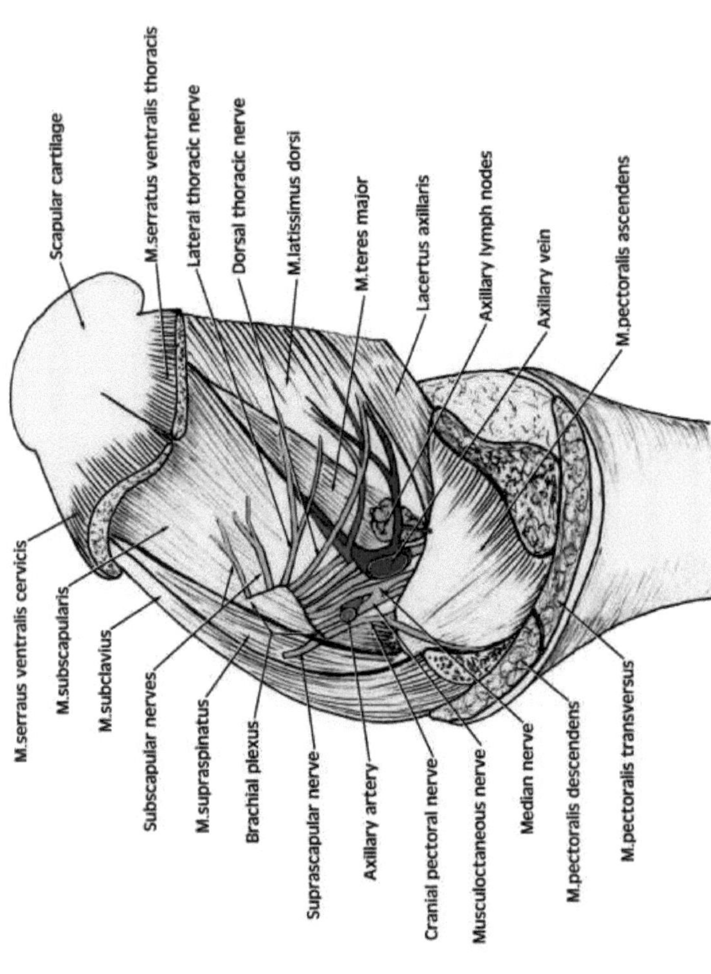

Fig.141. Dissection of the right shoulder and arm regions , medial view

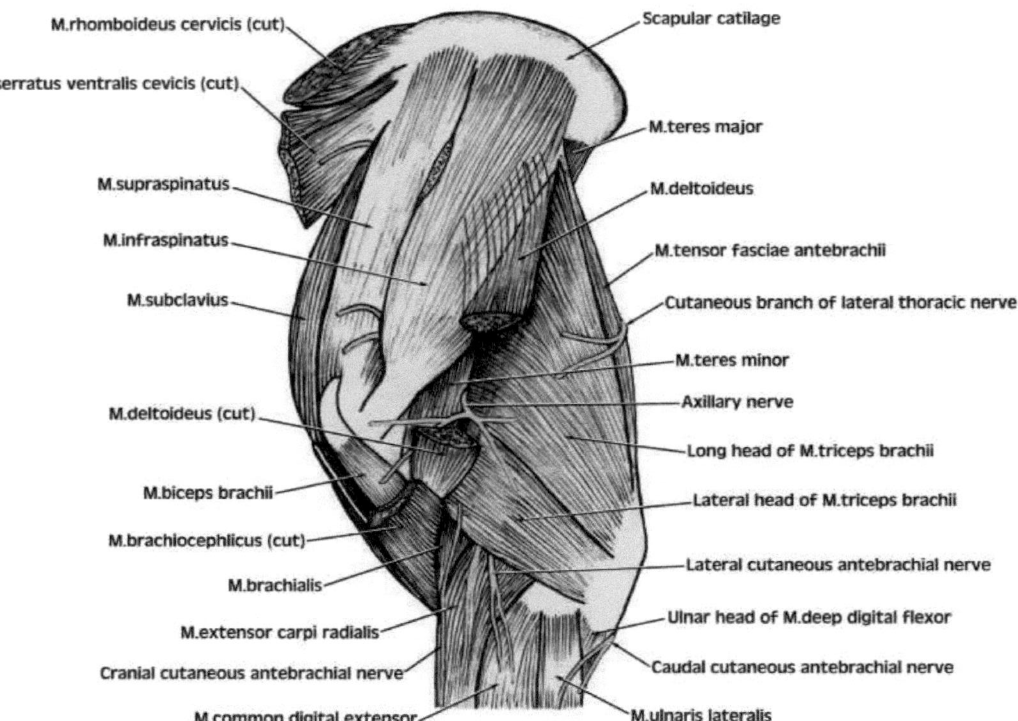

Fig.142. Dissection of the left shloulder and arm regions , lateral surface

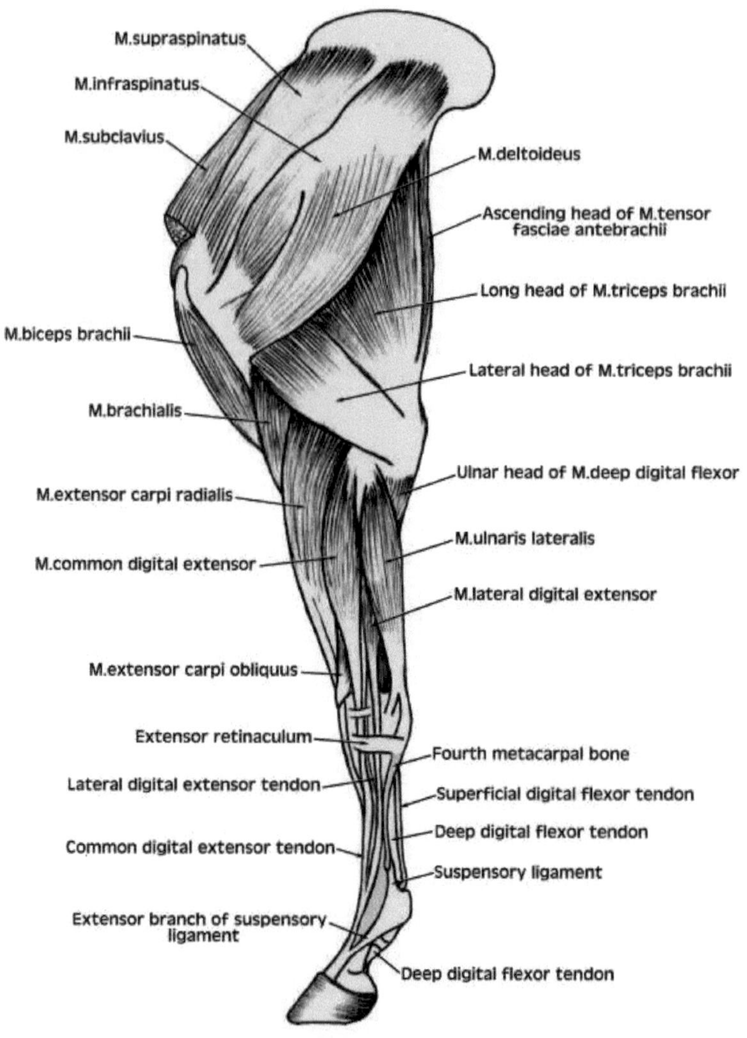

Fig.143.Dissection of left thoracic limb , lateral surface

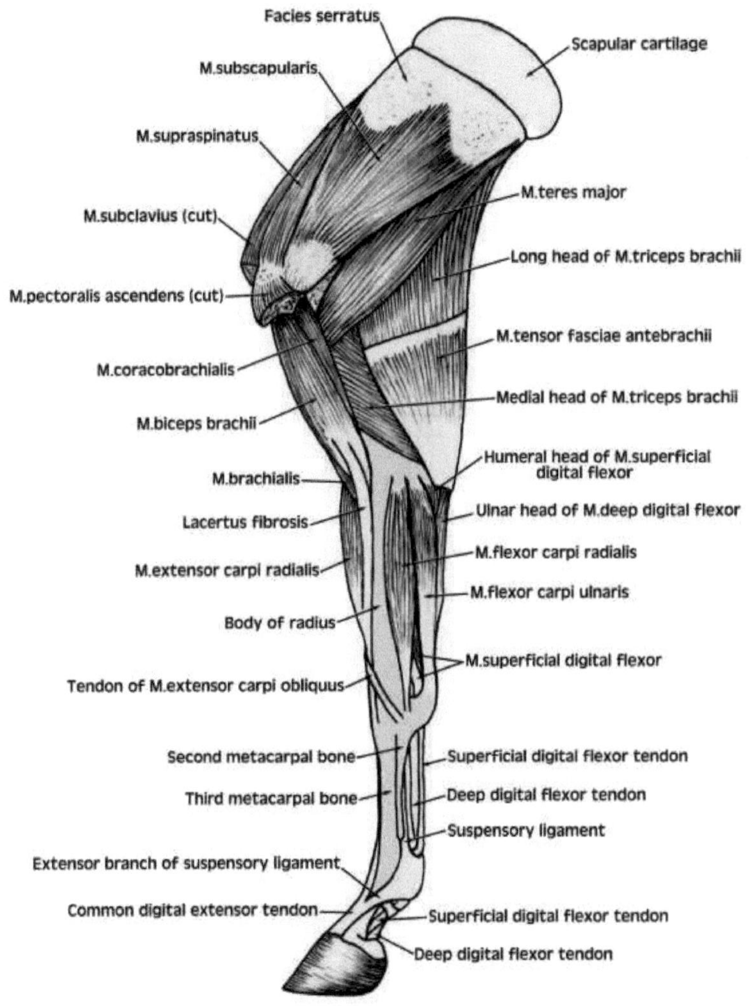

Fig.144.Dissection of right thoracic limb, medial surface

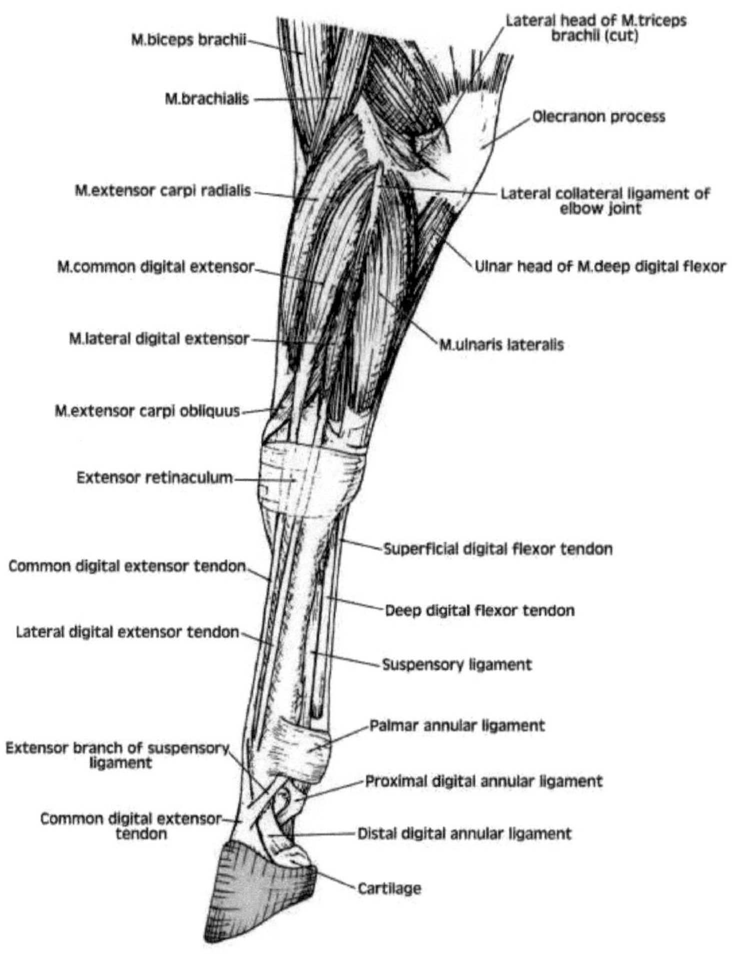

Fig 145. Dissection of forearm region and manus , lateral surface

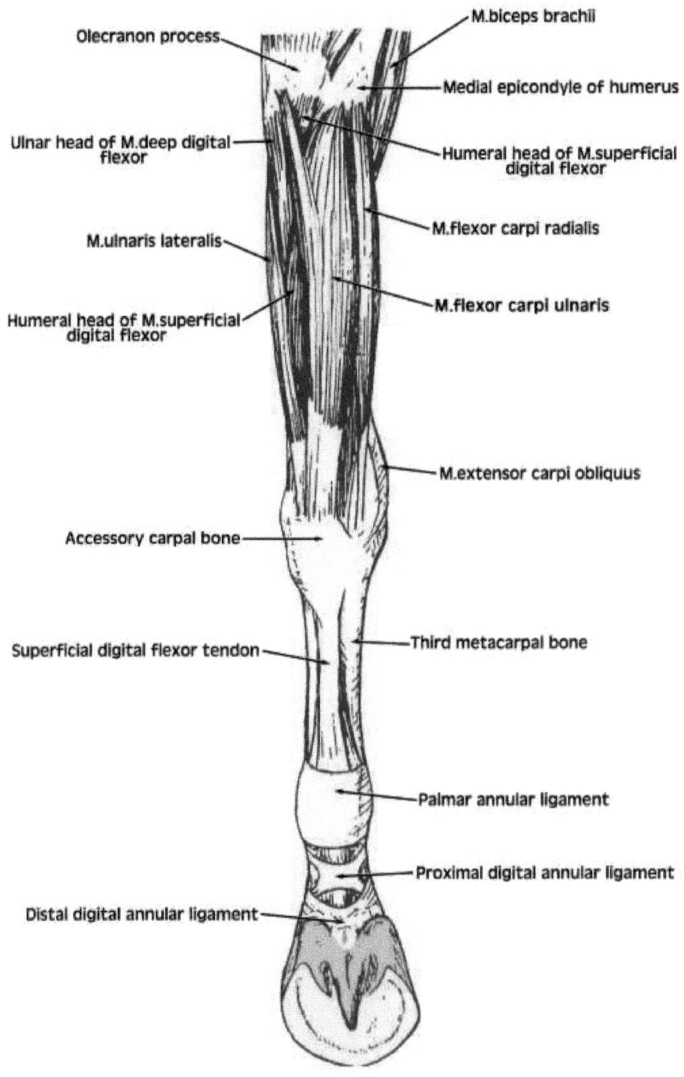

Fig.146. Dissection of left forearm region and manus , caudal surface

157

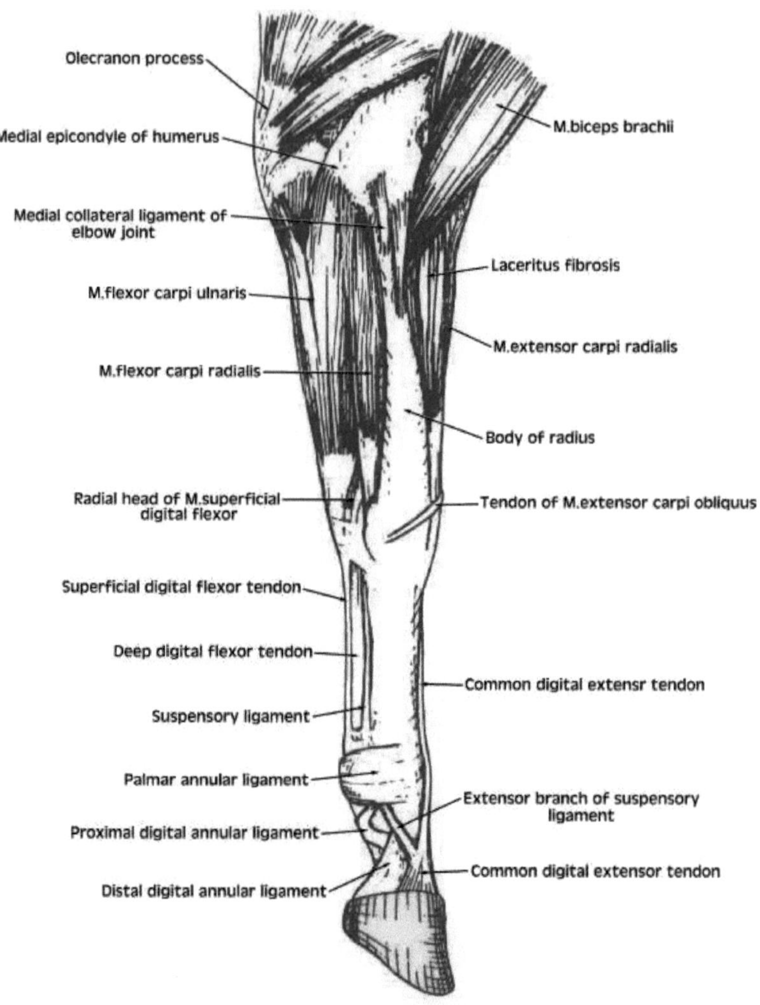

Fig.147. Dissection of left forearm region and manus , medial surface

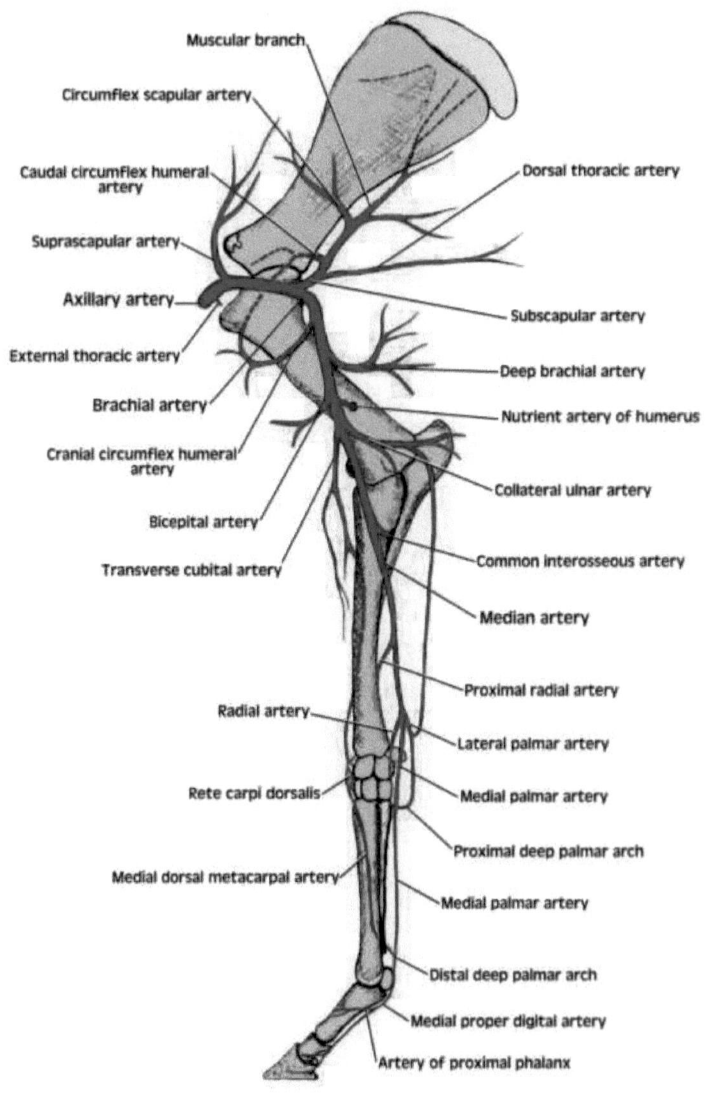

Fig.148. Arteries of right thoracic limb , medial view ; diagrammatic

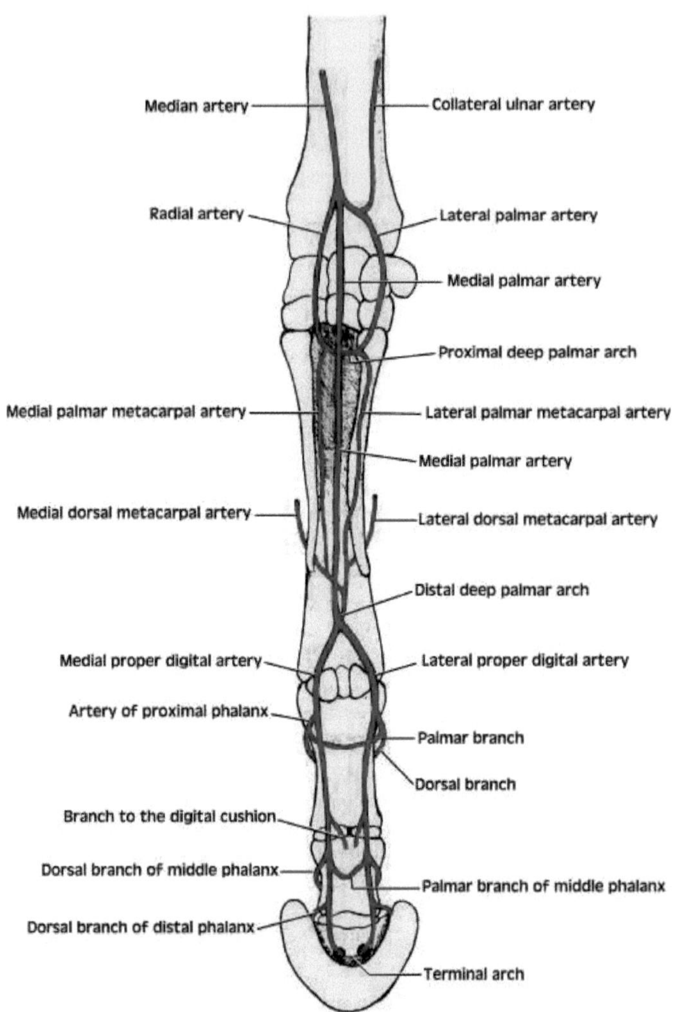

Fig.149. Arteries of the right manus , palmar surface ; diagrammatic

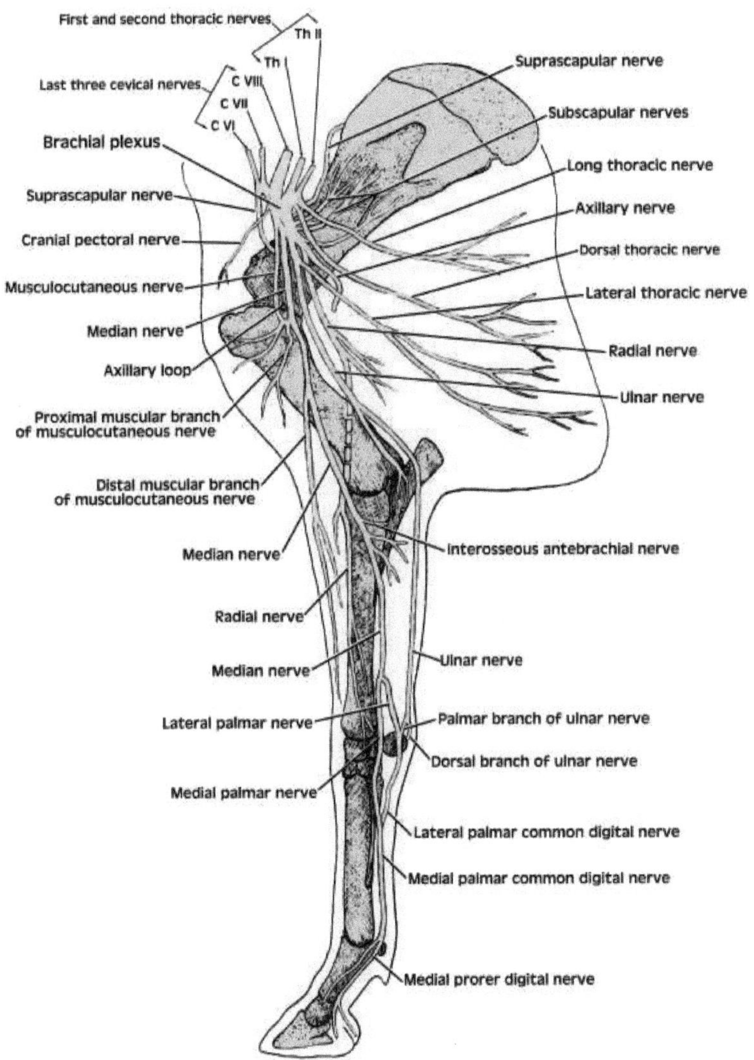

Fig.150. Nerves of thoracic limb (Brachial plexus) ,
medial view , diagrammatic

161

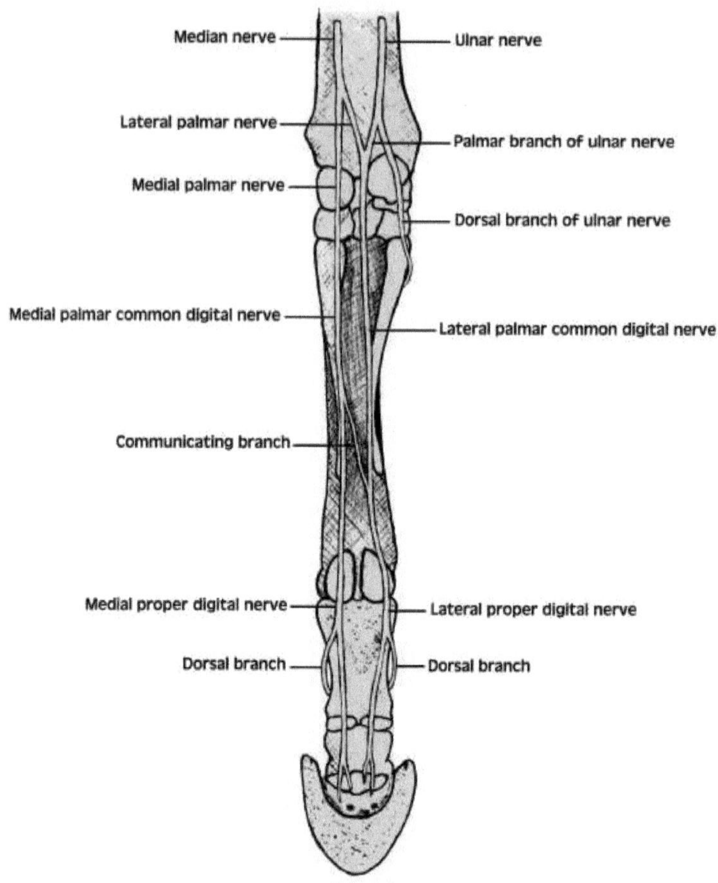

Fig.151. Nerve supply of right manus , palmar view

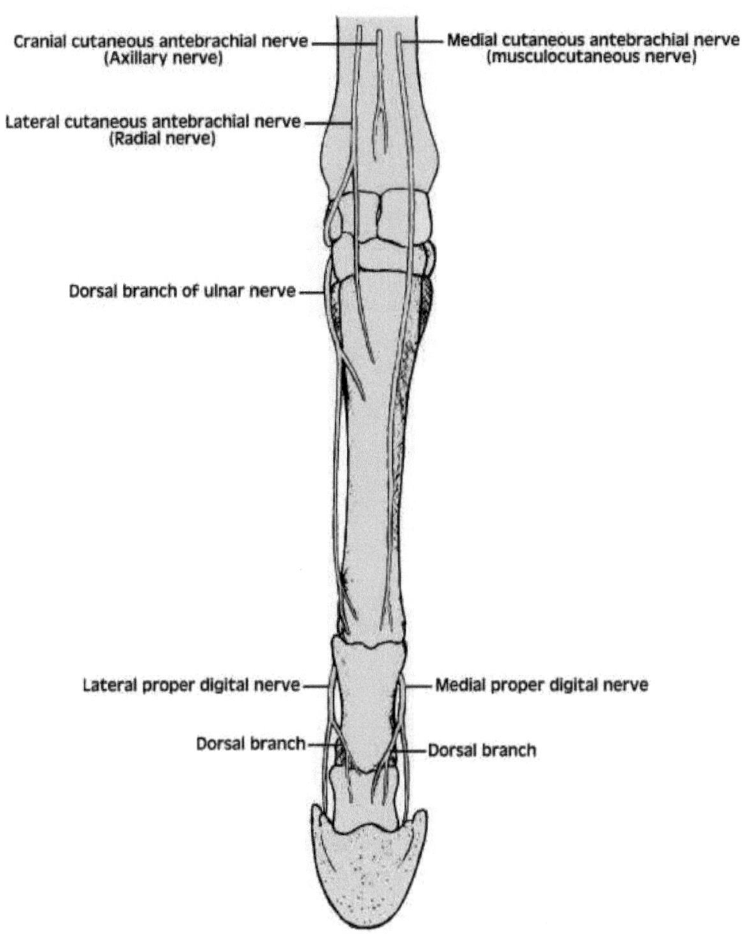

Fig.152. Nerve supply of right manus , dorsal view

163

Chapter 5
Pelvic Limb

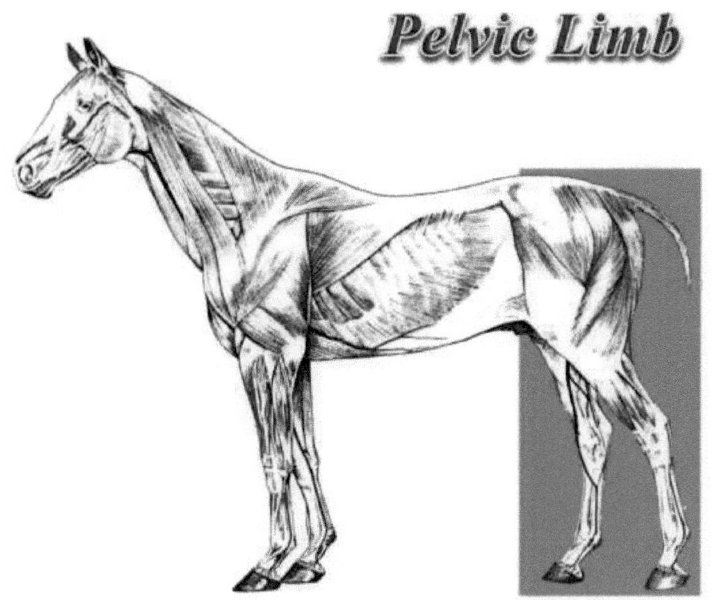

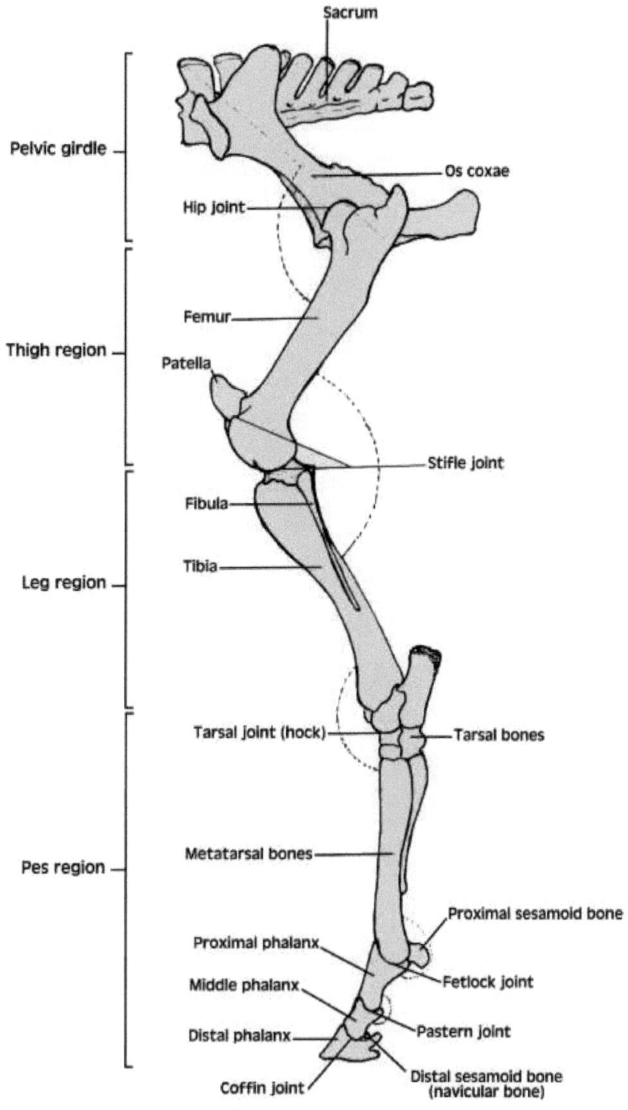

Fig.153. Bones and joints of the pelvic limb , lateral view

167

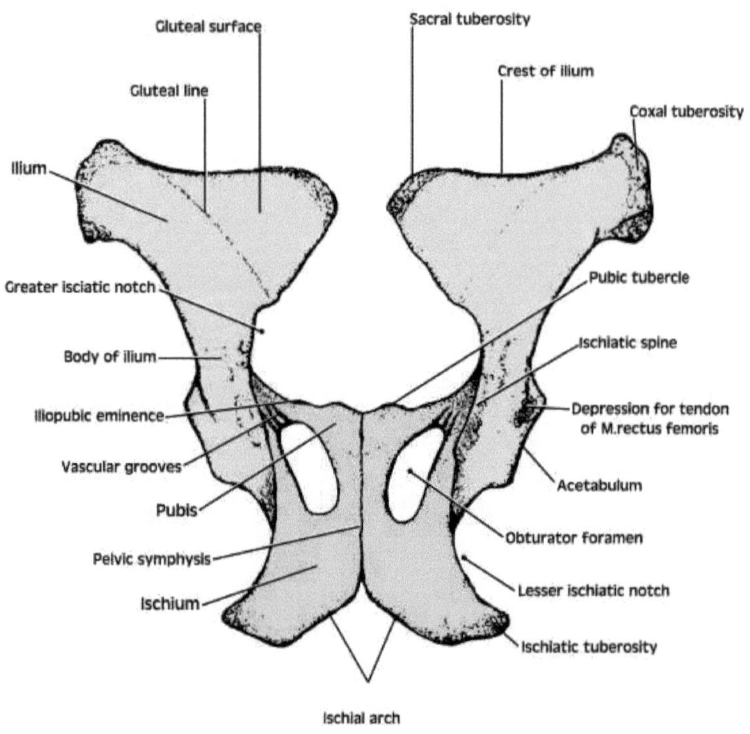

Fig 154. Ossa coxarum , dorsal view

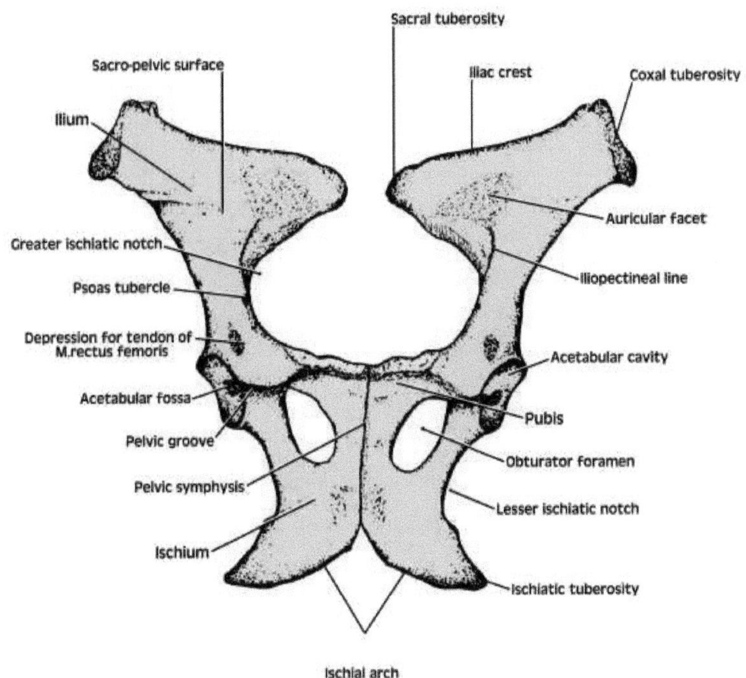

Fig.155. Ossa coxarum , ventral view

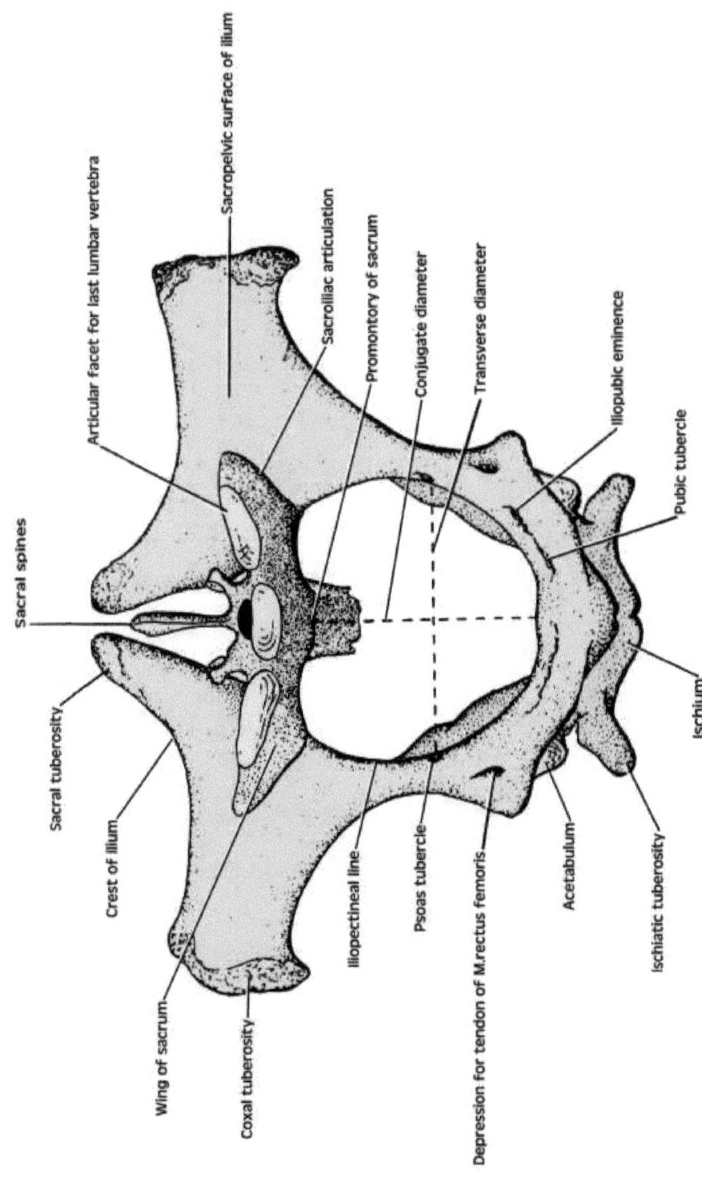

Fig.156. Pelvic bones and sacrum , cranioventral view

170

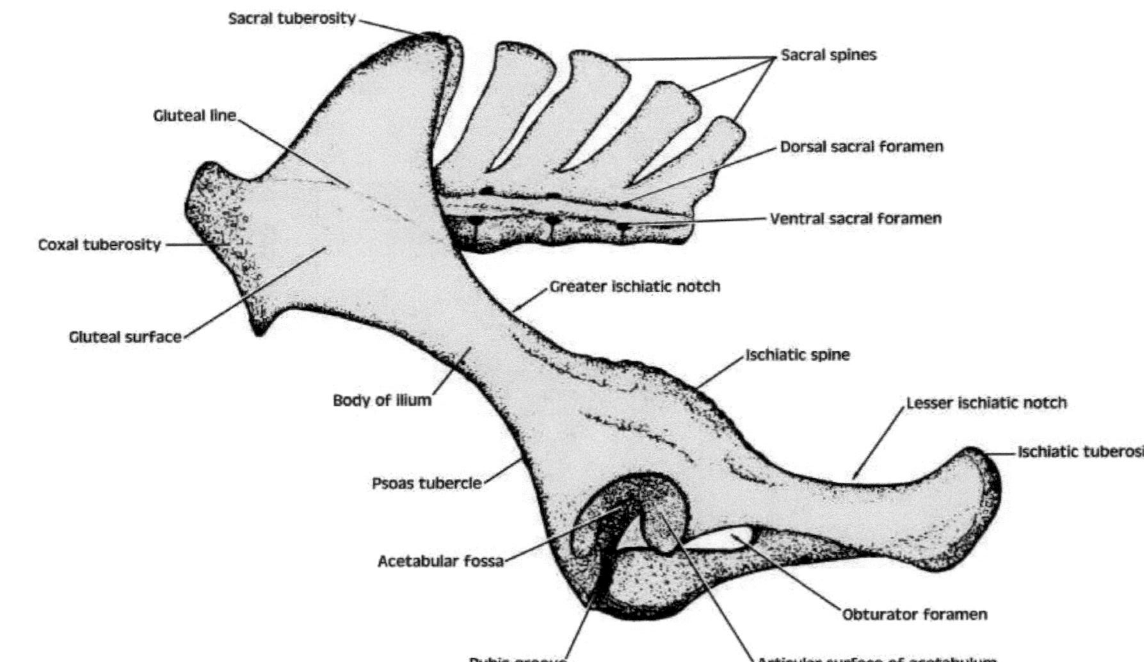

Fig.157. Left os coxae and sacrum , left lateral view

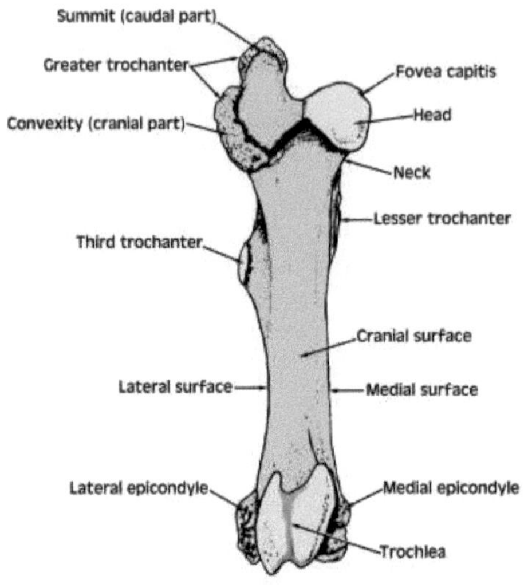

Cranial view

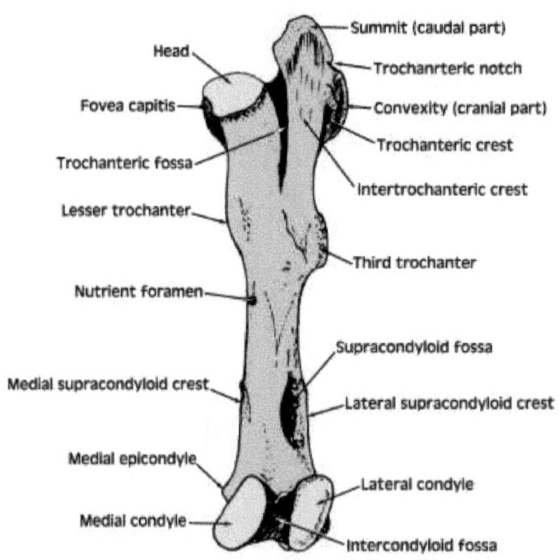

Caudal view

Fig.158. Right femur

172

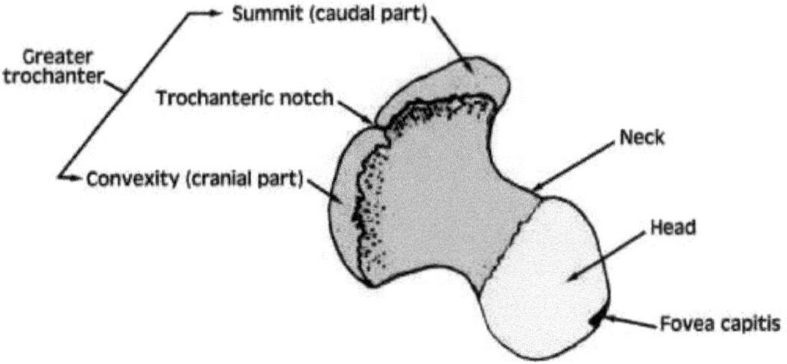

Proximal extremity

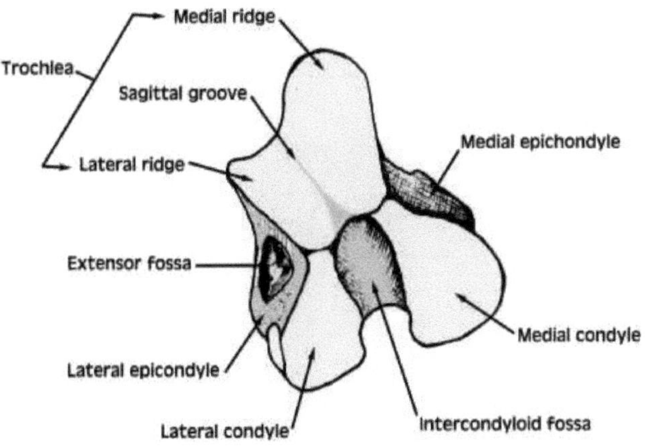

Distal extremity

Fig.159. Extremities of right femur

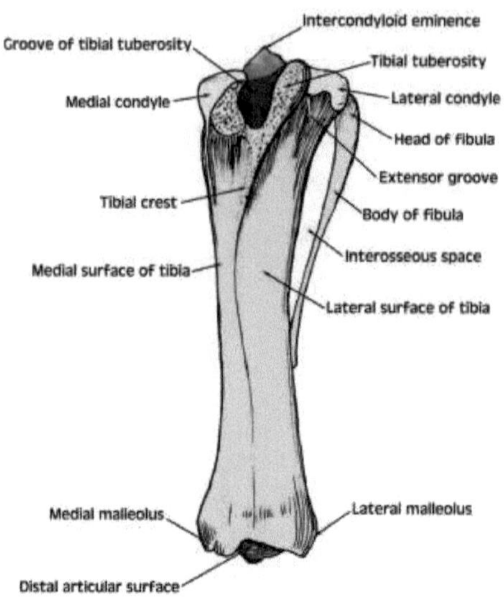

Cranial view

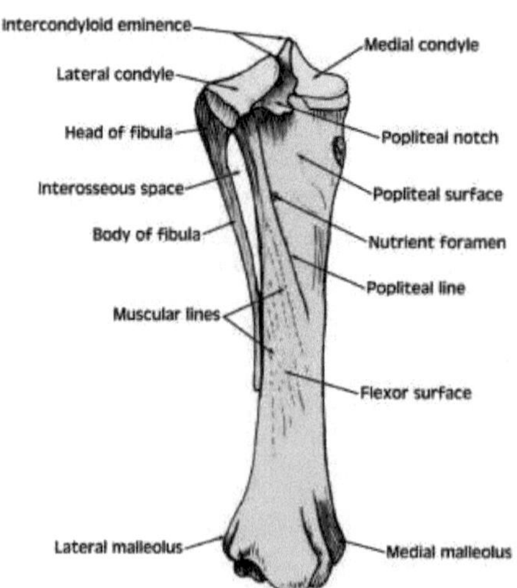

Caudal view

Fig.160. Left tibia and fibula

174

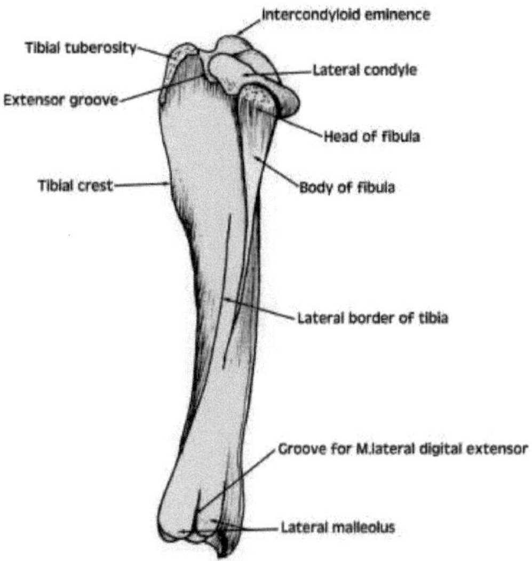

Fig.161. Left tibia and fibula , lateral view

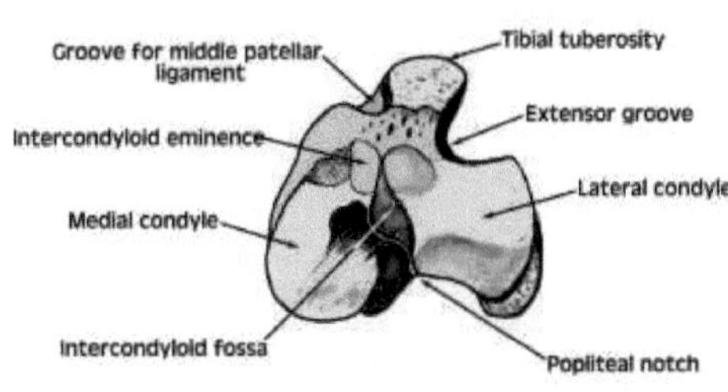

Proximal extremity

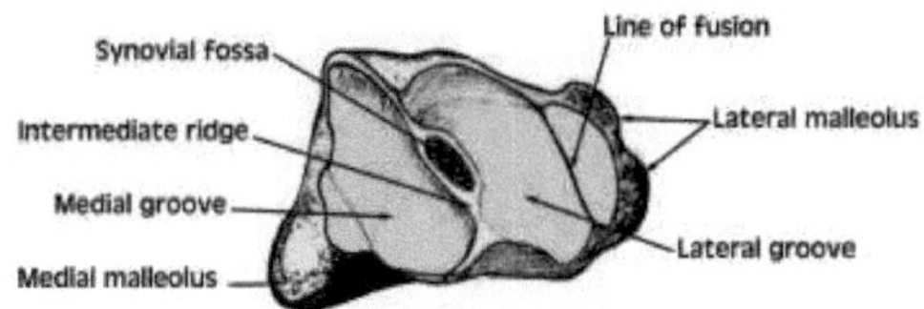

Distal extremity

Fig.162. Extremities of right tibia and fibula

175

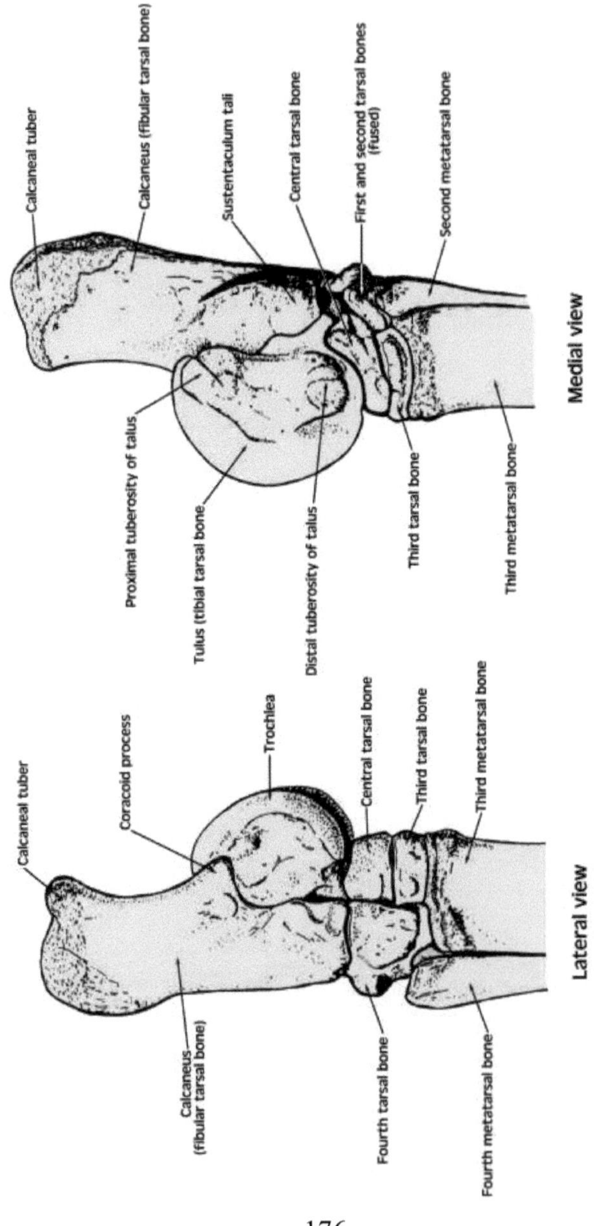

Fig.163. Right tarsus and proximal part of metatarsus

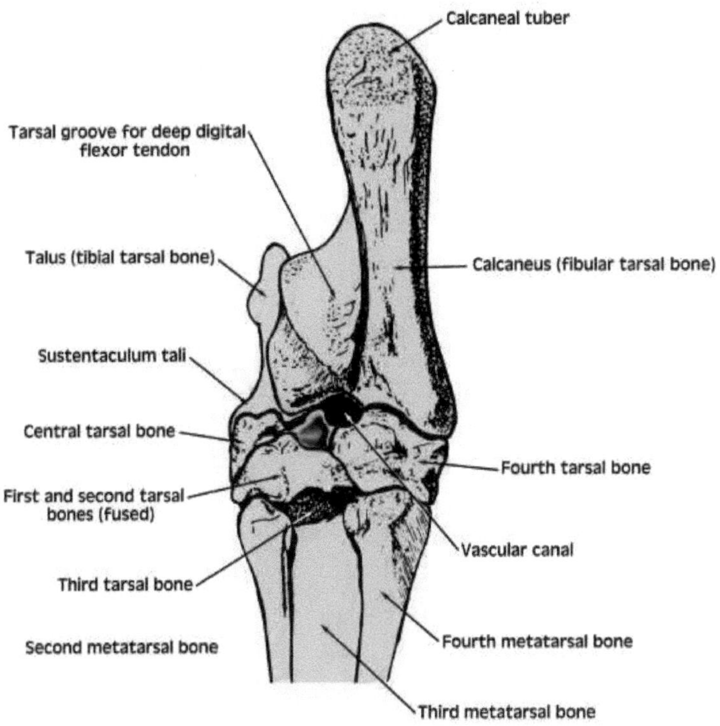

Fig.164. Right tarsus and proximal part of metatarsus , plantar view

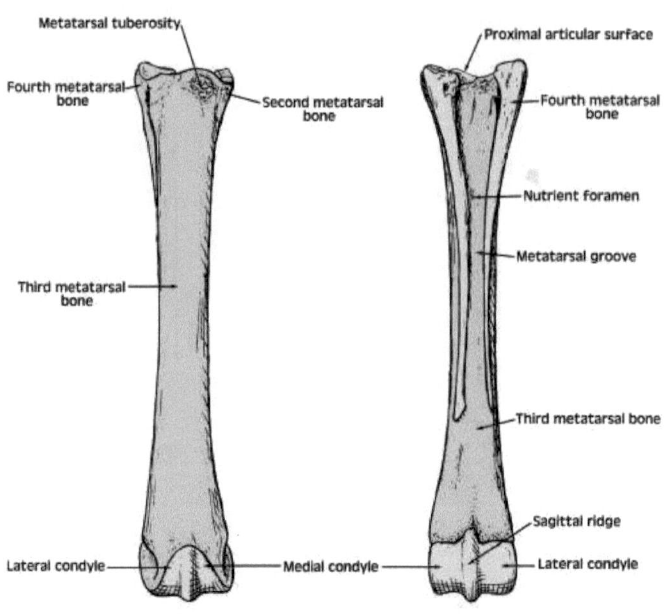

Right metatarsus , dorsal view

Right metatarsus , plantar view

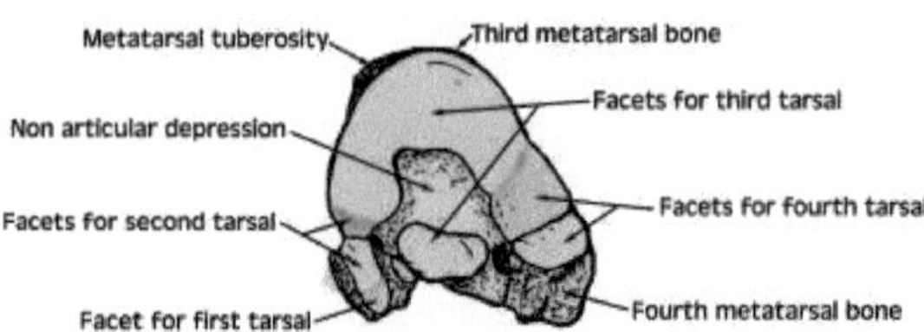

Proximal extremities of right metatarsal bones

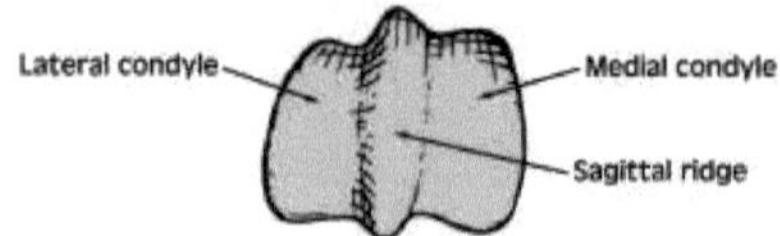

Distal articular surface of large metatarsal bone

Fig.165. Metatarsal bones

178

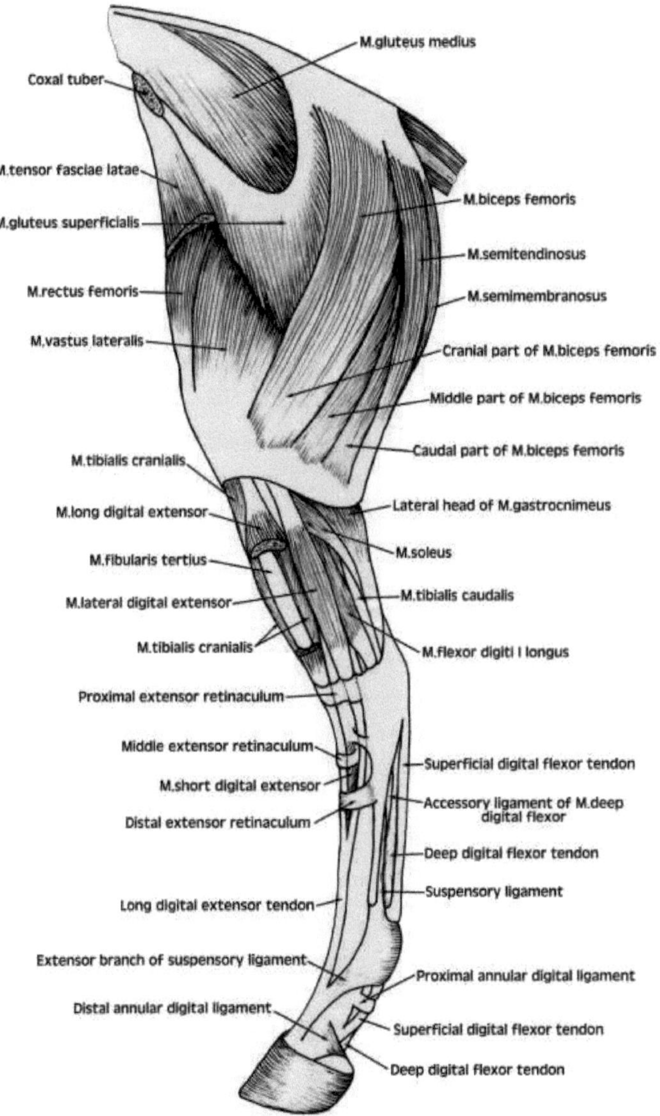

Fig.166. Dissection of left pelvic limb , lateral surface

179

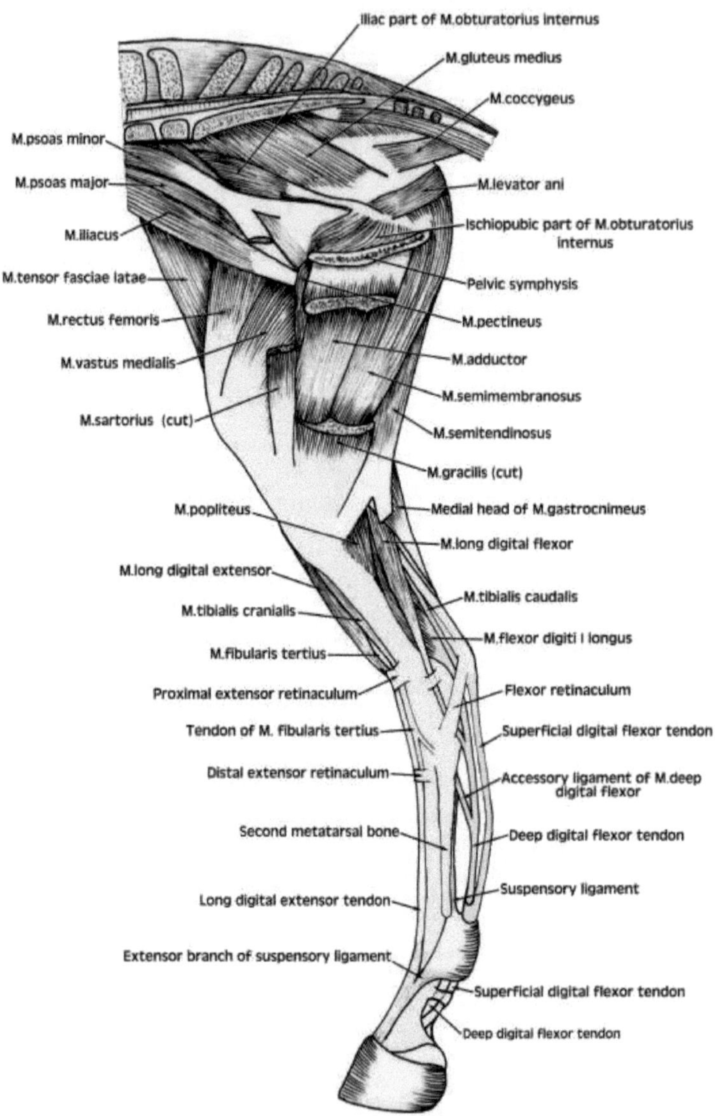

Fig.167. Dissection of right pelvic limb, medial surface

180

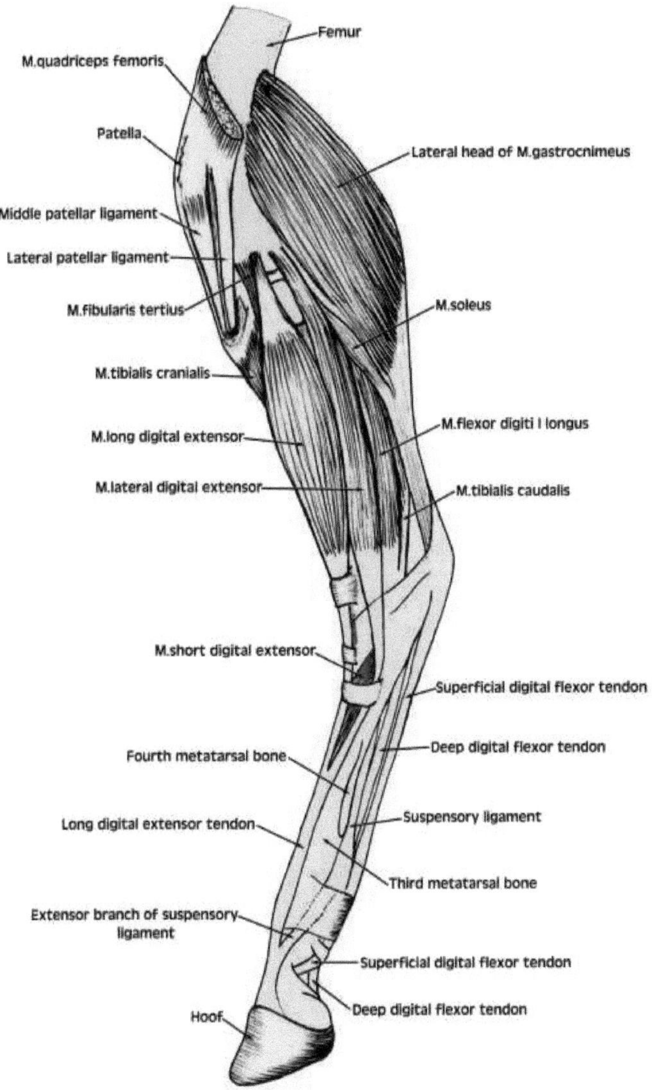

Fig.168. Dissection of the leg and pes regions ,
lateral surface

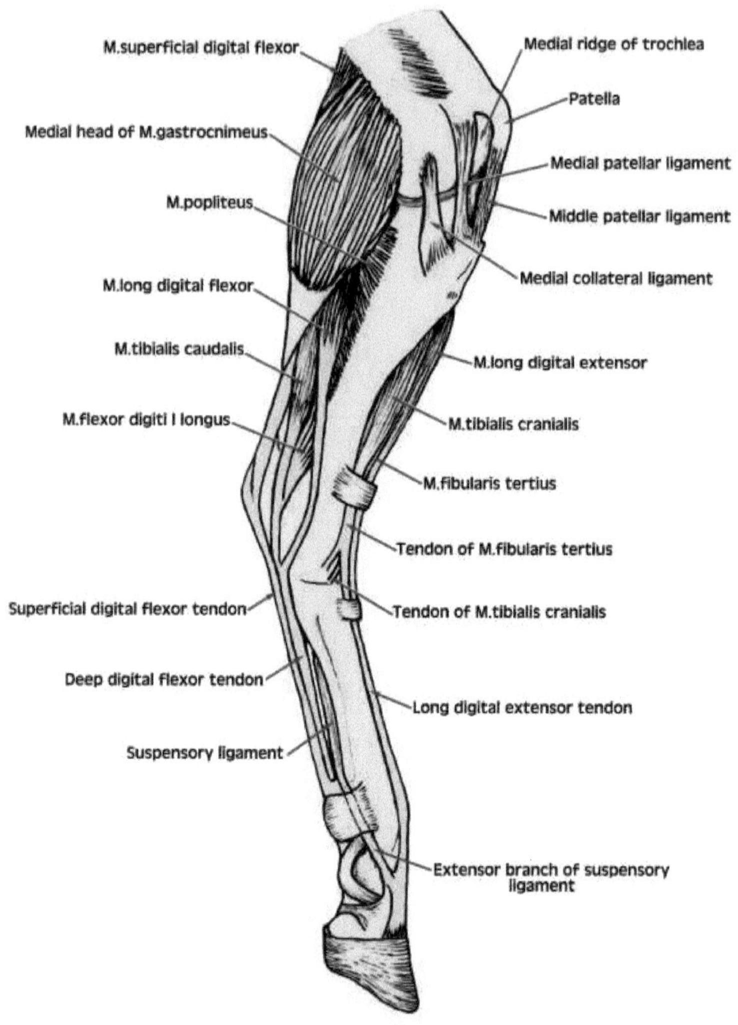

Fig.169. Dissection of the leg and pes regions , medial surface

182

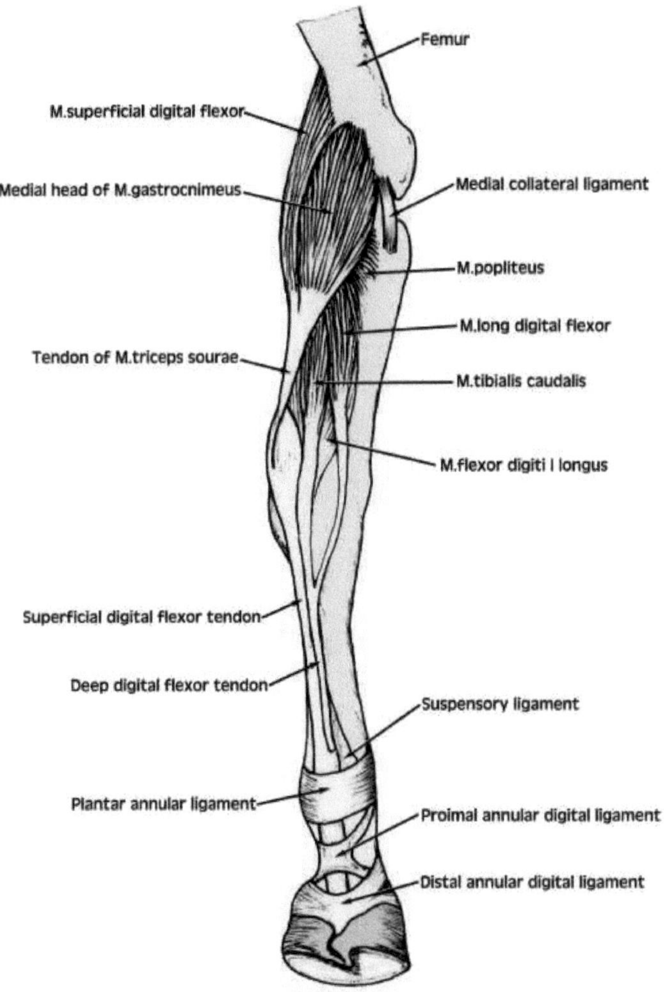

Fig.170. Dissection of the leg and pes regions , caudomedial view

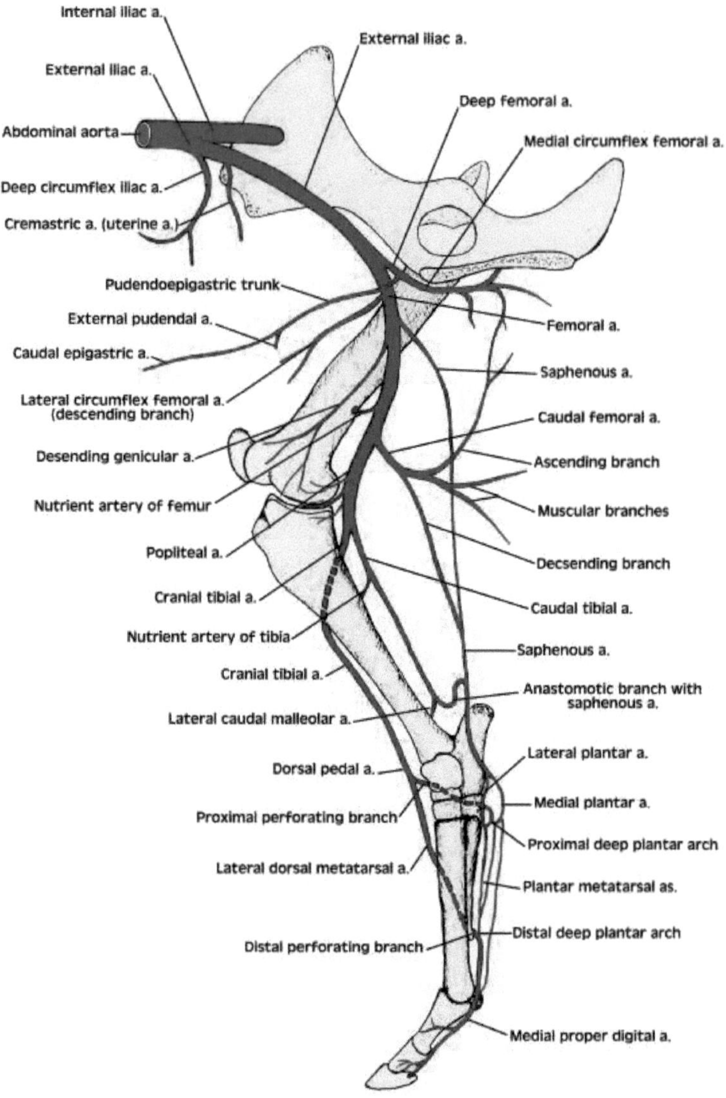

Fig 171. Arteries of right pelvic limb , medial view ; diagrammatic

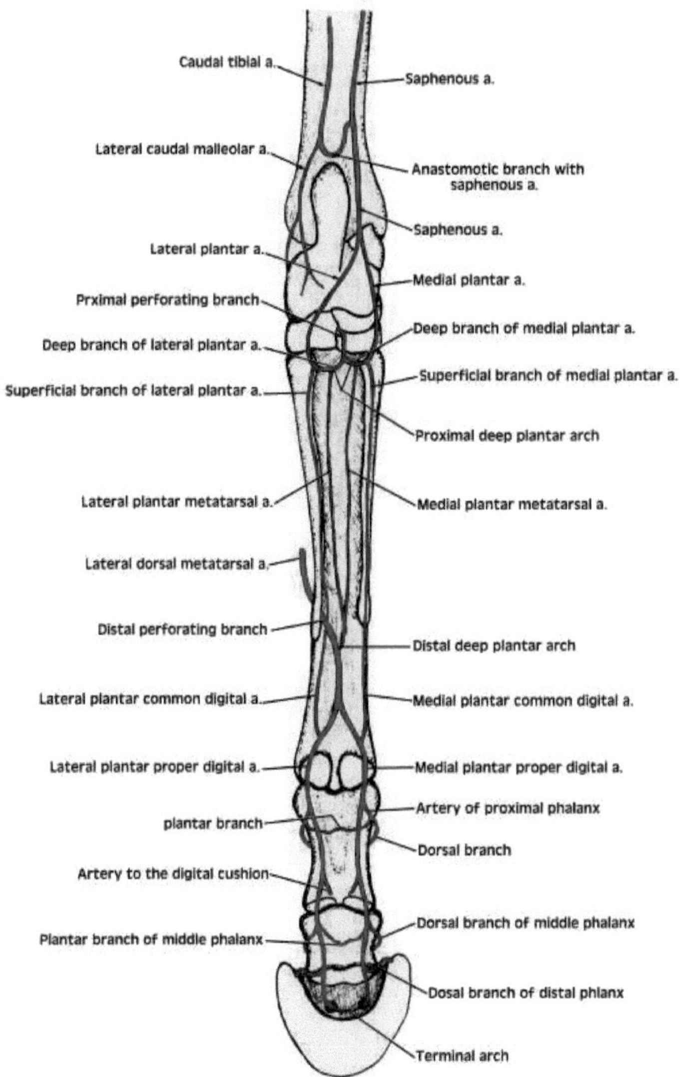

Fig.172. Arteries of the pes region , plantar view ; diagrammatic

185

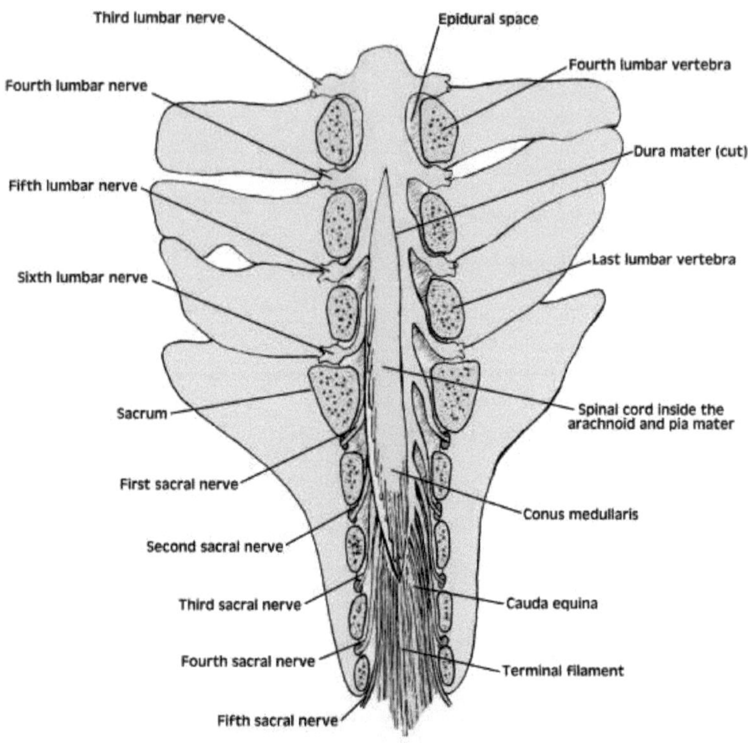

Fig.173. Terminal part of spinal cord inside the vertebral canal , dorsal view

186

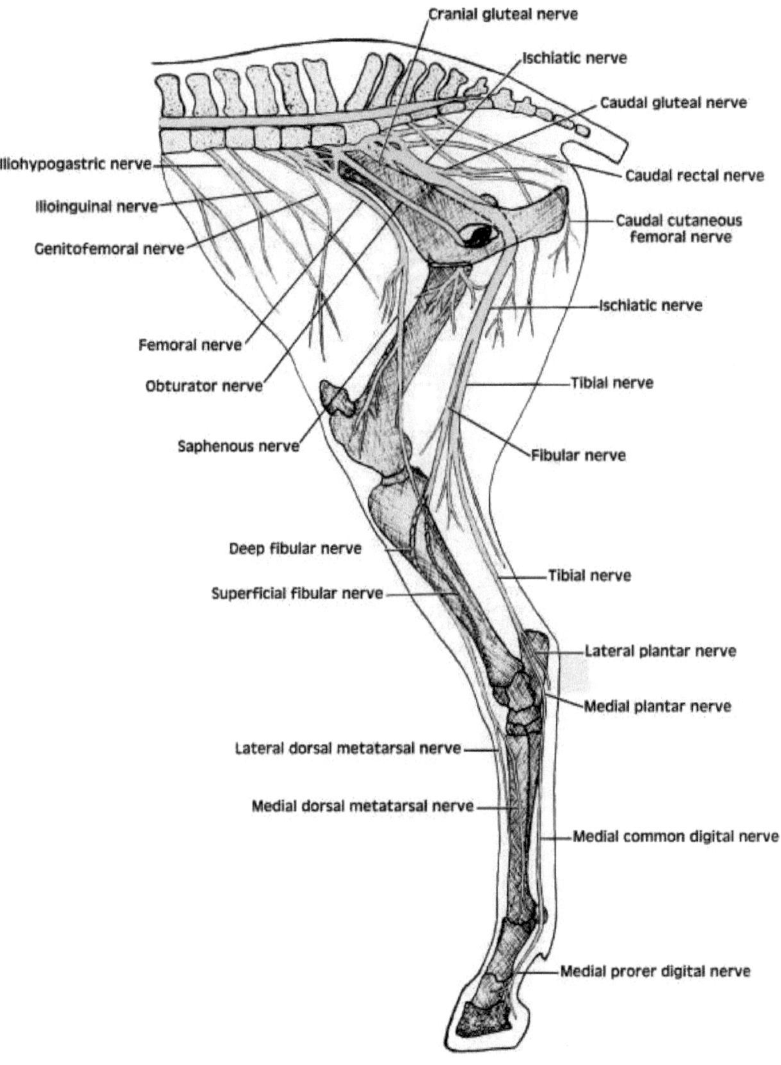

Fig.174. Nerves of right pelvic limb (lumbo-sacral plexus), medial surface

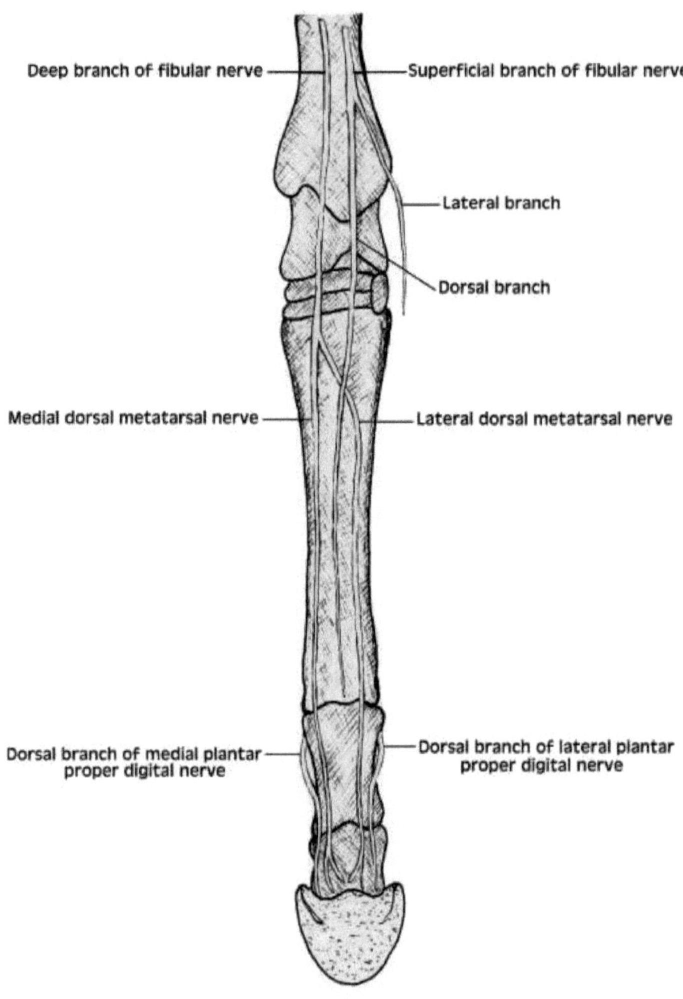

Fig.175. Nerves of left pes region , dorsal view

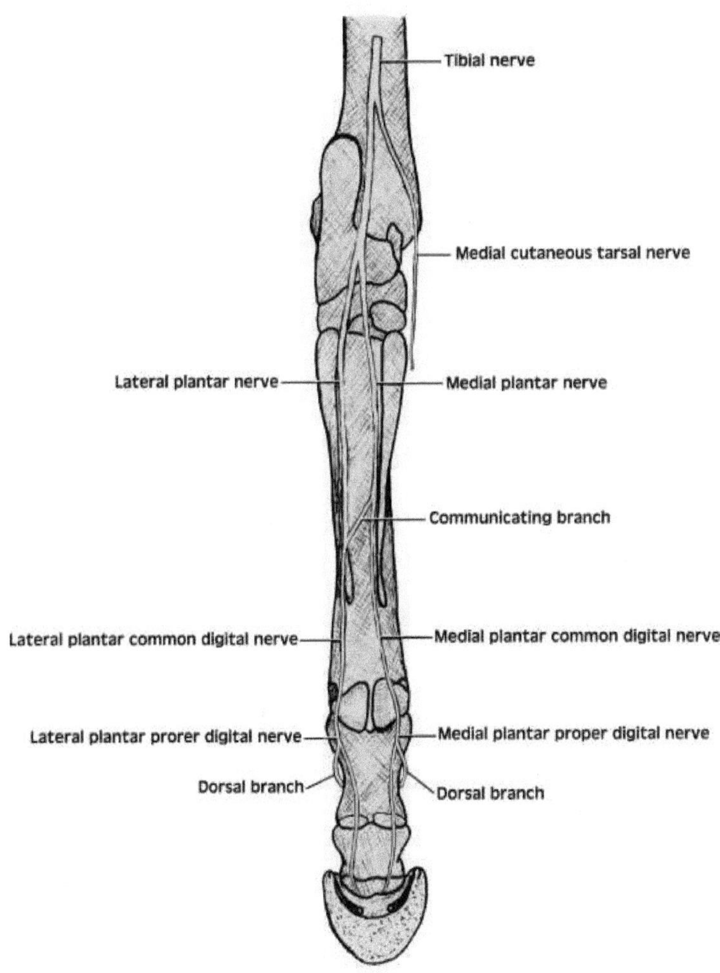

Fig.176. Nerves of left pes region , plantar view

189

Chapter 6
Joints and Ligaments of Limbs

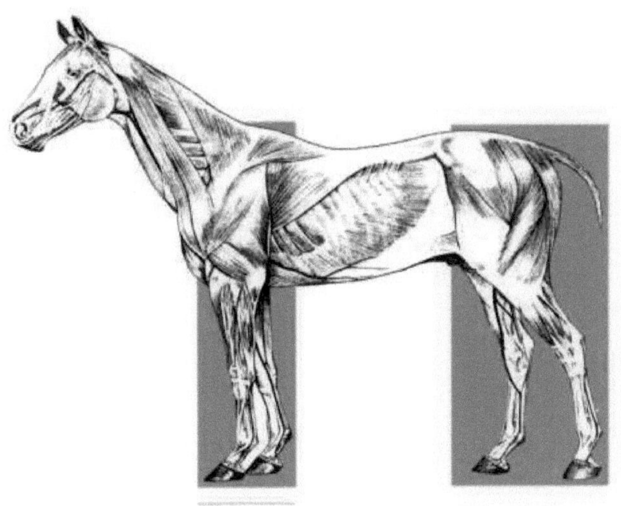

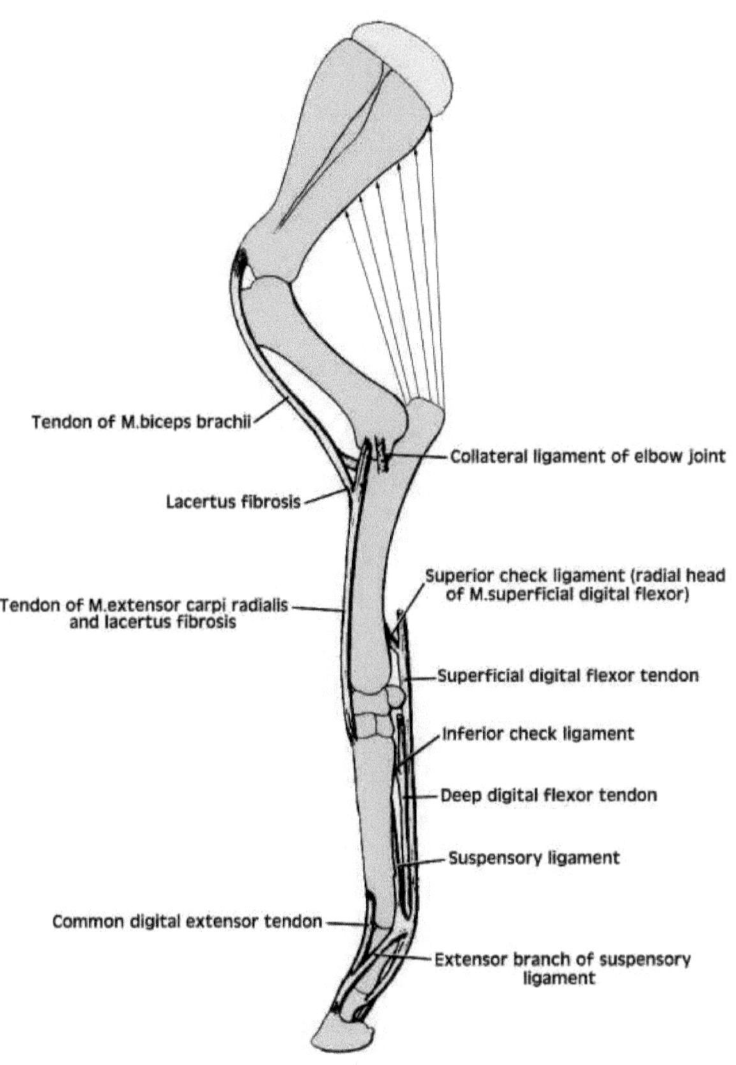

Fig.177. Structures making up the stay apparatus of the thoracic limb

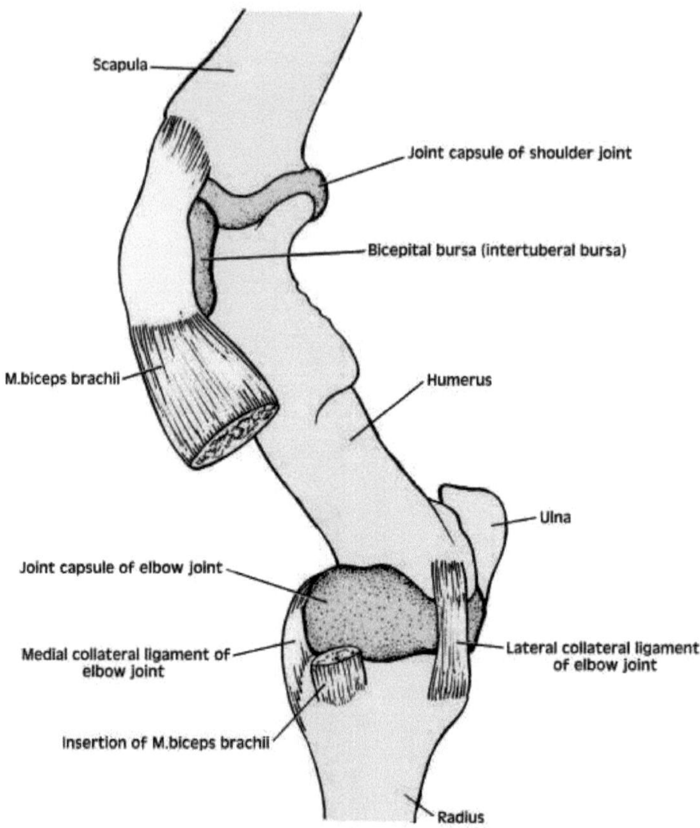

Fig.178. Shoulder and elbow joints , craniolateral view

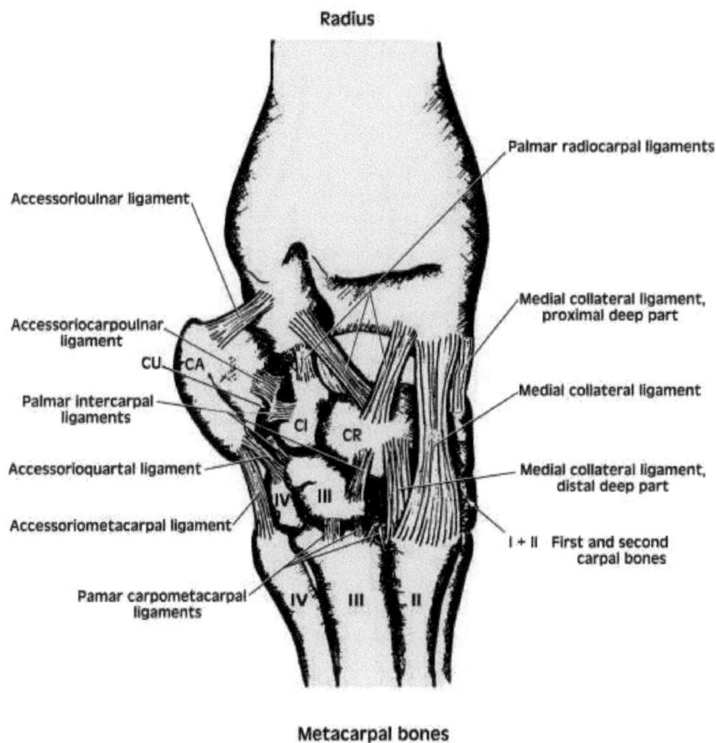

Fig.179. Carpal joint , palmar medial view

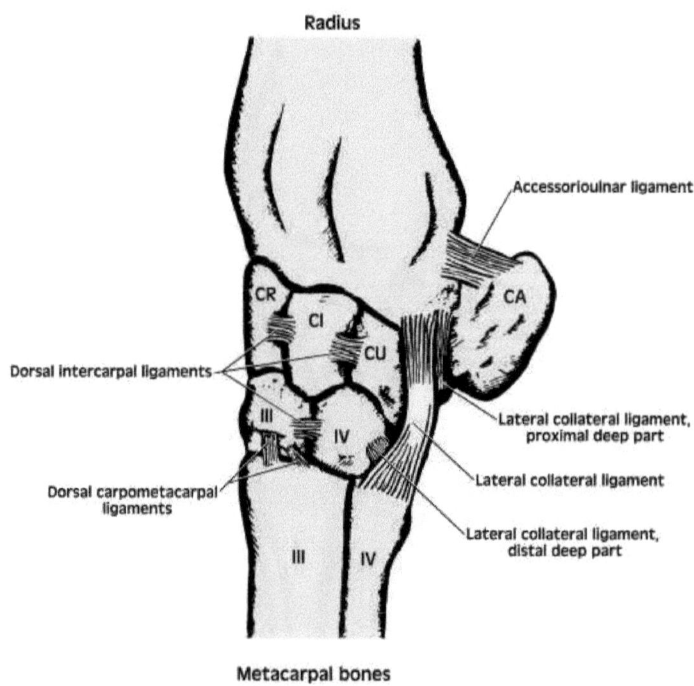

Fig.180. Carpal joint , dorsolateral view

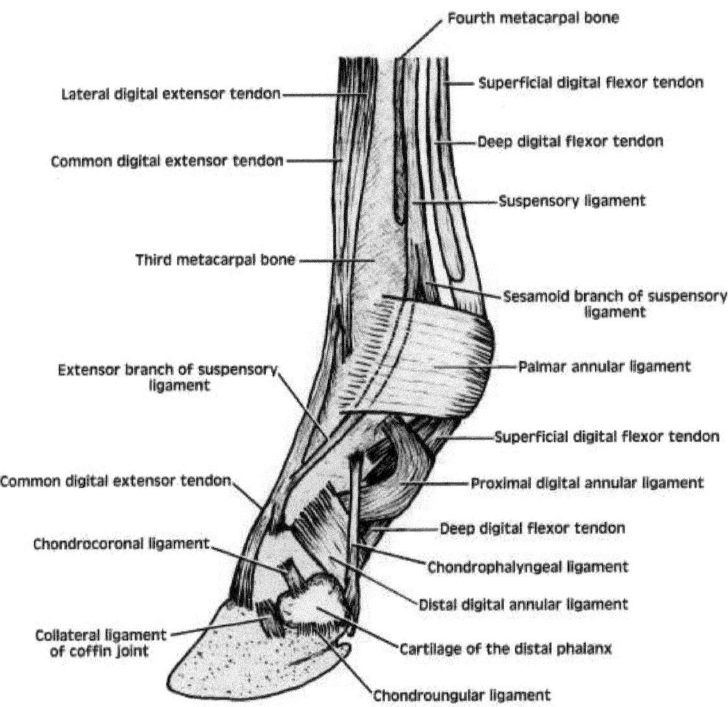

Fig.181. Dissection the distal part of thoracic limb, lateral surface

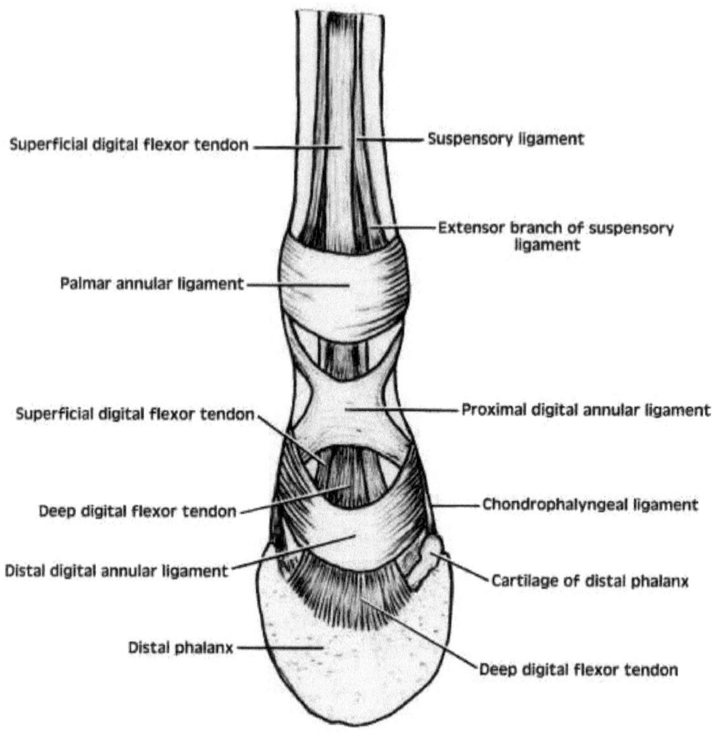

Fig.182. Dissection the distal part of thoracic limb, palmar surface

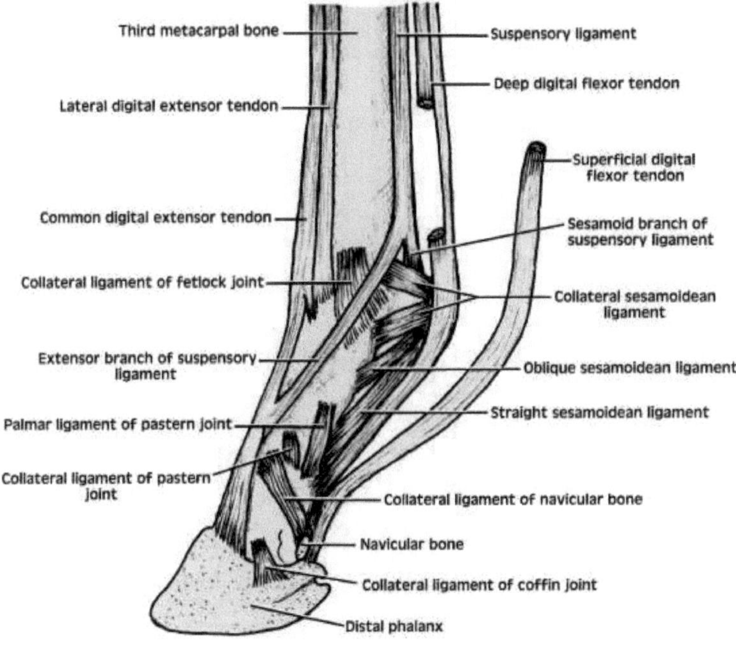

Fig.183. Deep dissection of the distal part of thoracic limb, lateral surface

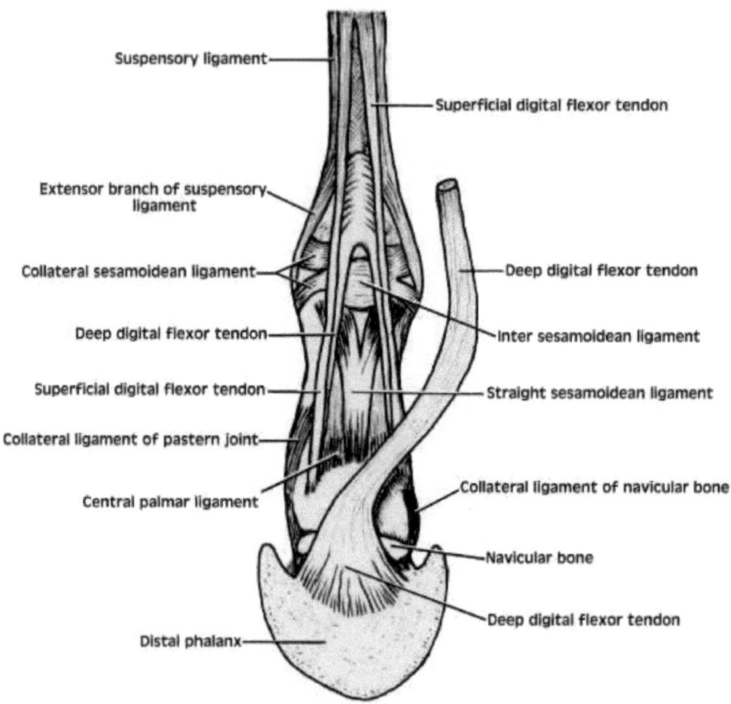

Fig.184. Deep dissection of the distal part of thoracic limb, palmar surface

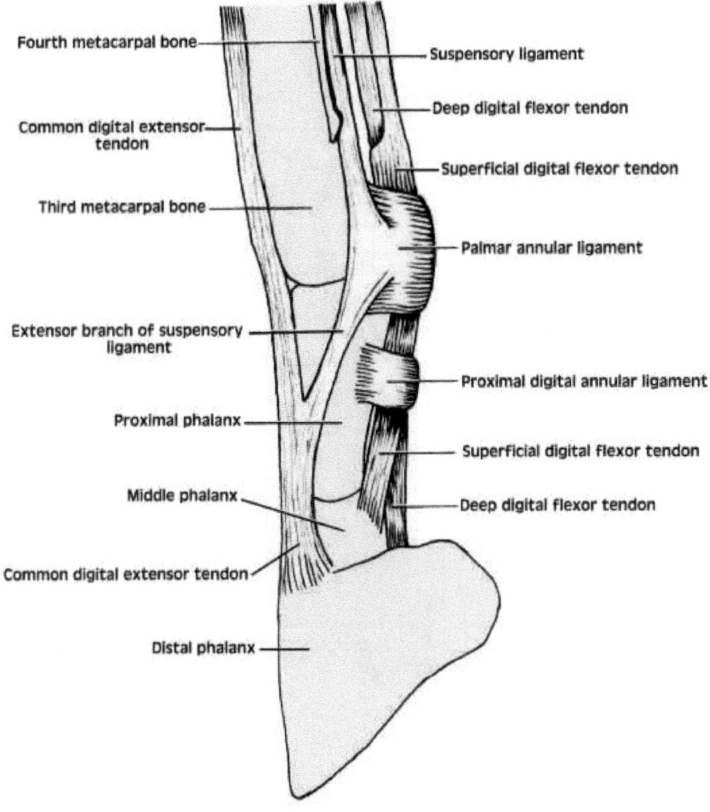

Fig.185. Ligaments and tendons of the left digit , lateral surface

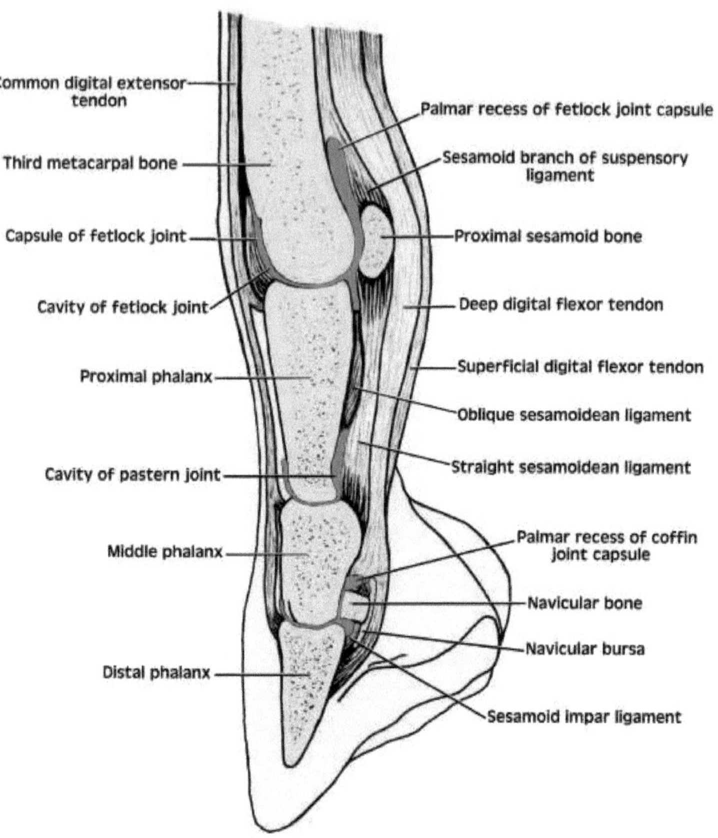

Fig.186. Sagittal section in the digit and distal part of metacarpus

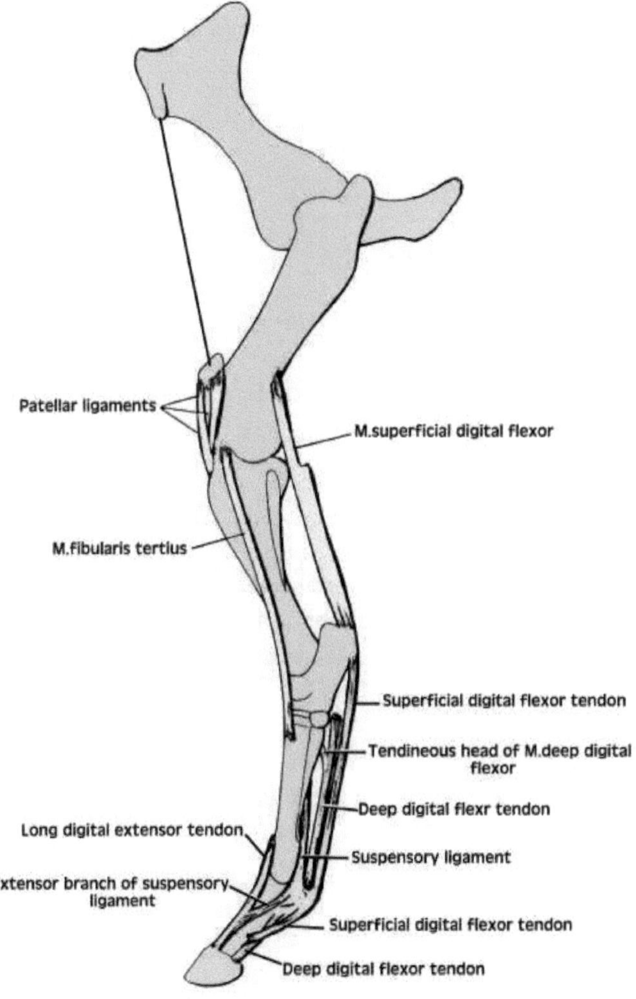

Fig.187. Structures making up the stay apparatus of the pelvic limb

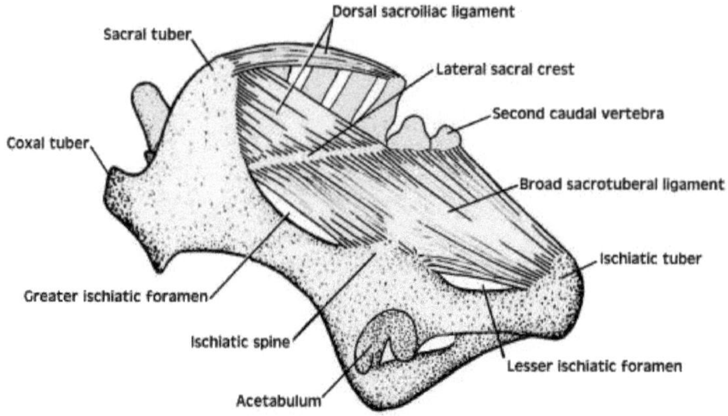

Fig.188. Pelvic ligaments , lateral view

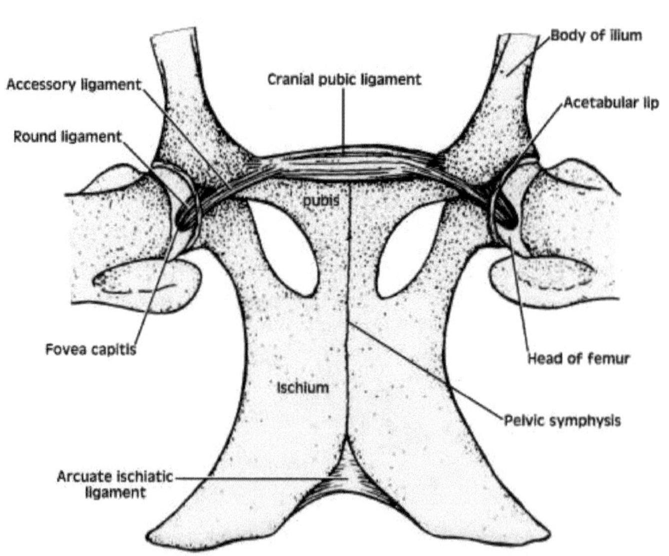

Fig.189. Ligaments of hip joint , ventral view

204

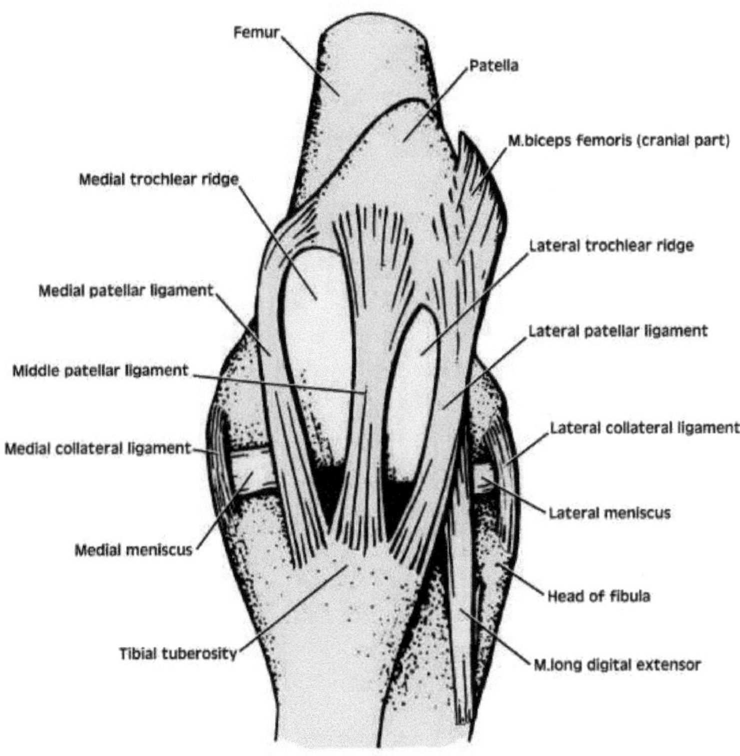

Fig.190. Ligaments of the stifle joint , cranial surface

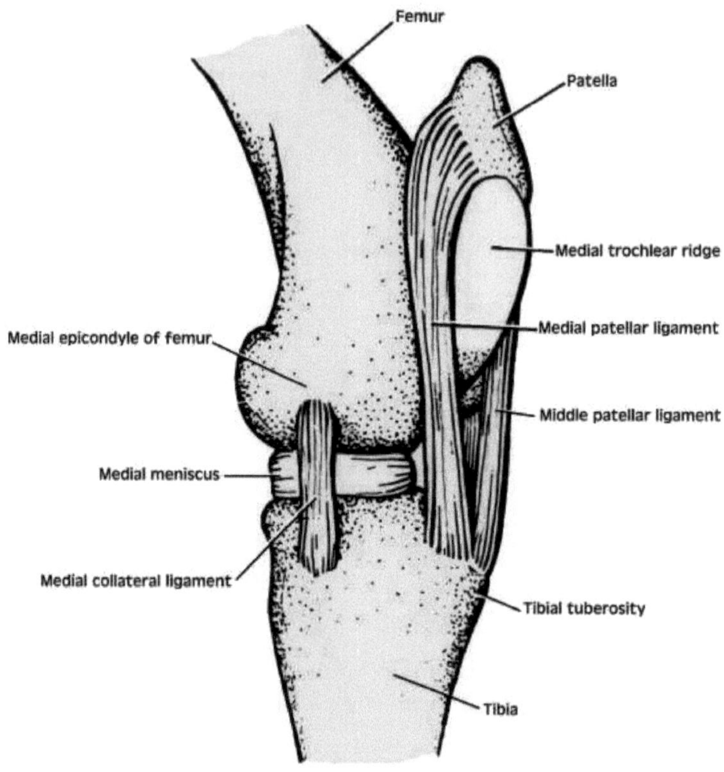

Fig.191. Ligaments of the stifle joint , medial surface

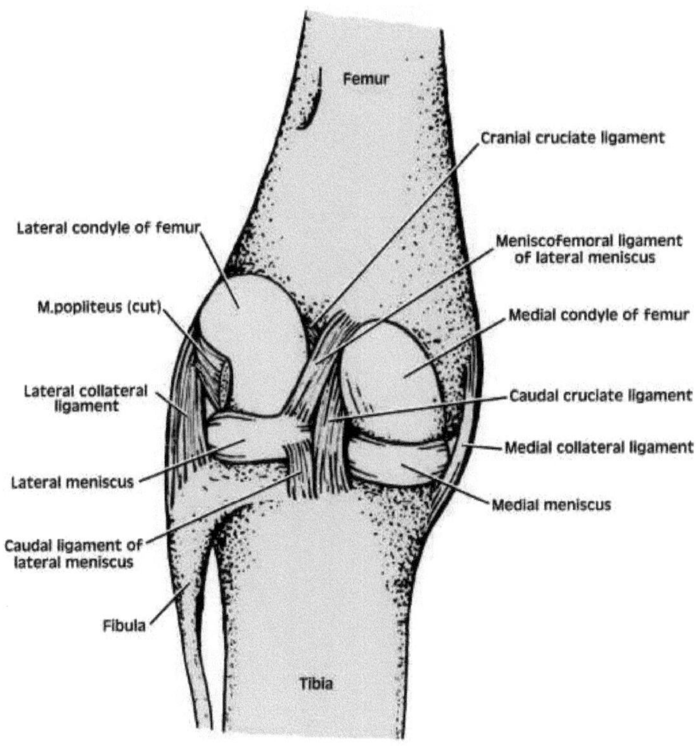

Fig.192. Ligaments of the stifle joint , caudal view

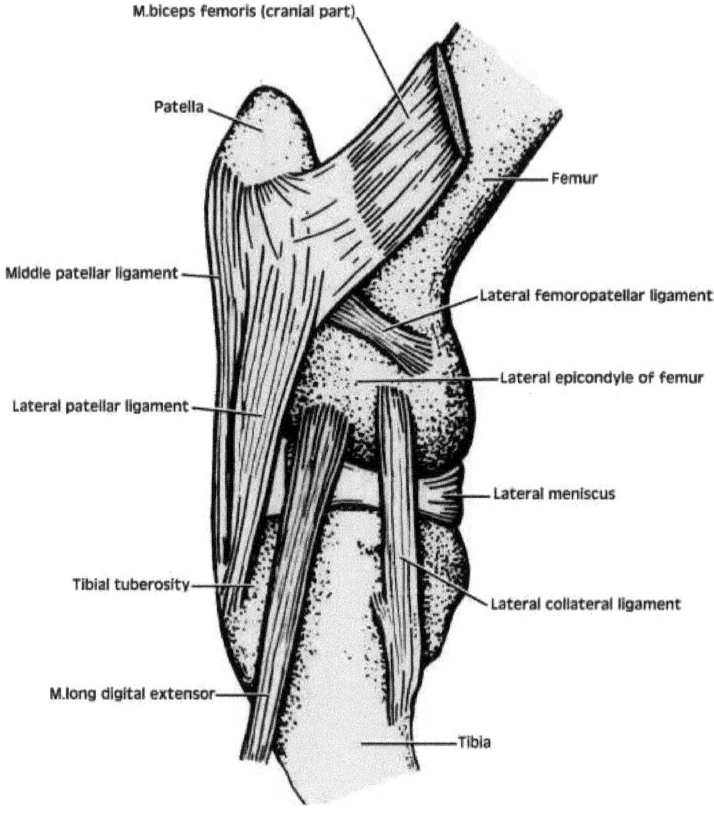

Fig.193. Ligaments of the stifle joint , lateral surface

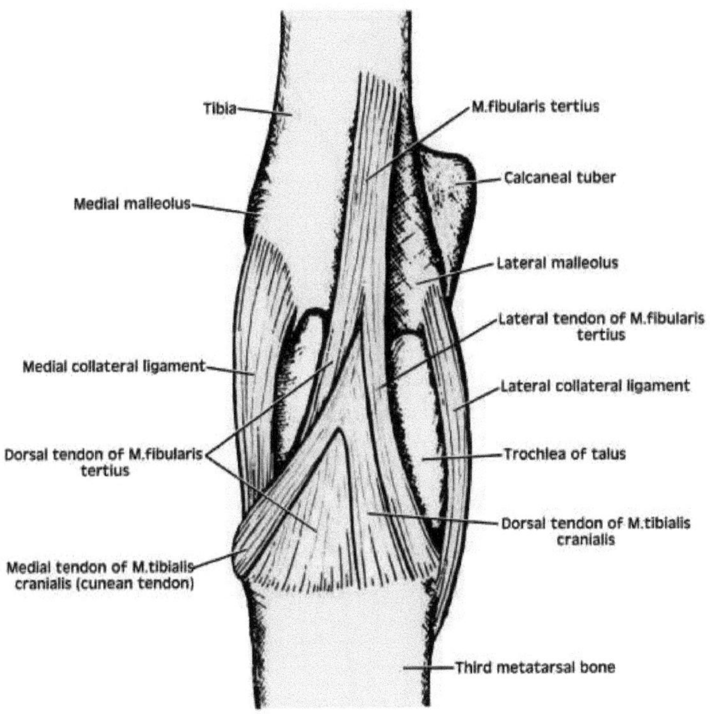

Fig.194. Ligaments of the hock joint , dorsal surface

209

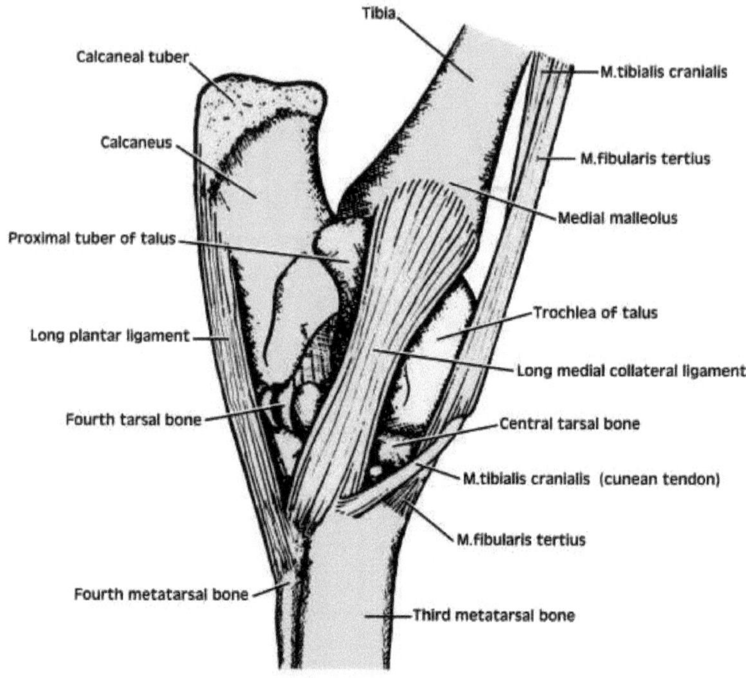

Fig.195. Ligaments of the hock joint , medial surface

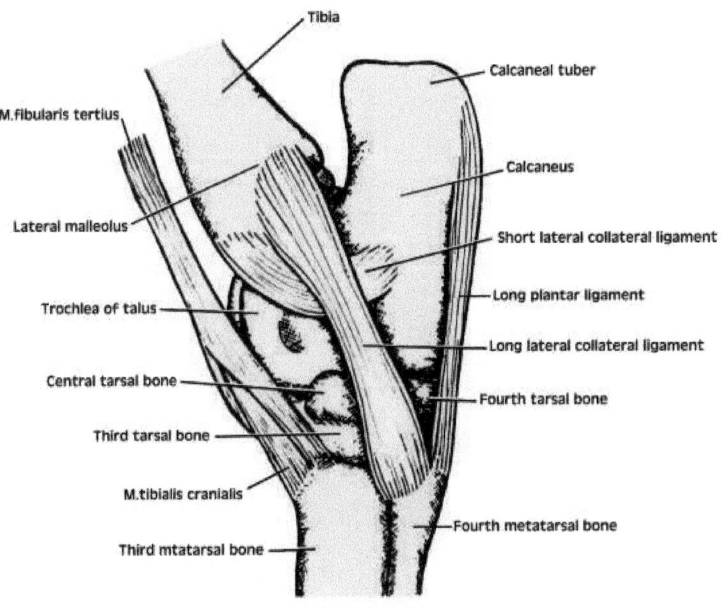

Fig.196. Ligaments of the hock joint , lateral surface

211

Part II

Tables of Muscles, Arteries and Nerves

Chapter 1

Head and Neck

Part I. Muscles of the head and neck

Table (1) Muscles of the muzzle, nostrils, lips and cheeks

Muscle	Origin	Insertion	Action	Innervation
Cutaneous faciei	Apart of platysma which covers the masseter muscle and intermandibular space, arises from the dorsal superficial fascia of the neck.	Its fibers blends with the M.orbicularis oris at the labial commissure (angle of the mouth)	Retracts the angle of the mouth after contraction of the M.orbicularis oris	Dorsal and ventral buccal branches of facial nerve
Transversus nasi (dilatator naris apicalis)	Unpaired , quadrilateral muscle, lies between the nostrils and consists of :- Superficial layer; from the superficial face of lamina of alar cartilage. Deep layer; from convex edge of the cornua of alar cartilage	The superficial and deep layers are attached to the lamina and cornua of the alar cartilage of the opposite side	Dilates the nostrils	Dorsal buccal branch of facial nerve
Levator nasolabialis	Thin muscle, lies on the lateral surface of the nasal region, arises from the frontal and nasal bones	Its belly is divided into two braches between which the M.caninus passes. The dorsal branch reaches the maxillary lip and lateral wing of nostril. The ventral branch blends with the labial commissure	Elevates the maxillary lip and dilates the nostril	Dorsal and ventral buccal branches of facial nerve
Caninus (dilatator naris lateralis)	Thin triangular muscle, passes between the two branches of levator nasolabialis. Arises from the maxilla close to the rostral end of facial crest	Lateral wing of the nostril	Dilates the nostril	Dorsal and ventral buccal branches of facial nerve
Levator labii maxillaris	The area of junction between the lacrimal, zygomatic and maxillary bones	The maxillary lip, by a common tendon with its fellow of the opposite side	Elevates the maxillary lip	Ventral buccal branch of facial nerve

Table (1) Muscles of the muzzle, nostrils, lips and cheeks (continued)

Muscle	Origin	Insertion	Action	Innervation
Depressor labii mandibularis	Alveolar border of the mandible near the coronoid process and maxillary tuber	Mandibular lip	Depresses and retracts the mandibular lip	Ventral buccal branch of facial nerve
Orbicularis oris	Sphincter muscle of the mouth consists of two parts. The labial part is continuous with the muscles blended with the lips. The marginal part is closely adherent to the skin and mucous membrane of lips	The muscle fibers form a circular sphincter muscle under the labial stroma	Closes the lips	Dorsal and ventral buccal branches of facial nerve
Buccinator	- Buccal part; from the alveolar borders of both maxilla and mandible - Molar part; longitudinal fibers arise from the maxillary tuber and alveolar border of the mandible near the coronoid process	The fibers of the buccal part are blended at the longitudinal raphe and with the molar part to the angle of the mouth, blending with the orbicularis oris	Control the food in the buccal vestibule between the teeth and retracts the angle of the muoth	Dorsal and ventral buccal branches of facial nerve
Zygomaticus	Facia covering of the massseter muscle under the facial crest	Labial commissure , blending with the buccinator muscle	Retracts and raises the angle of the muoth	Dorsal buucal branch of facial nerve
Incisivus maxillaris	Lies under the mucous membrane of the maxillary lip; arises from the alveolar border of incisive bone	The maxillary lip	Depresses the maxillary lip	Dorsal buccal branch of facial nerve
Incisivus mandibularis	Alveolar border of incisive part of the mandibular body	Skin of the mandibular lip and prominence of the chin	Raises the mandibular lip	ventral buccal branch of facial nerve
Mentalis	Lies in the prominence of the chin; arises from the each side of the body of the mandible	Skin of the chin	Raises and corrugates the skin of the chin	Mental nerve

Table (2) Muscles of mastication (mandibular muscles)

Muscle	Origin	Insertion	Action	Innervation
Masseter	Occupies the lateral surface of the mandibular ramus, arises from the zygomatic arch and facial crest	Lateral surface of the mandibular ramus	Closes the mandible	Mandibular nerve
Buccinatpr	Alveolar borders of maxilla and mandible and maxillary tuber	Longitudinal raphe of the buccal part and angle of the mouth, blending with the orbicularis oris	Controls the food in the oral vestibule	Buccal branches of facial nerve
Temporalis	Occupies the temporal fossa, arises from the temporal fossa and temporal crest	Coronoid process of the mandible	Raises the mandible	Mandibular nerve
Pterygoideus medialis	Occupies the concave medial surface of the mandibular ramus; arises from the pterygoid crest of the basisphenoid and palatine bones	Medial surface of the mandibular ramus	Pulls the mandible forwords or to the side	Mandibular nerve
Pterygoideus lateralis	Small muscle lies lateral to the dorsal part of pterygoideus medialis; arises from the lateral surface of the pterygoid process of the basisphenoid bone	Rostral border of the mandibular condyle and articular disc	Closes the jaw and pulls it to the side during chewing	Mandibular nerve
Digastricus	Composed of two fusiform flattened bellies, united by a round tendon, perforates the tendon of insertion of the stylohyoideus. The caudal belly; the larger dorsal part is the occipitomandibularis , extends from the jugular process to the caudal border of the mandibular ramus. The caudal belly arises from the jugular process of occipital bone.	Rostral belly; terminates by thin tendinous bundles in the medial surface of the ventral border of the molar part of the mandibular body	Depresses the mandible and opens the mouth	Facial nerve Mandibular nerve

Table (3) Muscles of the tongue (lingual muscles)

Muscle	Origin	Insertion	Action	Innervation
I. Extrinsic muscles	The group of muscles which arise from bony processes around the tongue and inserted, blending with the intrinsic muscles which form the architecture of the tongue. They play an important role in prehension, mastication by fixation of the food between the cheek teeth and aid the process of deglutition.			
1) Styloglossus	Long and thin muscle which lies along the lateral part of the tongue. It arises from the lateral surface of the stylohyoid bone by a thin flat tendon, near the articulation with ceratohyoid bone	Near the tip of the tongue, blending with the fellow of the opposite side	Retracts the tongue. Unilateral action draws the tongue toward the side of the muscle acting.	Hypoglossal nerve (XII)
2) Hyoglossus	Wide, flat and thick muscle lies on the lateral part of the root and body of tongue. It arises from the lateral surface of the basihyoid bone and lingual process	Root and caudal two thirds of the dorsum of tongue	Retracts and depresses the tongue	Hypoglossal nerve (XII)
3) Genioglossus	Fan shaped muscle, arises from the medial surface of the mandible just caudal to the symphysis by a clear tendon	The muscle fibers pass in a radiating manner to be inserted in the apex, body and root of tongue	Draws the tongue rostrally and downward	Hypoglossal nerve (XII)
II. Intrinsic muscles	Groups of muscular bundles which run longitudinally, vertically and transversely to form the architecture of the tongue. They blended with the extrinsic muscles and interspersed with considerable amount of fat. They arise from the different areas of the lingual mass.	The different areas of the lingual mass	Acts by a complex manner in different directions	Hypoglossal nerve (XII)

Table (4) Muscles of the pharynx

Muscle	Origin	Insertion	Action	Innervation
1.Rostral pharyngeal constrictors	Arise from the pterygoid region of skull. They run onto the rostral part of the roof of pharynx. They form with their fellows of the opposite side the rostral arch that encloses the rostral dorsal and lateral aspects of the pharyngeal cavity.			
a) Palatopharyngeus	Palatine and pterygoid bones by means of the apponeurosis of the soft palate. Rosrtral wide part of auditory tube.	Median fibrous pharyngeal raphe	Shorten the pharynx and draw it rostrally to receive the polus	Pharyngeal plexus
b) Pterygopharyngeus	Pterygoid bone dorsal to the origin of palatophryngeus	Median fibrous pharyngeal raphe		
2. Middle pharyngeal constrictors	Arise from the neighboring parts of hyoid bone. They form with their fellows of the opposite side the middle arch that encloses the middle dorsal and lateral aspects of the pharyngeal cavity.			
a)Stylopharyngeus cranialis	Medial surface of the ventral third of the stylohyoid bone	Median fibrous pharyngeal raphe	Constrict the middle part of pharynx during deglutition	Pharyngeal plexus
b) Hyopharyngeus	Thyrohyoid bone and the thyroid lamina	Median fibrous pharyngeal raphe		
3. Caudal pharyngeal constrictors	Arise from the thyroid and cricoid laryngeal cartilages. They form the caudal arch that conceals the caudal dorsal and lateral aspects of the pharyngeal cavity.			
a)Thyropharyngeus	Lateral surface of the thyroid lamina caudal to the oblique line	Median fibrous pharyngeal raphe	Constrict the caudal part of laryngopharynx to hurry the polus into the esophagus	Pharyngeal plexus
b) Cricopharyngeus	Lateral surface of the cricoid arch	Median fibrous pharyngeal raphe		
4. Pharyngeal dilator	Arise from the hyoid apparatus but runs more transversely to fan out in the pharyngeal wall.			
Stylopharyngeus caudalis	Medial surface of the dorsal third of the stylohyoid bone	Dorsal wall of the pharynx	Widens the rostral part of pharynx to accept the polus	Pharyngeal plexus

221

Table (5) Muscles of the soft palate

Muscle	Origin	Insertion	Action	Innervation
Palatinus	The muscle attached to the caudal border of hard palate by the median palatine aponeurosis	Extends along the median palatine aponeurosis to be inserted near the free border of soft palate	Shortens the soft palate	Pharyngeal plexus
Levator veli palatini	Muscular process of the petrous part of temporal bone and lateral lamina of the cartilage of auditory tube	The muscle fibers spread out to blend with that of the other side in an aponeurosis around the oral surface of the soft palate	Raises the soft palate to close the choanae during deglutition	Pharyngeal plexus
Tensor veli palatini	Fusiform and flat muscle, arises form the muscular process of the petrous part of temporal bone, pterygoid bone and lateral lamina of the auditory tube	The muscle passes rostrally across the medial surface of origin of the pterygoideus medialis. Its tendon of insertion is reflected around the hamulus of the pterygoid bone and lubricated by a bursa, turns inward and inserted in the median palatine aponeurosis	Tenses and flattens the soft palate	Mandibular nerve

Table (6) Muscles of the hyoid apparatus

Muscle	Origin	Insertion	Action	Innervation
Mylohyoideus	Medial surface of the alveolar border of the molar part of mandible (mylohyoid line)	Basihyoid bone and the median fibrous raphe extending from the mandibular symphysis to basihyoid bone between the two muscles	Sheet like muscle, acts as a sling for the tongue and floor of the mouth	Mylohyoid nerve of mandibular nerve
Geniohyoideus	A small depression on the medial surface of molar part of mandible, close to the symphysis	Lingual process of hyoid bone	Draws the hyoid bone and tongue rostrally	Hypoglossal and facial nerves

222

Table (6) Muscles of the hyoid apparatus (continued)

Muscle	Origin	Insertion	Action	Innervation
Sternohyoideus	A part of sterothyrohyoideus, arises from the manubrium of the sternum	Basihyoid bone and lingual process of hyoid bone	Retracts and depresses the hyoid bone during deglutition	Ventral branches of the first and second cervical nerves
Thyrohyoideus	Oblique line and lateral surface of the thyroid lamina	Caudal border of the thyrohyoid bone	Draws the larynx close to the tongue during deglutition	Hypoglossal nerve XII
Stylohyoideus	A small, fusiform muscle, arises from the muscular angle of the dorsal extremity of the stylohyoid bone	Rostral part of the thyrohyoid bone	Draws the base of the tongue and the larynx dorsally and caudally	Facial nerve VII
Occipitohyoideus	A small, triangular muscle, arises from the jugular process of the occipital bone	Proximal end of the stylohyoid bone	Retracts the hyoid apparatus	Facial nerve VII
Ceratohyoideus	Lies under cover of the hyoglossus, arises from the caudal border of ceratohyoid bone	Dorsal edge of thyrohyoid bone	Raises the thyroid bone and the larynx	Glossopharyngeal nerve IX
Hyoideus trasversus	A small, unpaired muscle arises from the medial face of ceratohyoid bone	The same point of the bone of the other side	Elevates the root of the tongue	Glossopharyngeal nerve IX
Omohyoideus	Subscapular fascia close to the shoulder joint	Basihyoid bone and the lingual process of the hyoid bone	Retracts the hyoid bone and the root of the tongue	Ventral branches of cervical nerves

Table (7) Muscles of the larynx

Muscle	Origin	Insertion	Action	Innervation
A. Extrinsic muscles	Group of muscles which attach between the laryngeal cartilages and the sternum and hyoid bone (bony prominences near or fare from the laryngeal cartilages). They move the larynx rostrally or caudally as one unite.			
1. Sternothyroideus	Manubrium of the sternum	Oblique line and lateral surface of the thyroid lamina	Depresses the larynx during deglutition	First and second cervical nerves
2. Thyrohyoideus	Lateral surface of the thyroid lamina, rostral to the oblique line	Caudal border of the thyrohyoid bone	Draws the larynx close to the tongue	Hypoglossal nerve (XII)
3. Hyoepiglotticus	Basihyoid bone	Basal part of the lingual surface of the epiglottis	Depresses the epiglottis onto the tongue	Hypoglossal nerve (XII)
B. Intrinsic muscles	Small paired muscles (except the fourth) that join the laryngeal cartilages and influence their mutual relations.			
1. Cricothyroideus	Caudal border and lateral surface of the cricoid arch	Caudal border and adjacent part of the lateral surface of the thyroid lamina	Tenses the vocal folds	Cranial laryngeal nerve
2. Cricoarytenoideus dorsalis	Muscular process and dorsal surface of the cricoid lamina	Muscular process of the arytenoid cartilage	Dilates the rima glottidis	Caudal laryngeal nerve
3. Cricoarytenoideus lateralis	Rostral border of the cricoid arch	Muscular process of the arytenoid cartilage	Closes the rima glottides	Caudal laryngeal nerve
4. Arytenoideus transversus	The dorsal surfaces of the two arytenoid cartilages	The median fibrous raphe between the right and left parts	Closes the intercartilagenous part of rima glottidis	Caudal laryngeal nerve
5. Thyroarytenoideus	The muscle consists of two parts; M.vestibularis, the cranial part and M.vocalis, the caudal part. The laryngeal saccule extends between the two parts of the M.thyroarytenoideus.			
• Vestibularis	Rostral part of the medial surface of the thyroid lamina	Muscular process of the arytenoid cartilage	Closes the laryngeal vestibule	Caudal laryngeal nerve
• vocalis	The thyroid body	The vocal process of the arytenoid cartilage	Slackens the vocal folds	Caudal laryngeal nerve

Table (8) Muscles of the eye lids (palpebral muscle)

Muscle	Origin	Insertion	Action	Innervation
Orbicularis aculi	Sphincter muscle situated in and around the eye lids. It arises from the skin and stroma of the lids	The skin of the lids, palpebral ligament at the medial canthus and lacrimal bone	Closes the eye lids	Auriculopalpebral nerve, branch of facial nerve
Levator palpebrae superioris	Flat muscle, placed entirely within the orbit. It arises from the pterygoid crest	By a thin tendon in the upper eye lid	Elevates the upper eye lid	Oculomotor nerve (III)
Corrugator supercillii (levator anguli oculi medialis)	Very thin, small muscle, arises form the root of the zygomatic process of frontal bone	Spreads out in the upper eye lid , blending with the orbicularis oculi	Raises the upper eye lid and wrinkles its skin	Auriculopalpebral nerve, branch of facial nerve
Malaris	Very thin, arises from the fascia rostral to the orbit	Spread out in the lower eye lid	Depresses the lower eye lid	Facial nerve (VII)

Table (9) Muscles of the eye ball (bulbar muscles)

Muscle	Origin	Insertion	Action	Innervation
1. Rectus dorsalis	Arise close to each other from the common fibrous ring around the optic foramen	Dorsal surface of the sclera, anterior to the equator	Rotate the eye ball about a transverse axis	Oculomotor nerve (III)
2. Rectus ventralis		Ventral surface of the sclera, anterior to the equator		Oculomotor nerve (III)
3. Rectus medialis		Medial surface of the sclera, anterior to the equator	Rotate the eye ball about a vertical axis	Oculomotor nerve (III)
4. Rectus lateralis		Lateral surface of the sclera, anterior to the equator		Abducent nerve (VI)
5. Obliquus ventralis	Medial wall of the orbit in a depression caudal to the lacrimal fossa	In the ventrolateral aspect of the sclera, near the equator	Rotate the eye ball about a longitudinal axis	Oculomotor nerve (III)
6. Obliquus dorsalis	Wall of the orbit, near the ethmoidal foramen. It passes around the trochlea	In the dorsolateral aspect of the sclera, near the equator		Trochlear nerve (IV)
7. Retractor bulbi	Surrounds the optic nerve, arise from the fibrous edge of the optic foramen	Sclera caudal to the equator	Draws the eye ball caudally	Abducent nerve (VI)

Table (10) Muscles of the ear and forehead

Muscle	Origin	Insertion	Action	Innervation
Auriculares rostrales	Group of eight muscles for each side, arise from the fascia over the scutiform cartilage and rostral part of the forehead	Rostral part of the dorsal surface on the base of conchal cartilage	Erect the ear and turn the opening rostrally	Auriculopalpebral nerve, branch of facial nerve (VII)
Auriculares caudales	Group of four muscles for each side, arise from the fascia of the neck, near the base of the base of the ear and nuchal crest	Scutiform cartilage, caudomedial and caudolateral parts of the base of the ear	Draw the auricular cartilage caudally	Auriculopalpebral nerve, branch of facial nerve (VII)
Auriculares dorsales	Two to three muscles for each side, arise from the fascia over the scutiform cartilage and dorsal part of the forehead	Scutiform cartilage and dorsal convex surface of the conchal cartilage	Adduction and create a symmetrical position of the ears	Auriculopalpebral nerve, branch of facial nerve (VII)
Auricularis ventralis (parotido-auricularis)	Ribbon like muscle, lies on the parotid salivary gland. It arises from the fascia over the ventral part of parotid gland	The conchal cartilage, ventral to the intertragic notch, into the antitragus	Draws the ear ventrally and caudally	Cervical branch of facial nerve (VII)
Stapideus	Mastoid wall of the middle ear	The neck of the stapes	One of the smallest of all muscles. It dampens ossicle oscillation by tensing the annular ligament	Stapedial nerve, branch of facial nerve (VII)
Tensor tempani	The upper wall of osseous auditory tube	The upper end of the handle of the malleus	Tenses the tympanic membrane	Trigeminal nerve (V) via the otic ganglion

Table (11) Muscles of the neck

Muscle	Origin	Insertion	Action	Innervation
Cutaneous colli	Apart of platysma which covers the ventral region of the neck. It arises from the manubrium of the sternum and a median fibrous raphe	Its fibers are directed cranially to the sides of the neck to be attached with the superficial cervical fascia	Twitches the skin to get rid of insects	Cervical nerves
A. Ventral cervical muscles	The group of muscles which lie on the ventral and lateral to the cervical vertebrae.			
1. Sternocephalicus (sternomandibularis)	Cartilage of the manubrium of the sternum	Caudal border of the mandibular ramus	Flexion the head and neck	Ventral branch of accessory nerve
2. Sternothyrohyoideus	Cartilage of the manubrium of the sternum	- Lateral surface and oblique line of the thyroid lamina - basihyoid and lingual process of the hyoid bone	Retracts and depresses the hyoid bone, root of tongue and larynx during deglutition	Ventral branches of the first and second cervical nerves
3. Omohyoideus	Subscapular fascia close to the shoulder joint	Basihyoid bone and lingual process of hyoid bone	Retracts the hyoid bone and root of the tongue	Ventral branch of the first cervical nerve
4. Scalenus medius	It is separated into two parts; small dorsal and large ventral, between which the cervical roots of brachial plexus emerge. It arises from the cranial border and lateral surface of the first rib	Transverse processes of the last four cervical vertebrae	Draws the first rib cranially and moves the neck on the side of contracting muscle	Ventral branches of the cervical nerves
5. Longus capitis	Transverse processes of the third, fourth and fifth cervical vertebrae	Basilar tubercle of the basioccipital bone	Flexes the head and a part of the neck	Ventral branches of the cervical nerves

Table (11) Muscles of the neck (continued)

Muscle	Origin	Insertion	Action	Innervation
6. Rectus capitis ventralis	The ventral arch of atlas	Basilar part of occipital bone, ventral to the Foramen magnum	Flexes the atlanto-occipital joint	Ventral branches of the cervical nerves
7. Rectus capitis lateralis	The ventral arch of atlas, next to the origin of Rectus capitis ventralis	Jugular process of the occipital bone	Flexes the atlanto-occipital joint	Ventral branches of the cervical nerves
8. Longus colli	The transverse processes of the cervical vertebrae	Bodies of the cervical vertebrae and ventral tubercle of the atlas	Flexes the neck	Ventral branches of the cervical nerves
9. Intertransversii cervicis	The muscle bundles occupy the spaces between the lateral surface of the vertebrae and the transverse and articular processes. Each bundle consists of dorsal and ventral parts.			
9a. Intertransversii dorsales cervicis	Dorsal surfaces of the transverse processes	The articular processes of the preceding vertebrae	They flex the neck laterally	Cervical nerves
9b. Intertransversii ventrales cervicis	Ventral surfaces of the transverse processes	The transverse processes of the preceding vertebrae	They flex the neck laterally	Cervical nerves
B. Dorsolateral cervical muscles	The group of the muscles which lie on the dorsal and lateral aspects of the neck.			
1. Brachiocephalicus	- Mastoid process of petrous temporal bone and nuchal crest - Wing of the atlas - Transverse processes of the second, third and fourth cervical vertebrae	Deltoid tuberosity, humeral crest, and the fascia of the shoulder and arm regions	The two muscles act together to extend the head and neck. It acts separately to incline the head and neck to the same side	Accessory nerve (XI) Cervical nerves Axillary nerve

Table (11) Muscles of the neck (continued)

Muscle	Origin	Insertion	Action	Innervation
2. Trapezius cervicis	The funicular part of nuchal ligament, from the level of the second cervical to the third thoracic vertebrae	Tuber of the scapular spine	Elevates the shoulder and draws the scapula cranially and dorsally	Dorsal branch of accessory nerve
3. Rhomboideus cervicis	The funicular part of nuchal ligament, from the level of the second cervical to the second thoracic vertebrae	Medial surface of the scapular cartilage	Elevates the neck	Dorsal branches of the sixth and seventh cervical nerves
4. Splenius	The dorsal scapular ligament and funicular part of nuchal ligament	Nuchal crest, mastoid process, wing of atlas and the transverse processes of the cervical vertebrae (3-5)	The two muscles elevate the head and neck. Single action inclines the head and neck to its side	Dorsal branches of the last six cervical nerves
5. Longissimus capitis	The transverse processes of the first and second thoracic vertebrae	Mastoid process of petrous temporal bone	Extension of the head	Dorsal branches of the last six cervical nerves
6. Longissimus atlantis	The articular processes of the cervical vertebrae	Wing of the atlas	Extension of the head Rotation of the atlas	Dorsal branches of the last six cervical nerves
7. Longissimus cervicis	The spinous processes of the first five thoracic vertebrae and supraspinous ligament	Transverse processes of the last four cervical vertebrae	Assists the extension of the head	Dorsal branches of the last five cervical nerves
8. Semispinalis capitis (Complexus)	The dorsal scapular ligament, and the articular processes of the cervical vertebrae	The rough area under the nuchal crest of the occipital bone	Principal muscle which extends the head and neck	Dorsal branches of the last six cervical nerves

Table (11) Muscles of the neck (continued)

Muscle	Origin	Insertion	Action	Innervation
9. Multifidus cervicis	Segmental muscle lies along the spinous processes of cervical vertebrae. It arises from the articular processes of the last five cervical and first thoracic vertebrae	Spinous and articular processes of the preceding cervical vertebrae	Extension of the neck in bilateral action	Dorsal branches of the last six cervical nerves
10. Spinalis	The apices of the spinous processes of cervical vertebrae	Caudal borders of the spinous processes of preceding cervical vertebrae	Assists the extension of the head	Dorsal branches of the cervical nerves
11. Obliquus capitis caudalis	The caudal articular and spinous processes of the axis	Dorsal surface of the wing of atlas	Rotation of the head with the atlas (acts on the atlanto-axial joint)	Dorsal branch of the second cervical nerve
12. Obliquus capitis cranialis	The ventral surface and cranial border of the atlas	Jugular process, mastoid process, and nuchal crest of occipital bone	Extension of the head (acts on the occipito-atlantal joint)	Dorsal branch of the first cervical nerve
13. Rectus capitis dorsalis major	The dorsal edge of the spinous process of the axis	Rough area under the nuchal crest, ventral to the insertion of M.semispinalis capitis	Extension of the head	Dorsal branch of the first cervical nerve
14. Rectus capitis dorsalis minor	The dorsal surface of atlas	Occipital bone, under the insertion of the preceding muscle	Assists the extension of the head	Dorsal branch of the first cervical nerve

Part II. Arteries of the head and neck
Table (12) Common carotid artery

Main trunk	Branches	Subdivisions	Distribution
Common carotid artery	The right and left common carotid arteries arise from the brachiocephalic trunk, at the level of the first rib, by a common trunk termed the bicarotid trunk. Each passes on the lateral surface of the trachea to reach the deep face of the mandibular salivary gland, where it swerves to the dorsal surface of the trachea and gives off the terminal branches. Along its course, it releases collateral branches.		
A. The collateral branches	**1. Muscular branches**		Branches of variable number and size, supply the muscles of the ventral aspect of the neck and skin
	2.Tracheal and esophageal branches		Ramify in the cervical parts of the trachea and esophagus
	3. Parotid artery		Enters the ventral part of parotid salivary gland. It sends twigs to the parotid lymph nodes and mandibular gland.
	4. Caudal thyroid artery		Sends branches to the caudal part of thyroid gland as well as small tracheal and muscular twigs
	5. Cranial thyroid artery	**a) Cranial thyroid branches**	Supply the cranial end of the thyroid gland
		b) Caudal laryngeal branch	- **Laryngeal branches** to the extrinsic, intrinsic muscles and mucous membrane of the larynx. - **Pharyngeal branch** supplies the constrictors of the pharynx.
	6. Ascending pharyngeal artery		Passes dorsally and cranially to the M.cricopharyngeus to give small branches to the caudal part of pharynx and origin of esophagus. It also supplies the trachea, esophagus, sternothyrohyoideus and omohyoideus.

Table (12) Common carotid artery (continued)

Main trunk	Branches	Subdivisions	Distribution
B. The terminal branches	The common carotid artery is divided, on the deep face of the manibular salivary gland, into internal carotid, occipital and external carotid arteries.		
I. External carotid artery	The external carotid artery is the direct continuation of the common carotid artery on the lateral surface of the pharynx at the ventral border of the guttural pouch. It ascends on the lateral face of the stylohyoid bone parallel to the caudal border of the ramus of the mandible and continues as maxillary artery. The chief collateral branches are:-		
	1. Masseteric artery		Passes rostrally under cover the parotid gland to the caudal border of the ramus of the mandible to enter the masseter muscle. It also sends branches to the pterygoideus medialis, occipitomandibular part of M.digastricus and parotid gland.
	2. Linguofacial trunk		Arises from the external carotid artery on the deep surface of the caudal belly of M.digastricus. It passes cranioventrally on the lateral wall of pharynx toward the stylohyoid bone, continues its course parallel to the caudal border of the later bone accompanied by the glossopharyngeal nerve cranially and hypoglossal nerve caudally. After giving off the lingual artery at the middle of the stylohyoid bone, the linguofacial trunk becomes the facial artery.
		a) Ascending palatine artery	Passes rostrally on the lateral wall of the pharynx to supply the pharynx, soft palate and palatine tonsils.
		b) Lingual artery	The large branch which supply the tongue. It dips in the tongue between the hyoglossus and genioglossus , courses as the deep lingual artery in a flexuous manner accompanied by the hypoglossal and lingual nerves. It is the chief artery of the tongue, and anastomoses with the opposite artery at the tip of the tongue.

Table (12) Common carotid artery (continued)

Main trunk	Branches	Subdivisions	Distribution
		c) Facial artery	The direct continuation of the linguofacial trunk beyond the origin of the lingual artery. It crosses over the hypoglossal nerve, mandibular duct and intermediate tendon of the digastricus to reach the vascular notch on the ventral border of molar part of the mandible.The facial artery ascends on the face, rostral to the masseter muscle, accompanied by the facial vein and parotid duct. It gives off the following branches:- **1) Sublingual artery;** to the mucous membrane of the floor of the mouth, sublingual salivary gland, muscles and skin of the rmandibular space and mandibular lymph nodes. **2) Mandibular labial artery;** supplies the mandibular lip, ventral buccal glands, skin and mucous membrane of the cheeks. **3) Maxillary labial artery;** to the maxillary lip and dorsal part of cheeks. **4) Lateral nasal artery;** ramifies in the lateral nasal region and nostril. **5) Dorsal nasal artery;** to the dorsal nasal region. **6) Artery of the angle of the eye;** to the medial canthus of the eye
	3. Caudal auricular artery	a) Medial auricular branch	Passes dorsally on the medial border of the external ear to the apex. It anastomoses with the intermediate auricular branch and ramifies in the muscles and skin of the external ear.
		b) Intermediate auricular branch	Ascends on the convex surface of the external ear, joins with the preceding branch to form an arch.
		c) Lateral auricular branch	Courses dorsally on the lateral border of the external ear and forms an arch with the intermediate auricular branch.
		d) Deep auricular branch	Inters the interval between the external acoustic meatus and mastoid process to the interior of the external ear to supply the skin. It also gives off; Stylomastoid artery; passes through the stylomastoid foramen to the tympanic membrane. Caudal tympanic artery; to the middle ear and its muscles.

Table (12) Common carotid artery (continued)

Main trunk	Branches	Subdivisions	Distribution
	4. Superficial temporal artery		A short artery passes dorsally on the deep face of the parotid gland, caudal to the caudal border of the mandibular ramus. It is divided ventral to the level of the mandibular condyle into rostral auricular and transverse facial arteries.
		a) Rostral auricular artery	Ascends caudal to the temporomandibular joint, accompanied by the auriculopalpebral nerve, to supply the rostral auricular and temporal muscles as well as the skin of the temporal region. Collateral small branches are detached to parotid gland.
		b) Transverse facial artery	Turns around the mandibular neck and emerges the deep face of the parotid gland, passes rostrally ventral to the zygomatic arch on the masseter muscle. It is accompanied by the transverse facial vein and nerve to enter the dorsal part of masseter muscle to supply it and the skin of the region.
Maxillary artery	5. maxillary artery		The direct continuation of the external carotid artery beyond the origin of the superficial temporal artery. It has a complex course and widely distributed branches, thus it must be described as a main trunk, divided into three segments according to their position from the alar canal.
A. First part of maxillary artery			The large part of maxillary artery which forms a double curve and lies in contact with the guttural pouch. It passes rostrally and dorsally on the medial surface of the mandible, then turns medially on the ventral surface of pterygoideus lateralis. It continues its course between the later muscle and tensor veli palatine to end at the alar foramen. This part gives off the following branches;-
	1. Mandibular alveolar artery	a) Mylohyoid branch	Supplies the mylohyoideus (the sling of the tongue)
		b) Alveolar branches	To the alveoli of the maxillary cheek teeth and gum.
		c) Mental artery	Emerges through the mental foramen to the chin and maxillary lip.
		d) Dental branches	Continues rostrally inside the body of incisive bone to the alveoli of the mandibular incisors, gum and canine tooth.

Table (12) Common carotid artery (continued)

Main trunk	Branches	Subdivisions	Distribution
	2. Pterygoid branches		Two to three branches, ramify in the pterygoideus, levator veli palatini and tensor veli palatini.
	3. Rostral tympanic artery		A very small artery, passes along the auditory tube to supply the middle ear.
	4. Middle meningeal artery		Passes caudally across the wing of the basisphenoid, enters the cranial cavity through the foramen spinosum to supply the dura mater. It anastomoses with the caudal meningeal artery.
	5. Caudal deep temporal artery		Courses dorsally and caudally in the temporal fossa to supply the temporalis. It sends a branch laterally to the masseter.
B. Second part of maxillary artery			This part lies inside the alar canal, about 2-3 cm. length. It gives off the rostral deep temporal and external ophthalmic arteries.
	1. Rostral deep temporal artery		Emerges from the alar canal through the small alar foramen. It ascends in the rostral part of temporal fossa to ramify in the temporalis and gives twigs to the orbital fat and skin of the frontal region
	2. external ophthalmic artery		Emerges from the alar canal through the round foramen and enters the apex of the periorbita. It forms a semicircular band under the rectus dorsalis and continues as external ethmoidal artery which enters the ethmoidal foramen. The external ophthalmic artery gives off :-
		a) Supraorbital artery	Passes along the medial wall of the orbit in company with the supraorbital nerve to leave the orbit trough the supraorbital foramen. It ramifies in the orbicularis oculi, corrugator supercillii and skin of the supraorbital region.
		b) Lacrimal artery	Runs dorsally and rostrally within the periorbita, along the lateral edge of the levator palpebrae superioris to ramify in the lacrimal gland.

Table (12) Common carotid artery (continued)

Main trunk	Branches	Subdivisions	Distribution
		c) Muscular branches	Supply the ocular muscles, periorbita, third eye lid and conjunctiva.
		d) Ciliary arteries	Two groups of small branches include:- **1) Anterior ciliary arteries;** pierce the sclera in front of of the equator and ramify in the ciliary body and the iris. **2) Posterior ciliary arteries;** pierce the posterior part of the sclera. This set can be divided into posterior short and long ciliary arteries. **- Posterior short ciliary arteries;** ramify in the chorioid coat. **- Posterior long ciliary arteries;** two branches of larger size, one on each side, passes between the sclera and chorioid to the fixid border of the iris. Here each divides into two branches, anastomose and form a circle termed **circulus iridis mojor**. From the later circle, secondary branches are detached toward the free border of the iris, anastomose and form a circle around the pupil termed **circulus iridis minor**.
		e) Central artery of the retina	Pierces the optic nerve a short distance posterior to the sclera. It runs in the center of the nerve to the lamina cribrosa, breaks up into 30-40 fine branches. They appear in the fundus of the eye at the margin of the optic papilla and radiate in the posterior part of retina.
		f) R.anastomoticus cum a.ophthalmica interna	A small branch accompanied the optic nerve inside the optic canal to the cranial cavity. It anastomoses with the internal ophthalmic artery
		g) External ethmoidal artery	Enters the cranial cavity through the ethmoidal foramen and joined the internal ethmoidal artery. It passes on the cribriform plate and divides into two branches:- **1) Rostral meningeal artery;** ramifies in the rostral part of dura mater and anastomoses with the common artery of the corpus callosum. **2) Nasal branch;** to the ethmoidal labyrinth and adjacent part of nasal septum.

Table (12) Common carotid artery (continued)

Main trunk	Branches	Subdivisions	Distribution
C. Third part of maxillary artery	The part which placed in front of the alar canal. It passes rostrally in the pterygopalatine fossa in company with the maxillary nerve. Its branches are:-		
	1. Infraorbital artery		Arises from the dorsal aspect of maxillary artery, gives off the malar artery and passes rostrally and dorsally to the maxillary foramen. It runs through the infraorbital canal in company with the infraorbital nerve and is continued within the maxillary and incisive bones to the maxillary incisors. It detaches a branch emerges from the infraorbital foramen which anastomoses with the lateral nasal and maxillary labial arteries.
		a) Malar artery	Passes along the floor of the orbit and gives off small branches to supply the lacrimal sac and the obliquus ventralis, then divides into medial superior and inferior palpebral arteries. It is finally ramified in the lower eye lid and anastomoses with the angularis aculii.
		b) Alveolar branches	Arise from the infraorbital artery inside the infraorbital canal to supply the alveoli of the maxillary cheek teeth and gums.
	2. Descending palatine artery	a) Sphenopalatine artery	Passes through the sphenopalatine foramen into the nasal cavity and divides into two arteries:- - **Caudal nasal artery**; to the mucous membrane of the nasal septum - **Lateral and septal nasal artery;** to the ventral concha, ventral meatus, choanae and maxillary and frontal sinuses.
		b) Greater palatine artery	Passes through the greater palatine canal to the palatine groove of the hard palate tell the body of the incisive bone. It curves medially to be joined with its fellow of the opposite side forming the palatolabial artery which passes through the interincisive canal to the maxillary lip. Along its course it gives of collateral branches to the hard palate, soft palate, gums and floor of the nasal cavity.
		c) Lesser palatine artery	A small branch which passes rostrally on the medial side of the maxillary tuber to ramify in the soft palate.

Table (12) Common carotid artery (continued)

Main trunk	Branches	Subdivisions	Distribution
	3. Buccal artery		Arises from the maxillary artery after its emergence from the alar canal, turns around the maxillary tuber, accompanied by the buucal nerve on the deep face of masseter muscle. It enters the cheek, divides into several branches to supply the cheek, dorsal buccal glands, masseter and pterygoideus.
II. Occipital artery	The second large terminal branch of the common carotid artery. It pursues a somewhat flexuous course to the atlantal fossa where it divides into cranial and caudal branches. It gives of collateral branches to the mandibular salivary gland, guttural pouch, longus capitis, rectus capitis ventralis and rectus capitis lateralis .		
	1. Condyloid artery	a) Meningeal branches	Enter the cranial cavity through the jugular and hypoglossal foramina to supply the dura mater.
		b) Muscular branch	To the longus capitis, rectus capitis lateralis and guttural pouch
	2. Occipital branch		Anastomoses with the vertebral artery in the atlantal fossa
	3. Caudal meningeal artery		Runs dorsally and rostrally between the obliquus capitis cranialis and jugular process, gives collateral branches to the atlanto-occipital joint and adjacent muscles. It passes through the mastoid foramen into the temporal canal, enters the cranial cavity to be distributed in the dura mater.

Table (12) Common carotid artery (continued)

Main trunk	Branches	Subdivisions	Distribution
III. Internal carotid artery			Arises from the common carotid artery just caudal to the origin of occipital artery, crosses its deep face and runs caudally and dorsally on the guttural pouch to the foramen lacerum (foramen caroticum) to enter the cranial cavity. It passes through the ventral petrosal sinus to the cavernous sinus, within which it forms an S-shaped curve and releases the caroticobasilar artery. It is connected with the opposite artery by the caudal intercarotid artery which lies in the intercavernous sinus caudal to the hypophysis and gives off the caudal hypophysial arteries. The internal carotid artery leaves the cavernous sinus, perforates the dura mater at the level of the hypophysis. It gives off the caudal communicating artery and continues rostrally to be terminated as the rostral and middle cerebral arteries.
	1.Caroticobasilar artery		Courses in a caudomedial direction and leaves the cavernous sinus to join the pontine segment of basilar artery on the ventral surface of pons. It gives off branches to the dorsolateral parts of pons and anastomosing branches to the labyrinthine artery.
	2. Hypophysial arteries	a) Anterior hypophysial arteries	Arise from the internal carotid artery just after its pierces the dural roof to leave the cavernous sinus. They course rostromedially to supply the tuber cinereum, infundibulum of the hypophysis and optic chiasma.
		b) Posterior hypophysial arteries	Arise from the caudal intercarotid artery, directed rostromedially to ramify in the neurohypophysis.
	3. Caudal communicating branch		Courses on the ventral surface of the cerebral crus, units with its fellow of the opposite side to join the rostral end of basilar artery. This structure forms the lateral and caudolateral quadrants of the cerebral arterial circle. The caudal communicating branch is divided into proximal and distal segments at the origin of the caudal cerebral artery. The distal segment of the caudal communicating branch gives off the mesencephalic artery to supply the different parts of the mesencephalon.

239

Table (12) Common carotid artery (continued)

Main trunk	Branches	Subdivisions	Distribution
	4. Caudal cerebral artery		A large branch arises at the junction of the proximal and distal segments of the caudal communicating branch rostral to the oculomotor nerve root. It releases the following branches:-
		a) Perforating branches	Arise at various levels to be distributed in the cerebral crus, optic tract and caudal part of piriform lobe.
		b) Caudal choroidal branch	Ascends dorsomedially around the cerebral crus, divides into fine branches to supply the thalamus, choroid plexus of the third ventricle, cerebral crus, pineal body, rostral and caudal colliculi.
		c) Cortical branches	Arise from the caudal cerebral artery during its course along the parahippocampal gyrus. They are distributed to the caudal, caudoventral and caudomedial parts of the cerebral hemisphere, piriform lobe and corpus callosum. The cortical branches anastomose with the cortical branches of the rostral and middle cerebral arteries.
	5. Middle cerebral artery		The largest branch of internal carotid artery, passes laterally on the ventral surface of the rostral piriform lobe. It ascends by crossing the lateral olfactory tract to reach the junction of the rosrtral and caudal parts of the lateral rhinal sulcus. It gives off the central, collateral and cortical branches.
		a) Central branches	Given off from the dorsal surface of the middle cerebral artery. They are distributed in the rostral perforate substance and rostral piriform lobe.
		b) Collateral branches	Two to three branches arise from the initial part of middle cerebral artery at varying levels and distribute in the piriform lobe, ventral rostrolateral and ventral caudolateral parts of the cerebral hemisphere.
		c) Cortical branches	Arise at the terminal course of the middle cerebral artery to be distributed in the lateral aspect of the cerebral hemisphere.

Table (12) Common carotid artery (continued)

Main trunk	Branches	Subdivisions	Distribution
	6. Rostral cerebral artery		The continuation of the internal carotid artery, courses rostromedially to the dorsal aspect of the optic chiasma. It reaches the longitudinal fissure and meets with its fellow of the opposite side to form the common artery of the corpus callosum. It gives off the following branches:-
		a) Rostral meningeal artery	Arises from the parent trunk dorsal to the optic chiasma. It passes rostrally and releases fine branches which distribute on the ventral surface of medial olfactory tract and the dura mater around the optic bulb. During its course it gives off :- • **Internal ethmoidal artery;** a large branch, continues rostrally on the ventral surface of the olfactory trigone toward the olfactory bulb to reach the ethmoidal foss. It anatsomoses with the branches of the external ethmoidal artery on the cribriform plate to form the ethmoidal rete. • **Ethmoidal rete;** detaches several branches to ramify in the olfactory bulb and olfactory mucosa of the nasal fundus.
		b) Common artery of the corpus callosum	Formed by the union of the rostral cerebral arteries of either side. It courses for a short distance in the longitudinal fissure, and then ascends to be divided into right and left arteries to the corresponding corpus callosum. The artery in its course gives off cortical branches to the rostral half of the medial surface of the cerebral hemispheres and other branches share in the formation of the ethmoidal rete.
		c) Internal ophthalmic artery	A small branch arises from the rostral cerebral artery lateral to the level of the optic chiasma. It courses on the dorsal aspect of the optic nerve to leave the cranial cavity through the optic foramen. It terminates by anastomosing with the external ophthalmic artery.

Table (13) Vertebral artery

Main trunk	Branches	Subdivisions	Distribution
Vertebral artery			Arises from the subclavian artery on the left side and brachiocephalic artery on the right side, opposite to the level of the first intercostal space. It emerges from the thorax to the neck to pass on the ventral to the transverse process of the seventh cervical vertebra and continues along the neck through the series of transverse foramina (transverse canal of cervical vertebrae), accompanied by the homonymous vein and nerve, to reach the atlantal fossa where it anastomoses with the occipital branch of occipital artery. The vertebral artery runs dorsally trough the alar foramen and enters the vertebral canal through the lateral vertebral foramen to the ventral aspect of the spinal cord. It joins its fellow of the opposite side and with the ventral spinal artery to form the basilar artery.
	1. Basilar artery		The basilar artery contributes the internal carotid artery in vascularization of the brain. It courses rostrally in the median groove on the ventral surface of medulla oblongata, trapezoid body and pons to join the cerebral arterial circle via the distal segments of caudal communicating arteries of both sides. Along its course, it gives off the following branches:-
		a) Medullary branches	Six to ten branches supply the dorsal and ventral surfaces of the medulla oblongata. They form a network on the dorsal aspect of medulla oblongata, anastomoses rostrally with the caudal cerebellar artery and caudally with the dorsal spinal artery.
		b) Caudal cerebellar artery	The first major branch, passes laterally around the medulla oblongata, caudal to the pons, to the cerebellum to be distributed in cerebellar cortex and vermis lobe. It gives off small branches to the pons, medulla oblongata, choroid plexus of fourth ventricle. It also release:- **The labyrinthine artery;** arises caudal to the root of the vestibulocochlear nerve. It gives an anastomosing branch with the caroticobasilar artery, and then enters the internal acoustic meatus accompanies the vestibulocochlear nerve to supply the internal ear.

242

Table (13) Vertebral artery (continued)

Main trunk	Branches	Subdivisions	Distribution
		c) Pontine branches	Two to four transverse branches, arise from the sides of the basilar artery to supply the rostral part of pons.
		d) Rostral cerebellar artery	Arises from the terminal part of basilar artery. It oases dorsolaterally and caudally rostral to the pons and around the cerebral crus. It curves medially to contact the caudal colliculus and cerebellar lobes. It gives off perforating branches to the cerebral crus, pons, cerebellar lobes, vermis lobe and caudal colliculus.
	2. Spinal branches		Arise from the vertebral artery at each intervertebral and lateral vertebral foramen of cervical vertebrae. Each spinal branch enters the vertebral canal and divides into dorsal and ventral branches, reinforcing the dorsal and ventral spinal arteries.
	3. Muscular branches	a) Dorsal muscular branches	Are the larger; they passed dorsally to supply nuchal ligament, splenius, semispinalis capitis, multifidus cervicis, obliquus capitis cranialis and obliquus capitis caudalis. They amastomose with the branches of the deep cervical artery.
		b) ventral muscular branches	They supply the scalenus medius, longus colli, intertransversii cervicis, and longus capitis.
	4. Descending branch		Emerges dorsally from the alar foramen and supplies the obliquus capitis cranialis and caudalis, rectus capitis dorsalis major and minor, semispinalis capitis and spinalis capitis.

Table (14) Deep cervical artery

Deep cervical artery	This artery supplies the neck as a muscular branch, emerges from the thoracic cavity to the neck by passing through the space caudal to the first costotransverse articulation. It continues craniodorsally on the deep face of the semispinalis capitis to reach the level of the axis where it anastomoses with the descending branch of vertebral artery. During its cervical course, it supplies the dorsolateral cervical muscles, nuchal ligament and skin.

Part III. Nerves of the head and neck
Table (15) Cranial nerves

Nerve	Type	Origin	Foramina of emergence	Branches	Distribution
I. Olfactory nerves	Sensory nerves (sense of olfaction)	Olfactory bulb inside the ethmoidal fossa	Foramina of the cribriform plate of the ethmoid bone		The nerve fibers of the olfactory nerves are not aggregated to form a trunk as the other cranial nerves. The olfactory cells are situated in the mucous membrane of the nasal fundus (olfactory region). The central processes of the olfactory nerves are nonmyelinated, formed of small bundles and enclosed in sheathes derived from the cerebral meninges. They pass through the foramina of the cribriform plate to join the convex surface of the olfactory bulb.
				Terminal nerves	Closely related to the olfactory nerves. Their olfactory cells are placed on the caudal portion of the nasal septum. The terminal nerves pass through the cribriform plate of the ethmoid bone to be attached by several rootlets to an area of the brain medial to the olfactory tract.
				Vomeronasal nerve	Emerges the dorsal aspect of the vomeronasal organ by means of several fine twigs which course caudally on the nasal septum. They unite in one or two trunks and pierce the cribriform plate to reach the cranial cavity. The vomeronasal nerve terminates on the caudal surface of the olfactory bulb.

Table (15) Cranial nerves(continued)

Nerve	Type	Origin	Foramina of emergence	Branches		Distribution
II. Optic nerve	Sensory nerve (sense of vision)	Optic chiasma	Optic foramen			Composed of fibers which are the central processes of ganglion cells of the retina. The fibers converge within the eye ball to the optic papilla to form a round trunk, the optic nerve. The nerve pierces the choroid and sclera, emerges from the posterior part of the eye ball and passes slightly flexuous, surrounded by the retractor bulbi muscle to the optic canal. After traversing the latter, it decussates with its fellow of the opposite side to form the optic chiasma.
III. Oculomotor nerve	Motor nerve	Basal surface of the cerebral crus, lateral to the intercrural fossa	Orbital fissure	**1. Dorsal branch**		Short and divides into two twigs to supply the rectus dorsalis and levator palpebrae superioris.
				2. Ventral branch		Larger and longer branch and carries the ciliary ganglion. It supplies motor and parasympathetic fibers to the ciliary ganglion. It also ramifies in the rectus medialis, rectus ventralis and obliquus ventralis. The ciliary ganglion gives off the short ciliary nerves to the ciliary and constrictor pupilae muscles
IV. Trochlear nerve	Motor nerve	Dorsal surface of the cerebral crus, just caudal to the caudal colliculus	Orbital fissure			The smallest of the cranial nerves. It pierces the tentorium cerebelli and passes rostrally along the lateral border of the maxillary nerve. It leaves the cranial cavity through the orbital fissure and courses rostrally along the medial wall of the orbit to end in the caudal part of the obliquus dorsalis.

Table (15) Cranial nerves(continued)

Nerve	Type	Origin	Foramina of emergence	Branches	Distribution
V. Trigeminal nerve	Mixed nerve	Lateral part of pons by a large sensory root and a small motor root	Leaves the cranial cavity dividing into three branches, emerging through three foramina		The trigeminal nerve is formed of three branches and a ganglion termed the trigeminal or semilunar ganglion embedded in the dens fibrous tissue which occupies the rostrolateral part foramen lacerum. The semilunar ganglion receives the sensory root of the trigeminal nerve from the pons and its convex face gives rise the ophthalmic and maxillary nerves and the sensory part of the mandibular nerve. The motor root of the last mixed nerve is detached directly from the lateral part of pons.
1.Ophthalmic nerve	Purely sensory nerve	Convex surface of the semilunar ganglion	Orbital fissure	**1. Lacrimal nerve**	The smallest branch of ophthalmic nerve passes rosrtrally in the orbital cavity on the rectus dorsalis and levator palpebrae superioris; it ramifies in the lacrimal gland and upper eye lid.
				2.Zygomaticotempor al nerve	Arises from the ophthalmic nerve alone or in a common trunk with the lacrimal nerve. It perforates the periorbita to the lacrimal fossa and emerges from the orbital cavity caudal to the supraorbital process and ramifies in the skin of the temporal region. It forms the rostral auricular plexus with the auriculopalpebral and frontal nerves.
				3. Frontal nerve	Passes rostrally parallel with the obliquus dorsalis, then perforates the periorbita to pass dorsally through the supraorbital foramen as supraorbital nerve to ramify in the skin of the forehead. It shares in the formation of the rostral auricular plexus.

246

Table (15) Cranial nerves(continued)

Nerve	Type	Origin	Foramina of emergence	Branches	Distribution
				4. Nasociliary nerve	Passes rostrally and medially under the rectus dorsalis and divides into two terminal branches:- **a) Ethmoidal nerve;** enters the cranial cavity accompanied by the ethmoidal artery through the ethmoidal foramen. It crosses the ventral part of the ethmoidal fossa, leaves the cranial cavity through the cribriform plate to the nasal cavity to ramify in the mucous membrane of the nasal septum and dorsal nasal concha. **b) Infratrochlear nerve;** supplies the third eye lid, medial canthus, conjunctiva, lacrimal caruncle, lacrimal duct and lacrimal sac. During its course inside the orbit, the nasociliary nerve gives off :- **- Communicating branch;** to the ciliary ganglion which carries sympathetic fibers to join the short ciliary nerves. **- Long ciliary nerves;** perforate the sclera to the ciliary body.
2. Maxillary nerve	Purely sensory nerve	Convex surface of the semilunar ganglion	Round foramen	**1. Zygomaticofacial branch**	Arises from the maxillary nerve before it reaches the pterygopalatine fossa. It pierces the periorbita and divides into two to three branches which pass along the rectus lateralis muscle to the lateral canthus. It ramifies in the lower eye lid and adjacent skin.

Table (15) Cranial nerves(continued)

Nerve	Type	Origin	Foramina of emergence	Branches	Distribution
				2. Pterygopalatine nerve	Arises from the maxillary nerve in the pterygopalatine fossa. It formes a plexus with the pterygopalatine ganglia and the nerve of pterygoid canal and gives these branches: **a) Caudal nasal nerve;** passes through the sphenopalatine foramen to the nasal cavity. It divides into medial and lateral branches to supply the mucous membrane of the nasal septum, vomeronasal organ, ventral nasal concha and nasal meatuses. **b) Greater palatine nerve;** the largest branch of the pterygopalatine nerve, runs rostrally in the greater palatine canal and palatine groove to ramify in the hard palate, gums and floor of the nasal cavity. **c) Lesser palatine nerve;** the smallest branch, supplies the soft palate.
				3. Infraorbital nerve	Traverses the infraorbital canal, where it gives off the maxillary alveolar branches, then emerges from the infraorbital foramen and divides into external nasal, internal nasal and maxillary labial branches. **a) Maxillary alveolar branches;** supply the alveoli of the maxillary cheek teeth and the gums. **b) External nasal branches;** two to three branches, ramify in the nasal region. **c) Internal nasal branches;** large, supply the maxillary lip, nostril and nasal vestibule. **d) Maxillary labial branch;** the largest and ramify in the skin and mucous membrane of maxillary lip and cheeks.

Table (15) Cranial nerves(continued)

Nerve	Type	Origin	Foramina of emergence	Branches	Distribution
3. Mandibular nerve	Mixed nerve	The sensory root from the convex surface of the semilunar ganglion The motor root from the motor nucleus of pons	Oval foramen (foramen lacerum)		The mandibular nerve is formed by union of two roots; the larger sensory root comes from the semilunar ganglion and the motor root is the smaller part of the trigeminal nerve. It emerges from the cranial cavity and passes between the wing of the basisphenoid bone and the muscular process of petrous part of temporal bone. It continues its course on the lateral surface of guttural pouch and, on reaching the lateral surface of pterygoideus medialis, divides into two terminal branches; the mandibular alveolar and lingual nerves. The mandibular nerve gives off the following branches:-
				1. Masseteric nerve	Passes laterally through the mandibular notch across the rostral surface of the temporomandibular articulation, turns ventrally to enter the deep face of masseter muscle.
				2. Deep temporal nerves	Two to three in number, arise by a common trunk from the mandibular nerve with the masseteric nerve to supply the temporalis muscle.
				3. Buccal nerve	Passes rostroventrally to cross the medial surface of temporomandibular articulation to the lateral surface of the maxillary tuber. It continues rosrterally in the submucosa of the cheek till the labial commissure to ramify in the buccal glands, mucous membrane of the lips and labial glands. Along its course, it gives off:- **a) Lateral pterygoid nerve;** to the pterygoideus lateralis and release collateral twigs to cheek and buccal glands. **b) Medial pterygoid nerve;** passes through the otic ganglion and gives off nerves to the tensor veli palatini and tensor tympani muscles, then penetrates the caudal part of the pterygoideus medialis to ramify in it.

Table (15) Cranial nerves (continued)

Nerve	Type	Origin	Foramina of emergence	Branches	Distribution
				4. Auriculotemporal nerve	Passes laterally between the parotid gland and the neck of the mandibular ramus, turns around the latter and divides into two branches:- **a) Transverse facial branch;** accompanies the transverse facial vessels and ramifies in the skin of the cheek. **b) Rostral auricular nerves;** supply the external ear, skin of the external acoustic meatus, tympanic membrane, guttural pouch and parotid gland.
				5. Mandibularalveolar nerve	Enters the mandibular canal through the mandibular foramen and emerges the canal at the mental foramen as the mental nerve. Along its course, it gives off :- **a) Mylohyoid nerve;** arises from the mandibular alveolar nerve before its entering the canal. It passes between the mandibular ramus and the mylohyoideus to supply the muscle, rostral belly of digastricus and skin of the intermandibular space. **b) Mandibular alveolar branches;** to the alveoli of the mandibular cheek teeth and mandibular incisors. **c) Mandibular labial branches;** supply the mandibular lip. **d) Mental nerve;** ramifies in the chin.
				6. Lingual nerve	Runs on the medial face of mylohyoideus to reach the root of the tongue where it releases the sublingual nerve to the mucous membrane of the tongue and floor of the mouth. The nerve continues it course rostrally between the hyoglossus and genioglossus to the tip of the tongue. It gives branches to the fungiform papillae and mucous m.

Table (15) Cranial nerves (continued)

Nerve	Type	Origin	Foramina of emergence	Branches	Distribution
IV. Abducent nerve	Motor nerve	Lateral aspect of medullary pyramid, just caudal to pons	Orbital fissure		It passes rostrally across the pons, pierces the dura mater and accompanies the oculomotor and ophthalmic nerves to the orbit. It gives off very short branches to innervate the rectus lateralis and retractor bulbi.
IIV. Facial nerve	Mixed nerve	Lateral part of trapezoid body, just caudal to the pons	Internal acoustic meatus to the facial canal, emerges from the canal through the stylomastoid foramen		The facial nerve passes inside the facial canal of the petrous part of temporal bone. The nerve and canal are at first directed laterally between the vestibule and the cochlea, then curved caudally and ventrally at the knee in the caudal wall of the tympanic cavity to end at the stylomastoid foramen. The bend formed by the nerve at the knee bears the geniculate ganglion. After its emergence though the stylomastoid foramen, the extracanalicular part of facial nerve passes rostroventrally on the lateral aspect of guttural pouch and covered by the parotid gland. It crosses the caudal border of the mandibular ramus and continues rostrally to leave the deep face of the parotid gland, at the level of the transverse facial vessels, where it terminates into the dorsal and ventral buccal branches. The facial nerve detaches the first five branches inside the facial canal and the others between the stylomastoid foramen and its termination.
				1. Greater petrosal nerve	Arises from the geniculate ganglion, leaves the facial canal and contributes a filament to the tympanic plexus. It receives the deep petrosal nerve from the carotid plexus of sympathetic, emerges through the foramen lacerum and continues as the nerve of the pterygoid canal. It passes inside the pterygoid canal and terminates in the pterygopalatine plexus and ganglia.

Table (15) Cranial nerves (continued)

Nerve	Type	Origin	Foramina of emergence	Branches	Distribution
				2. lesser petrosal nerve	This nerve is formed by a delicate branch emerges from the geniculate ganglion and united with the filament from the tympanic plexus. The lesser petrosal nerve ends in the otic ganglion.
				3. Stapedial nerve	A short nerve, detaches from the facial nerve as it curves down in the facial canal. It innervates the stapedius muscle.
				4. Chorda tympani	Reaches the tympanic cavity through a small canal in the mastoid part of temporal bone. It traverses the tympanic cavity between the malleus and incus and emerges through the petrotympanic fissure to reach the lateral aspect of guttural pouch. It joins the lingual nerve and furnishes gustatory fibers to the taste buds of the rostral two thirds of the tongue.
				5. Anastomotic branches with vagus nerve	Are united with the auricular branch of vagus nerve near the stylomastoid foramen.
				6. Caudal auricular nerve	Arises from the facial nerve at its emergence from the facial canal. It passes caudodorsally with the caudal auricular artery on the deep surface of the parotid gland to supply the dorsal and caudal auricular muscles and the skin of the convex surface of the external ear. It connects with the branches of the first and second cervical nerves.
				7. Internal auricular branch	Ascends in the parotid gland just caudal to the auricular cartilage, passes through an opening in the auricular base to ramify in the skin of convex surface of the external ear.

Table (15) Cranial nerves (continued)

Nerve	Type	Origin	Foramina of emergence	Branches	Distribution
				8. Digastric branch	Descends on the deep face of the parotid gland. Its branches supply the caudal belly of digastricus muscle and its occipitomandibular part, stylohyoideus and occipitohyoideus.
				9. Auriculopalpebral nerve	Arises from the facial nerve near the caudal border of the mandibular ramus. It ascends inside the parotid gland, caudal to the superficial temporal nerve and divides into:- **a) Rostral auricular branches;** supply the auriculares rostrales and parotidoauricularis muscles. **b) Zygomatic branch;** runs over the temporalis muscle to the medial angle of the eye, forms a plexus with the ophthalmic never. Its branches ramify in the orbicularis oculi and corrugator supercilii.
				10. Cervical branch	Passes caudoventrally through the parotid gland, pierces the parotidoauricularis to reach the area near the jugular vein. It continues caudally along the neck in the subcutaneous tissue and reinforced by cutaneous branches of the second to the sixth cervical nerves to innervate the skin.
				11. Dorsal buccal branch	Passes rostrally on the dorsal part of masseter, dips under the zygomaticus and reaches the ventral border of caninus. It continues under cover the levator nasolabialis and ramifies in the muscles of the upper lip and nostril.
				12. Ventral buccal branch	Crosses obliquely the masseter and continues rostrally along the depressor labii mandibularis. It ramifies in the latter muscle, cutaneous faciei and buccinator. It is joined with the dorsal buccal nerve by variable branches.

Table (15) Cranial nerves (continued)

Nerve	Type	Origin	Foramina of emergence	Branches	Distribution
VIII. Vestibulocochlear nerve (Acoustic nerve)	Sensory nerve	Lateral part of trapezoid body, caudal to the facial nerve	Internal acoustic meatus		This nerve consists of two separate roots which form two functionally separate parts; vestibular and cochlear nerves. The cochlear nerve mediates the sense of hearing. The vestibular nerve is concerned in the mechanism of equilibration (sense of the position of the body). The nerve passes laterally to enter the internal acoustic meatus where it divides into two parts; the dorsal is the vestibular nerve and the ventral is the cochlear nerve.
				1.Vestibular part	The vestibular nerve bears the vestibular ganglion at the bottom of the internal acoustic meatus. The ganglion gives off the fibers of the nerve which are distributed to the utricle, saccule, and ampullae of the semicircular ducts of the internal ear. The vestibular nerve is connected by filaments with the geniculate ganglion of facial nerve
				2. Cochlear part	The cochlear nerve detaches a filament to the saccule, then passes through the lamina cribrosa of the cochlea to be distributed in the spiral cochlear duct (organ of Corti).
IX. Glossopharyngeal nerve	Mixed nerve	Rostral part of the lateral aspect of medulla oblongata	Jugular foramen		The glossopharyngeal nerve bears the jugular and petrous ganglia at its emergence from the jugular foramen. It is curved ventrally and rostrally over the guttural pouch and caudal to the thyrohyoid bone. It crosses the deep face of external carotid artery and divides into pharyngeal and lingual branches. Along its course, it gives off the following branches:-

Table (15) Cranial nerves (continued)

Nerve	Type	Origin	Foramina of emergence	Branches	Distribution
				1.Tympanic nerve	Arises from the petrous ganglion and passes between the pertous and tympanic parts of temporal bone to the tympanic cavity where it forms the tympanic plexus with the sympathetic carotid plexus. The branches of the tympanic plexus innervate the mucous membrane of tympanum and auditory tube.
				2. Branch of carotid sinus	A branch of considerable size runs caudally on the guttural pouch, concurs with twigs from vagus and sympathetic fibers from the cranial cervical ganglion to form the carotid plexus in the terminal part of common carotid artery.
				3. Pharyngeal branch	Courses rostrally across the deep face of the stylohyoid bone. It is joined with the branches of vagus, spinal accessory, hypoglossal nerves and sympathetic filaments from the cranial cervical ganglion to form the pharyngeal plexus. The plexus supplies the muscles and mucous membrane of the pharynx.
				4. Lingual branch	Runs along the caudal border of the stylohyoid bone, rostral to the linguofacial trunk and dips under the hyoglossus muscle. It ends in the mucous membrane of the caudal one third of the tongue where it supplies gustatory fibers to the taste buds. It gives off collateral branches to the soft palate, isthmus faucium and tonsils.

Table (15) Cranial nerves (continued)

Nerve	Type	Origin	Foramina of emergence	Branches	Distribution
X. Vagus nerve	Mixed nerve	Lateral aspect of medulla oblongata just caudal to the preceding nerve	Jugular foramen		Is the longest and widely distributed of the cranial nerves. It bears the jugular ganglion at its emergence from the jugular foramen. It runs caudally and ventrally with the accessory nerve in a fold of the guttural pouch, then descends with the internal carotid artery and crosses the medial face of origin of the occipital artery. Here it is accompanied by the cervical sympathetic trunk in a common sheath to form the vagosympathetic trunk which continues along the dorsal aspect of common carotid artery till the root of the neck. The vagus nerve is separated from the sympathetic trunk at the thoracic inlet and from this point the course and relations of the right and left vagi differ. **-The right vagus nerve;** enters the thorax at the origin of the bicarotid trunk, then passes caudodorsally to cross the lateral surface of the brachiocephalic trunk and the right face of trachea. It reaches the dorsal surface of the trachea and near the tracheal bifurcation divides into dorsal and ventral branches. **-The left vagus nerve;** enters the thorax on the ventral face of the esophagus, crossing obliquely under the left subclavian artery and passes caudally on its lateral surface. It continues caudally on the lateral surface of the aorta, inclines to the dorsal surface of the left principal bronchus and divides into dorsal and ventral branches. The dorsal and ventral branches unite with the corresponding branches of the opposite side to form **the dorsal and ventral vagal trunks**. The trunks run caudally in the caudal mediastinum, dorsal and ventral to the esophagus respectively tell the hiatus esophageus of the diaphragm,through which they leave to the abdominal cavity. Along the course of vagus nerve gives off the following branches:-

Table (15) Cranial nerves (continued)

Nerve	Type	Origin	Foramina of emergence	Branches	Distribution
				1. Pharyngeal branch	Courses cranioventrally on the guttural pouch to the dorsal wall of the pharynx. Here, it is joined with the branches of glossopharyngeal, spinal accessory, hypoglossal nerves and sympathetic filaments from the cranial cervical ganglion to form the pharyngeal plexus. The plexus supplies the muscles and mucous membrane of the pharynx. The plexus also gives a large esophageal branch to the cervical part of the esophagus.
				2. Cranial laryngeal branch	Runs cranioventrally over the lateral wall of the pharynx and caudal to the hypoglossal nerve. It passes through the the thyroid foramen to the interior of the larynx, where it divides into external and internal branches. The external branch descends to supply the cricothyroideus and cricopharyngeus, while the internal branch ramifies in the mucous membrane of the larynx, floor of the pharynx and entrance of the esophagus.
				3. Recurrent laryngeal nerve (caudal laryngeal nerve)	Differs on the two sides in its point of origin and in the first part of its course. The right nerve is detached opposite the second rib, turns around the costocervical trunk to run cranially on the right ventral surface of the trachea and ascends in the neck on the ventral surface of right common carotid artery. The left nerve arises from the vagus nerve where the latter begins to cross the aortic arch. It passes back over the arterial ligament, winds around the concavity of the aortic arch to run cranially on the left ventral surface of the trachea and continues on the ventral surface of the left common carotid artery.

Table (15) Cranial nerves (continued)

Nerve	Type	Origin	Foramina of emergence	Branches	Distribution
					Along the course of the recurrent laryngeal nerve, it gives off branches to the cardiac plexus, trachea and esophagus. The terminal part receives fibers from the accessory nerve, then passes between the cricoarytenoideus dorsalis and cricopharyngeus as the caudal laryngeal nerve to enter the larynx at the medial side of the thyroid lamina. It supplies all intrinsic muscles of the larynx except the cricothyroideus.
				4. Cardiac branches	Arise from the right and left vagi to join with the cardiac branches of sympathetic and recurrent laryngeal nerves to form the cardiac plexus.
				5. Bronchial branches	Are detached at the root of the lung and united with the sympathetic filaments in forming the pulmonary plexus. From the plexus, numerous branches proceed along the bronchi.
				6. Dorsal vagal trunk	Enters the abdominal cavity, passes to the left of the cardia and divides into gastric and celiac branches. **a) Gastric branch;** gives branches to the visceral surface of the stomach forming the caudal gastric plexus. **b) Celiac branch;** ends in the celiacomesentric ganglion and intermesentric plexus.
				7.Ventral vagal trunk	Smaller than the dorsal one, passes to the lesser curvature of the stomach and ramifies on the parietal surface of the stomach forming the cranial gastric plexus. The latter plexus gives off branches to supply the liver, pancreas and cranial part of duodenum.

Table (15) Cranial nerves (continued)

Nerve	Type	Origin	Foramina of emergence	Branches	Distribution
XI. Accessory nerve	Purely motor	Spinal roots; from the first five spinal cervical segments Cranial roots; from the lateral aspect of medulla oblongata	Jugular foramen		The spinal roots represent the external branch of the accessory nerve. The trunk which is very small at its origin at the fifth segment, increased in size when traced within the spinal subarachnoid space toward the brain because it receives accessions of fibers. It passes through the foramen magnum and joins the cranial roots (internal branch) forming the trunk of the accessory nerve. It emerges from cranial cavity through the jugular foramen and divides into internal and external branches. The internal branch passes with the vagus and shares in the formation of the pharyngeal plexus. The external branch runs caudally crossing the deep face of mandibular gland to the atlantal fossa where it divides into dorsal and ventral branches.
				1. Dorsal branch	Passes caudally through the brachiocephalicus and continues on the serratus ventralis cervicis, then enters the deep face of the trapezius, in which it ramifies.
				2. ventral branch	Passes caudoventrally to enter the deep face of the sternocephalicus at the tendon of insertion.
XII. Hypoglossal nerve	Purely motor	Ventral surface of medulla oblongata lateral to the caudal half of the pyramids	Hypoglossal canal		The bundles of the hypoglossal nerve are united to form a trunk which leaves the cranial cavity though the hypoglossal canal. It passes caudally and ventrally on the guttural pouch between the vagus and accessory nerves, turns ventrally and rostrally over the pharynx parallel with the stylohyoid bone and caudal to the linguofacial artery. It crosses beneath the latter and runs rostrally on the lateral surface of the hyoglossus muscle and divides into the terminal lingual branches:-
				1. Smaller branch	Supplies the styloglossus , hyoglossus and intrinsic muscles of the tongue.
				2. larger branch	Ramifies in the genioglossus and geniohyoideus muscles

Table (16) Cervical spinal nerves

Nerve	Foramen of emergence	Branches	Distribution
First cervical nerve	Lateral vertebral foramen of the atlas	**1. Dorsal branch (suboccipital nerve)**	Passes dorsolaterally between the obliquus capitis cranialis and recti capitis dorsales and supplies these muscles, the caudal auricular muscles and ramifies in the skin of the poll.
		2. Ventral branch	Descends through the alar foramen of the atlas to the deep surface of the parotid gland and divides into cranial and caudal branches. **a) Cranial branch;** enters the omohyoideus muscle **b) Caudal branch;** passes caudally and ventrally on the deep face of omohyoideus to join with a branch of the ventral division of the second cervical nerve to supply the sterothyrohyoideus muscle.
Second cervical nerve	Lateral vertebral foramen of the axis	**1. Dorsal branch (major occipital nerve)**	Ascends between the semispinalis capitis and the nuchal ligament to ramify in the skin of the poll.
		2. Ventral branch	Detaches muscular branches to the longus capitis amd communicating branches to the accessory nerve and the ventral branches of the first and third cervical nerve, then becomes superficial by passing between the two parts of the brachiocephalicus muscle. The ventral branch divides into:- **a) Great auricular nerve;** passes dorsally on the parotid gland parallel with the caudal border of the parotido-auricularis to ramify on the convex surface of the external ear. **b) Transverse cervical nerve;** courses caudally to be connected with the cervical branch of facial nerve and continues along the jugular groove. It gives off twigs to the cutaneus colli, skin of the parotid and laryngeal region and the mandibular space.

Table (16) Cervical spinal nerves (continued)

Nerve	Foramen of emergence	Branches	Distribution
Third cervical nerve	Intervertebral foramen between second and third cervical vertebrae	**1. Dorsal branch**	Emerges between two bundles of the intertransversii cervicis, accompanied by the corresponding dorsal muscular branch of vertebral nerve, runs dorsally to supply the mulifidus cervicis, semispinalis capitis and skin of the region.
		2.Ventral branch	Courses ventrally to supply the longus capitis, longissimus capitis,longissimus atlantis and skin of the region
Fourth and fifth cervical nerves	Intervertebral foramina; between the third and fourth cervical vertebrae for the fourth nerve, between the forth and fifth cervical vertebrae for the fifth nerve	**1. Dorsal branches**	Their distribution is similar to that of the third cervical nerve. The dorsal cervical plexus is formed by the communicating twigs of the dorsal branches from the third to sixth nerves.
		2. Ventral branches	Supply supply the longus capitis, longissimus capitis,longissimus atlantis, longus colli and skin of the region. The ventral branch of the fifth cervical nerve contributes a small branch to share in the formation of the phrenic nerve.
Sixth cervical nerve	Intervertebral foramen between the fifth and sixth cervical vertebrae	**1. Dorsal branch**	A small branch supplies the multifidus cervicis.
		2. Ventral branch	Contributes branches to the phrenic nerve and brachial plexus as well as other muscular and cutaneous branches. **a) Muscular branches;** to the longus colli, intertransversii cervicis, brachiocephlicus, serratus ventralis cervicis and rhomboideus cervicis. **b) Supraclavicular nerve;** sends twigs to the skin over the shoulder joint and descends to the skin over the pectoralis descendens and pectoralis transverses muscles.

Table (16) Cervical spinal nerves (continued)

Nerve	Foramen of emergence	Branches	Distribution
Seventh and eighth cervical nerves	Intervertebral foramina; between the sixth and seventh cervical vertebrae for the seventh nerve, between the seventh cervical and first thoracic vertebrae for the eighth nerve	**1. Dorsal branches**	Small braches ascend between the longissimus cervicis and multifidus cervicis to supply the latter muscles, spinalis, semspinalis capitis, rhomboideus cervicis and skin of the lateral aspect of the caudal part of the neck.
		2. Ventral branches	Very large branches go almost entirely to the brachial plexus. The ventral branch of the seventh cervical nerve contributes the caudal root of the phrenic nerve.
Vertebral nerve			The vertebral nerve represents the postganglionic sympathetic fibers arising from the caudal cervical (stellate) or cervicothoracic ganglion, as it courses through the transverse canal, gives off communicating branches to the cervical nerves from the second to the sixth. It accompanies the vertebral artery and vein in the transverse canal of the cervical vertebrae.
Phrenic nerve			The motor nerve to the diaphragm. It is formed by the union of three roots derived from the ventral branches of the fifth, sixth and seventh cervical nerves. The root derived from the fifth cervical nerve is small and inconstant, while the root from the seventh cervical comes by the way of brachial plexus. The phrenic nerve crosses the ventral border of the scalenus medius muscle just cranial to the thoracic inlet and enters the thorax between the subclavian artery and cranial vena cava. Beyond this the course of the right and left phrenic nerves are not the same. - **The right nerve** passes caudally over the right face of the cranial vena cava, crosses the pericardium and continues along the right face of the caudal vena cava in a special fold, the plica venae cavae. It inclines to the ventral face of the caudal vena cava to ramify in the right part of diaphragm. - **The left phrenic nerve** runs on the lateral side of the subclavian artery and ventral to the left vagus in the cranial mediastinum. It passes over the dorsal part of pericardium and continues caudally in the caudal mediastinum to reach the tendinous center of the diaphragm.

Chapter 2

Trunk and pelvis

Part I. Muscles of the trunk
Table (17) Muscles of the back, loins and tail

Muscle	Origin	Insertion	Action	Innervation
Trapezius thoracis	Supraspinous ligament extending between the spinous processes of the thoracic vertebrae from the third to tenth.	The tuber of the spine of the scapula	Elevates the shoulder and draws the scapula caudally	- Dorsal branch of accessory nerve - Dorsal branches of thoracic nerves
Latissimus dorsi	Thoracolumbar fascia which attached to the spinous processes of the thoracic and lumbar vertebrae	Teres major tuberosity of the humerus	Flexes the shoulder joint and draws the trunk cranially	Dorsal thoracic nerve
Rhomboideus thoracis	Supraspinous ligament extending between the spinous processes of the thoracic vertebrae from the second to seventh.	Medial surface of the scapular cartilage	Draws the scapula dorsally and cranially	Dorsal branches of the thoracic nerves
Serratus dorsalis cranialis	Thoracolumbar fascia and dorsal scapular ligament. The muscle fibers pass caudally and ventrally, attached to the ribs by seven or eight digitations.	Lateral surfaces of the ribs from the sixth to twelfth	Draws the ribs cranially and laterally to assist the inspiration	Thoracic nerves
Serratus dorsalis caudalis	Thoracolumbar fascia. The muscle fibers course cranially and ventrally, attached to the ribs by seven to eight digitations.	Lateral surfaces of the last seven ribs.	Draws the ribs caudally to assist in expiration	Thoracic nerves
Iliocostalis thoracis and lumborum	- Deep layer of thoracolumbar fascia - Cranial borders and lateral surfaces of the last fifteen ribs	Caudal borders of the ribs and transverse process of the last cervical vertebra	Depresses and retracts the ribs to help the expiration	Thoracic nerves

Table (17) Muscles of the back, loins and tail (continued)

Muscle	Origin	Insertion	Action	Innervation
Longissimus thorcis and lumborum	The largest and longest muscle in the body, arises from the iliac crest, supraspinous ligament and spinous processes of the thoracic and lumbar vertebrae	- Transverse processes of the thoracic and lumbar vertebrae - Lateral surfaces of the vertebral end of the ribs except the first	Powerful extensor of the back and loins, and assists in expiration	Dorsal branches of the thoracic and lumbar nerves
Multifidi	Long series of segmental muscles which lie along the sides of the spinous processes of the thoracic and lumbar vertebrae. They arise from the transverse processes of thoracic vertebrae and articular processes of lumbar vertebrae.	The muscle bundles are directed craniodorsally to be inserted into the summits of the spinous processes of the preceding thoracic and lumbar vertebrae.	Extends the dorsum by extension of the spines	Dorsal branches of the thoracic and lumbar nerves
Intertransversii lumborum	Very thin muscular and tendinous bands occupy the spaces between the transverse processes of lumbar vertebrae except the last. Each arises from the cranial border of the transverse process.	They extend cranially to be inserted in the caudal border of the preceding transverse process	Protection and increases the rigidity of the lumbar region	Lumbar nerves
Quadratus lumborum	Caudal border of the first rib and transverse processes of the lumbar vertebrae	Ventral surface of the wing of sacrum	Draws the last rib caudally to assist the expiration	Costoabdominal and lumbar nerves
Coccygeus	Flat triangular muscle, arises from the pelvic surface of the broad sacrotuberal ligament near the ischiatic spine.	The first four caudal vertebrae and fascia of the tail	Depresses or flexes the tail	Caudal rectal nerve

266

Table (17) Muscles of the back, loins and tail (continued)

Muscle	Origin	Insertion	Action	Innervation
Sacrocaudalis dorsalis medialis	Lies along the dorsomedian aspect of the tail, arises from the last three sacral spines and some of the first caudal vertebrae	Dorsal surface of the caudal vertebrae	Elevates or extends the tail	Ventral caudal plexus
Sacrocaudalis dorsalis lateralis	Sides of the sacral spines, immediately lateral to the preceding	Lateral surface of the caudal vertebrae, except the first four	Assists the elevation of the tail	Ventral caudal plexus
Sacrocaudalis ventralis lateralis	Lie on the ventral aspect of the sacrum and caudal vertebrae. It is composed of two parts:- - Lateral part; arises from the lateral part of the ventral surface of sacrum - Medial part; from the ventral surface of the sacrum medial to the lateral part	Transverse processes and ventral surfaces of the caudal vertebrae	Depress or flex the tail and move the tail to the sides	Ventral caudal plexus
Sacrocaudalis ventralis medialis				
Intertransversii dorsales et ventrales caudae	Muscular bundles lie on the lateral aspect of the tail between the sacrocaudalis dorsalis latralis and sacrocaudalis ventralis lateralis. They arise from the lateral edge of sacrum	The spaces between the transverse processes of the caudal vertebrae in the form of dorsal and ventral segments	They fix the caudal vertebrae	Ventral caudal plexus

Table (18) Muscles of the thorax (respiration)

Muscle	Origin	Insertion	Action	Innervation
Levatores costarum	Sets of small muscles occupy the dorsal ends of the intercostal spaces and arise from the transverse processes of the thoracic vertebrae	Lateral surfaces and cranial borders of the dorsal ends of the ribs caudal to the vertebral origin	Draw the ribs cranially in inspiration	Intercostal nerves
Intercostales externi	Occupy the intercostal spaces, from the levatores costarum to the sternal extremity of the ribs and absent in the intercartilagenous spaces. Arise from the caudal border of the ribs	The muscle fibers are directed caudoventrally to insert in the cranial borders and lateral surfaces of the succeeding ribs	Draw the ribs cranially in inspiration	Intercostal nerves
Intercostales interni	Occupy the intercostal spaces including the intercartilagenous spaces and arise from the cranial borders of the ribs	The muscle fibers are directed cranioventrally to insert in the caudal borders of the preceding ribs and costal cartilages	Draw the ribs caudally in expiration	Intercostal nerves
Retractor costae	Lies caudal to the last rib, undercover the serratus dorsalis caudalis. It arises from the transverse processes of the first three lumbar vertebrae by means of the lumbar fascia	The caudal border of the last rib	Draw the last rib caudally to assist the expiration	Lumbar nerves
Rectus thoracis	Thin and oblique muscle crosses the ventral part of the first three intercostal spaces and arises from the lateral surface of the first rib	Cartilage of the first rib and the aponeurosis usually joins the rectus abdominis	Assists in inspiration	Intercostal nerves
Transversus thoracis	Situated on the thoracic surface of the sternum and the cartilages of sternal ribs, arises from the sternal ligament, meeting the opposite muscles	Costal cartilages from the second to eighth and adjacent parts of the sternal ends of the ribs	Draws the ribs and the cartilages caudally in expiration	Intercostal nerves

268

Table (18) Muscles of the thorax (respiration) (continued)

Muscle	Origin	Insertion	Action	Innervation
Diaphragm	The most important muscle of respiration which is broad unpaired, forms a partition between the thoracic and abdominal cavities. It is dome shaped and compressed laterally. The thoracic surface is strongly convex and covered by the pleura; the abdominal surface is deeply concave and covered by the peritoneum. The diaphragm is formed of a fleshy rim which subdivided into the two crura of the lumbar, costal and sternal parts; and a tendinous center. The fleshy parts are inserted by radiating fibers in different directions which blended together to form the tendinous center.			
1. Lumbar part	Right and left crura of the lumbar part arises by the ventral longitudinal ligament; from the first four lumbar vertebrae for the right crus, from the first and second lumbar vertebrae for the left one	Tendinous center	It is the main inspiratory muscle and regulates the pressure in the thorax and abdomen	Right and left phrenic nerves and Intercostal nerves
2. Costal part	Costal cartilages of the 8th, 9th, and 10th ribs. Caudal the tenth rib the costal part is attached to the medial surfaces of the ribs at increasing distance above the costo-chondral junction.	Tendinous center		
3. sternal part	Dorsal surface of the xiphoid cartilage	Tendinous center		

Table (19) Abdominal muscles

Muscle	Origin	Insertion	Action	Innervation
Obliquus externus abdominis	The most extensive, forms a broad sheet which is irregularly triangular in shape. Its fibers are directed ventrally and caudally. It arises from the lateral surface of the ribs caudal to the fourth rib and the thoracolumbar fascia.	- Ventrally, the aponeurosis is blended with the that of the internal abdominal oblique forming the external rectal sheath, inserted in the linea alba - Dorsally and caudally in the inguinal region, the aponeurosis stretches to form the inguinal ligament which is inserted into the coxal tuber and prepubic tendon.	Compress the abdominal viscera during defecation, micturition, parturition and expiration	Intercostal nerves
Obliquus internus abdominis	Forms a triangular sheet lies under the preceding muscle in the flank region. Its fibers are directed ventrally and cranially. It arises from the coxal tuber and adjacent part of inguinal ligament	Ventrally and medially, the aponeurosis is blended with that of the external abdominal oblique foming the external rectal sheath, inserted in the linea alba and the prepubic tendon		Ventral branches of lumbar nerves
Transversus abdominis	A triangular curved sheet and its fibers are transversely placed. It arises from the transverse processes of lumbar vertebrae and medial surface of costal arch	Caudally and ventrally the aponeurosis covers the deep face of the rectus abdominis and formes the internal rectal sheath which is inserted in the linea alba		Intercostal nerves and Ventral branches of lumbar nerves
Rectus abdominis	Formes the ventral part of the abdominal wall extends from the sternum to the pubis. It arises from the last four true costal cartilages and adjacent part of the sternum	Cranial border of the pubis by means of the prepubic tendon		Intercostal nerves and Ventral branches of lumbar nerves

Part II. Arteries of the trunk

Table (20) Arteries of the thoracic viscera and wall

Main trunk	Branches	Subdivisions	Distribution
Pulmonary trunk			Springs from the conus arteriosus at the left side of the base of right ventricle. The trunk is bulbous at its origin and forms three sinuses which correspond to the three semilunar cusps of the pulmonary orifice. The trunk courses caudodorsally and medially to be divided caudal to the aortic arch into right and left pulmonary arteries. Near the bifurcation it is connected with the aortic arch by the ligamentum arteriosum, a remnant of the ductus arteriosus in the fetal life. The pulmonary trunk carries the nonoxygenated blood from the right ventricle to the respiratory tissue of the lungs where the exchange of gases takes place and the oxygenated blood returns through the pulmonary veins to the left atrium of the heart.
	1. Right pulmonary artery		Is longer and wider than the left one. It passes on the ventral aspect of the tracheal bifurcation to the hilus of the right lung. It enters the root of the lung on the ventral surface of the right principal bronchus. In the lung it passes to the ventrolateral side of the principal bronchus and branched to follow the ramification of the bronchi and their subdivisions.
	2. Left pulmonary artery		Is very short, passes caudally to enter the root of the left lung ventral to the principal bronchus. Its branches within the lung are arranged like that of the right one.
Aorta			The main arterial trunk which carries the oxygenated blood from the base of the left ventricle to all parts of the body and could be divided into three parts. **The ascending aorta** begins at the bulbous aorticus which contains three sinuses correspond to the three semilunar cusps of the aortic orifice. The cranial and left sinuses give off the right and left coronary arteries respectively. The ascending aorta passes craniodorsally between the pulmonary trunk and right atrium till the heart base. **The aortic arch** curves sharply caudodorsally and inclines to the left. **The descending aorta** courses caudally on the ventral aspect of the bodies of the thoracic vertebrae in the caudal mediastinum as **thoracic aorta**. It traverses the aortic hiatus of the diaphragm to the abdominal cavity where it lies ventral to the vertebral bodies as **abdominal aorta**. Ventral to the sixth lumbar vertebra it divides into the terminal branches.

Table (20) Arteries of the thoracic viscera and wall (continued)

Main trunk	Branches	Subdivisions	Distribution
I. Ascending aorta	1. Right coronary artery		Very long, arises from the cranial aortic sinus. It passes cranially between the conus arteriosus and the right auricle to the coronary groove in which it curves around the cranial border to the right and continues to reach the basal end of the interventricular subsinosal groove where it divides into two branches:-
		a) Interventricular subsinosal branch	Descends in the interventricular subsinosal groove to the apex of the heart. It supplies the right surface of the ventricular mass and the right border of the interventricular septum by the **septal branches**.
		b) Right circumflex branch	Courses caudally in the coronary groove and anastomoses with the corresponding branch of the left coronary artery. They supply the base of the ventricular mass and the left atrium while the right atrium is supplied by the **atrial branches** of the right coronary artery.
	2. Left coronary artery		Very short, arises from the left aortic sinus. It passes laterally between conus arteriosus and left auricle to the coronary groove at the basal end of the interventricular paraconal groove where it divides into two branches:-
		a) Interventricular paraconal branch	Descends in the interventricular paraconal groove till the vascular notch on the right ventricular border near the apex. Its branches supply the left surface of the ventricular mass and the left border of the interventricular septum by the **septal branches**.
		b) Left circumflex branch	Passes caudally in the coronary groove, winds around the left ventricular border to the right side and anastomoses with the corresponding branch of the right coronary artery. It supplies the base of the ventricular mass and the left atrium.

Table (20) Arteries of the thoracic viscera and wall (continued)

Main trunk	Branches	Subdivisions	Distribution
II. Aortic arch			The short sharply curved part connects the ascending and descending parts of the aorta. It gives off a very large vessel, the **brachiocephalic trunk**, form the convexity of the arch within the pericardium. It is directed cranially and dorsally in the cranial mediastinum between the left vagus and the trachea. Opposite to the second rib, it gives off the **left subclavian artery** and continues cranially ventral to the trachea till the level of the first rib where it divides into the **right subclavian artery and the bicarotid trunk.**
Brachiocephalic trunk	1. left subclavian artery	a) Costocervical trunk	Passes dorsally across the left face of the trachea and esophagus toward the second intercostals space. On reaching the thoracic part of longus colli, it divides into two branches:- **1) Supreme intercostal artery**; passes caudally along the lateral border with the sympathetic trunk. It detaches **the second, third, fourth and fifth dorsal intercostal arteries.** **2) Dorsal scapular artery**; emerges through the dorsal end of the second intercostal space to supply the muscles and skin of the withers.
		b) Deep cervical artery	Leaves the thoracic cavity through the first intercostal space where it releases **the first dorsal intercostal artery.** It continues craniodorsally in the neck between the lamellar part of the nuchal ligament and semispinalis capitis to supply the muscles of the neck.
		c) Vertebral artery	To the extensors of the head and neck, the cervical part of the spinal cord, cerebellum, brain stem and the muscles of the poll. (the artery was fully described in tables of the head and neck).
		d) Superficial cervical artery	Arises from the dorsal surface of subclavian artery opposite to the first rib. It supplies the subclavius, brachiocephalicus, omohyoideus, and superficial cervical and caudal deep cervical lymph nodes.

273

Table (20) Arteries of the thoracic viscera and wall (continued)

Main trunk	Branches	Subdivisions	Distribution
		e) Internal thoracic artery	Arises from the ventral aspect of the subclavian artery opposite to the first rib. It curves ventrally and caudally to cross the ventral part of the first intercostal space and continues caudally under the transversus thoracis over the costosternal articulations to the eighth costal cartilage where it divides into musculophreic and cranial epigastric arteries. Along its course it gives off the following branches:- **1) Ventral intercostal branches**; eight in number, ascend in the corresponding intercostal spaces to anastomose with the dorsal intercostal arteries. They detach small twigs to the transversus thoracis, sternum, pericardium and perforating branches to the pectoral muscles and skin. **2) Pericardiacophrenic artery**; ascends in the mediastinum or plica vena cavae, gives twigs to the pericardium and pleura and accompanies the phrenic nerve to the diaphragm. **3) Musculophrenic artery**; passes along the costal attachment of the transversus abdominis till the last rib. It gives off the remaining ventral intercostal branches from nine to seventeen. **4) Cranial epigastric artery**; passes caudally to emerge from the thoracic cavity between the ninth costal cartilage and xiphoid cartilage and continues on the abdominal surface of rectus abdominis. It supplies the ventral abdominal wall and anastomoses with the caudal epigastric artery.
		f) Axillary artery	The course and branches will be described with the arteries of the thoracic limb.

Table (20) Arteries of the thoracic viscera and wall (continued)

Main trunk	Branches	Subdivisions	Distribution
III. Descending aorta			The descending aorta can be divided regionally into thoracic and abdominal parts. **The thoracic aorta** passes caudally between the two pleural sacs. The initial part is crossed on the right side by the esophagus and trachea cause it to deviate left to the median plane, then continues in the median plane on the ventral aspect of the bodies of thoracic vertebrae till the aortic hiatus of the diaphragm. **The abdominal aorta** extends caudally on the ventral surface of the lumbar vertebrae, ventral longitudinal ligament and psoas minor till the sixth lumbar vertebra where it terminates.
A. Thoracic aorta	**1. Bronchoesophageal artery**	**a) Bronchial artery**	Crosses the left surface of the esophagus to reach the dorsal surface of the tracheal bifurcation where it divides into right and left bronchial arteries. Each enters the hilus of the corresponding lung on the dorsal aspect of the principal bronchus, gives off lobar, segmental and subsegmental branches to follow the ramification of the bronchus. The bronchial artery supplies the lung tissue, tracheobronchial lymph nodes and mediastinum.
		b) Esophageal branch	A small branch passes caudally on the dorsal surface of the esophagus in the caudal mediastinum and anastomoses with the esophageal branch of the left gastric artery. it supplies the thoracic part of the esophagus, mediastinal lymph nodes and pleura.
	2. Dorsal intercostal arteries (The last 12 pairs)	**a) Dorsal branches**	Each dorsal branch is divided into:- **1) Spinal branch**; passes through the intervertebral foramen , gives twigs to the spinal meninges and perforates the dura mater to reinforce the ventral spinal artery. **2) Muscular branch**; to the epaxial muscles and skin of dorsum.
		b) Ventral branches	Each ventral branch is divided into:- **1) Dorsal intercostal artery**; descends in the intercostal space, and then gains the caudal border of the rib. It supplies the intercostal muscles, the rib and pleura. At the ventral part of the intercostal space it anastomoses with the corresponding ventral intercostal artery.

Table (20) Arteries of the thoracic viscera and wall (continued)

Main trunk	Branches	Subdivisions	Distribution
			2) Lateral cutaneous branches; perforate the serratus ventralis thoracis and abdominal muscles to ramify in the skin of the lateral thoracic wall.
	3. Dorsal costoabdominal artery		Descends caudal to the last rib. Its branches are closely resembled to that of the dorsal intercostal artery.
	4. Cranial phrenic artery		Arises from the ventral aspect of the thoracic aorta at the aortic hiatus. The artery spites into two to three branches to supply the crura of the lumbar part of the diaphragm.

Table (21) Arteries of the abdominal viscera and walls

Main trunk	Branches	Subdivisions	Distribution
B. Abdominal aorta	**1. Celiac artery (unpaired)**	**a) Splenic artery**	The largest branch of celiac artery, passes to the left on the left border of pancreas and crosses the saccus cecus of the stomach. It enters the splenic hilus through the gastrosplenic ligament to reach the apex of the spleen, beyond which it continues as the left gastroepiploic artery. It gives off the following branches: **1) Pancreatic branches**; to the left lobe of pancreas. **2) Short gastric branches**; pass in the gastrosplenic ligament to the greater curvature of the stomach, bifurcate and anastomose with the branches of the left and right gastric arteries. **3) Short splenic branches**; spring along the splenic hilus to enter the splenic parenchyma. **4) Left gastroepiploic artery**; follows the greater curvature of the stomach in the greater omentum and anastomoses with the right gastroepiploic artery of the hepatic. It gives off branches to the greater curvature of the stomach and twigs to the greater omentum

Table (21) Arteries of the abdominal viscera and wall (continued)

Main trunk	Branches	Subdivisions	Distribution
		b) Left gastric artery	Passes ventrally and cranially in the gastrophrenic ligament to the cardia of the stomach where it divides into parietal and visceral gastric branches. It gives off the following branches:- 1) **Pancreatic branches**; ramify in the body of the pancreas. 2) **Esophageal branch**; to the abdominal part of the esophagus and passes through the esophageal hiatus to anastomose with the esophageal branch of the bronchoesophageal artery. 3) **Parietal gastric branch**; crosses the lesser curvature and ramifies on the parietal surface of the stomach. Its branches are flexuous and anastomose with the short gastric arteries. 4) **Visceral gastric branch**; is distributed in the visceral surface of the stomach by the same manner as the parietal gastric branch.
		c) Hepatic artery	Passes cranially and to the right on the dorsal surface of pancreas, covered by the gastropancreatic fold and reaches the medial border of portal vein near the hepatic porta. The hepatic artery divides into 3-4 branches, enter the hepatic porta accompanied by the portal vein and hepatic duct to follow their divisions and subdivisions inside the hepatic lobes. Along its course, the hepatic artery gives off :- 1) **Pancreatic branches**; supply the body and right lobe of pancreas. 2) **Right gastric artery**; descends to the pylorus, gives off branches to the pylorus and first part of the duodenum. 3) **Gastroduodenal artery**; a short trunk passes to the cranial duodenal flexure and divided into two branches:- • **Right gastroepiploic artery**; crosses the caudal surface of the duodenum and enters the greater omentum. It follows the greater curvature to the left and anastomoses with the left gastroepiploic artery.

Table (21) Arteries of the abdominal viscera and wall (continued)

Main trunk	Branches	Subdivisions	Distribution
			• **Cranial pancreaticoduodenal artery**; divides into:- - **Pancreatic branch**; to the body of the pancreas. - **Duodenal branch**; to the cranial part of the duodenum and anastomoses with the caudal pancreaticoduodenal artery
	2. Cranial mesenteric artery (unpaired)	**a) Caudal pancreaticoduodenal artery**	A small branch, supplies the right lobe of the pancreas and cranial part of the duodenum. It anastomoses with the duodenal branch of the cranial pancreaticoduodenal artery.
		b) Jejunal arteries	About 15-20 arise close together from the origin of the parent trunk and pass in divergent manner between the layers of the mesentery toward the fixed border of the jejunum. Each jejunal artery divides into two branches which anastomose with the adjacent branches to form a series of primary arches. From the convexity of the primary arches, other branches are given off which united to form another set of secondary intestinal arches near the attached border of the jejunum. From the convex side of these arches terminal branches issue to ramify in the wall of the jejunum.
		c) Ileocecocolic artery	Passes cranially and to the right from the base of cecum and gives off:- **1) Ileal artery**; passes along the terminal part of the ileum and united with the last jejunal artery. **2) Lateral cecal artery**; passes between the cecum and the right ventral colon and continues on the lateral cecal band to the apex of the cecum. **3) Medial cecal artery**; courses along the medial cecal band to the apex of the cecum, where it anastomoses with the lateral cecal artery. **4) Colic branch**; runs along the dorsomedial bands of the ventral colon to the pelvic flexure where it joins with the right colic artery. It supplies the ventral colon and sends a branch to the base of the cecum.

Table (21) Arteries of the abdominal viscera and wall (continued)

Main trunk	Branches	Subdivisions	Distribution
		d) **Right and middle colic arteries**	Arise by a short common trunk and divides into:- 1) **Right colic artery**; a large branch passes along the dorsal part of the ascending colon to the pelvic flexure where it unites with the colic branch of ileocecocolic artery. 2) **Middle colic artery**; a small branch enters the descending mesocolon and supplies the transverse colon. It anastomoses with the right and left colic arteries.
	3. Caudal mesenteric artery (unpaired)	a) **Left colic artery**	Gives off 3-4 branches which divide and form colic arches inside the descending mesocolon and close to the descending colon. The colic arches supply the descending colon and the first arch unites with the middle colic artery.
		b) **Cranial rectal artery**	Passes caudally inside the mesocolon and mesorectum to terminate near the anus. It gives off 3-4 branches to form arches which supply the cranial part of the rectum and anastomoses with the caudal rectal artery
	4. Renal arteries (paired)		The right renal artery is the longer, crosses over the dorsal surface of the caudal vena cava to the hilus of the right kidney where it divides into 5-8 branches. The left renal artery is short, passes laterally to the hilus of the left kidney and divides like the right one. Each renal artery gives off the following branches inside the corresponding kidney:-
		a) **Interlobar arteries**	Arise from the division of the renal artery at the renal hilus. They pass between the renal pyramids to reach the subcortical zone.
		b) **Arcuate arteries (intralobar arteries)**	The continuation of the interlobar arteries that curve over the bases of the medullary pyramids in the subcortical zone. Each gives off:- 1) **Interlobular arteries**; divide the cortical zone into lobules centered by collecting tubules. Each artery gives off a large number of afferent arterioles which supply the individual renal corpuscles. 2) **Medullary branches**; descend inside the medullary pyramids.

Table (21) Arteries of the abdominal viscera and wall (continued)

Main trunk	Branches	Subdivisions	Distribution
	5a. Testicular arteries (males)		The right and left testicular arteries supply the corresponding testicles, epididymis and ductus deferens. Each is long slender vessel, arises from the abdominal aorta at the level of the fourth lumbar vertebra. It passes caudally in a narrow peritoneal fold to the deep inguinal ring and descends in the cranial border of the spermatic cord to form numerous coils, surrounded by the pampiniform plexus of the testicular vein and associated closely with the testicular nerves, lymphatics and smooth muscle fibers. It continues in a flexuous manner between the epididymis and attached border of the testicle to the tail pole. It is curved cranially to run along the free border of the testicle to the head extremity. The largest branches arise from its ventral part ascend inside the tunica albuginea on the either side of the gland and gives off fine branches to the parenchyma of the testicle. Collateral branches are detached to supply the ureter, epididymis and spermatic cord.
	5b. Ovarian arteries (females)		Two large and short arteries correspond to the testicular arteries in male. Each is placed in the cranial part of the broad ligament of the uterus and courses in a flexuous manner to enter the hilus of the ovary through the mesovarium. Along its course it gives off the following branches:-
		a) Tubal branches	Short branches arise by a common trunk. They form arterial arches inside the mesosalpinx which release small branches to supply the uterine tube.
		b) Uterine branch (cranial uterine artery)	Passes to the concave border of the uterine horn to ramify in the cranial part of the uterine horn. It anastomoses with the uterine artery (middle uterine artery); the branch of external iliac artery.

Table (21) Arteries of the abdominal viscera and wall (continued)

Main trunk	Branches	Subdivisions	Distribution
	6. Internal iliac artery		Results from the bifurcation of the abdominal aorta under the sixth lumbar vertebra where it gives off the last pair of lumbar arteries. It passes caudally under the wing of the sacrum and then inclines ventrally on the pelvic surface of the body of ilium. It continues along the ventral border of the obturatorius internus and divides ventral to the lumbosacral articulation into the caudal gluteal and internal pudendal arteries. The chief branches are:-
		a) Last pair of lumbar arteries	Each passes dorsally through the intervertebral foramen between the last lumbar vertebra and sacrum to be distributed as the other lumbar arteries (page 87)
		b) Caudal gluteal artery	Courses caudally and divides into the following branches:- **1) Sacral branches**; four branches enter the sacral canal through the pelvic sacral foramina. Each divides into two branches:- **i) Spinal branches**; ramify in the sacral part of the spinal cord and its meninges and reinforce the ventral spinal artery. **ii) Dorsal branches**; leave the sacral canal through the dorsal sacral foramina to supply the epaxial muscles and skin of the croup. **2) Median caudal artery**; unpaired vessel arises from the right or left caudal gluteal artery. It passes caudally on the pelvic surface of the sacrum in a median position and continues along the tail between the sacrocaudales ventrales mediales to supply them and the skin. **3) Ventrolateral caudal artery**; passes caudally between the sacrocaudalis ventralis lateralis and intertransversii ventrales, divides into caudal branches to supply the muscles and skin of the tail. **4) Cranial gluteal artery**; the largest branch of caudal gluteal artery. It gives off several gluteal branches to supply the gluteal muscles and leaves the pelvic cavity through the greater ischiatic foramen. During its course it gives off the following branches:-

Table (21) Arteries of the abdominal viscera and wall (continued)

Main trunk	Branches	Subdivisions	Distribution
			i) **Iliolumbar artery**; passes laterally caudal to the sacroiliac articulation and continues its course on the deep face of iliacus, then curved around the wing of ilium to be distributed in the gluteus medius and tensor fasciae latae. ii) **Obturator artery**; courses on the pelvic surface of the body of ilium accompanied by the obturator nerve and vein to reach the lateral part of the obturator foramen. It descends obliquely to leave the pelvic cavity through the latter foramen caudal to the obturatorius externus and continues on the ventral surface of ischium, where it detaches branches to supply the muscles of the medial aspect of the thigh. Along its course it gives off the following branches:- • **Iliacofemoral artery**; passes ventrolaterally between the body of ilium and gluteus medius and dips between the vastus lateralis and rectus femoris to supply the quadriceps femoris. • **Middle artery of the penis (in males)**; ramifies in the major part of the body of penis and anastomoses with the cranial artery of penis, the branch of external pudendal and the dorsal artery of penis, the branch of internal pudendal. • **Middle artery of the clitoris (in females)**; enters the root of the clitoris, where it divides into the **deep and dorsal** artery of the clitoris.
		c) Internal pudendal artery	Passes caudoventrally along the dorsal border of the iliac head of obturatorius internus, then dorsal to the ischiatic spine on the deep face of broad sacrotuberal ligament. It leaves the pelvic cavity and runs on the lateral surface of the latter ligament for a short distance. It reenters the pelvic cavity and passes caudally to the ischiatic arch and divides into the ventral perineal, artery of the penis in male; ventral perineal and artery of the vestibular bulb in female. The chief branches of internal pudendal artery are:-

Table (21) Arteries of the abdominal viscera and wall (continued)

Main trunk	Branches	Subdivisions	Distribution

			1) **Umbilical artery**; is converted into the round ligament of the urinary bladder where its lumen is almost obliterated. It passes on cranial edge of lateral vesicular ligament to the apex of the urinary bladder. From its reduced lumen at the apex, it gives off small branches to the urinary bladder (cranial vesicular artery), ductus deferens and ureter.
			2) **Urogenital artery** (prostatic artery in male and vaginal artery in female);
			• **Prostatic artery**; arises near the prostate and passes caudally lateral to the rectum. It detaches the following branches:-
			  - **Middle rectal artery**; to the middle part of the rectum.
			  - **Caudal vesicular artery**; to the caudal part of the urinary bladder.
			  - **Ureteric branch**; to the pelvic part of the ureter.
			  - **Urethral branch**; to the pelvic urethra.
			  - **Branch to ductus deferens**; to the abdominal part of ductus deferens.
			  - **Branches to the accessory genital glands**.
			• **Vaginal artery**; much larger in female and gives off :-
			  - **Uterine branch** (caudal uterine artery); supplies the uterine body, cervix and vaginal wall. It anastomoses with the uterine artery, the branch of external iliac artery.
			  - **Vestibular branch**; to the vaginal vestibule.
			3) **Ventral perineal artery**; small branch in male, supplies the bulbospongiosus and skin of the perineum. It is relatively large in female and distributed in the vulva and vestibular bulb. In both sexes, the ventral perineal artery detaches the **caudal rectal artery** to the caudal part of the rectum.
			4a) **Artery of the penis**; the direct continuation of the internal pudendal artery in male. It lies at the side of the urethra dorsal to the ischiatic arch. It dips under the bulbospongiosus and gives off the following branches:-

Table (21) Arteries of the abdominal viscera and wall (continued)

Main trunk	Branches	Subdivisions	Distribution
			i) **Deep artery of the penis**; to the corpus cavernosum penis. ii) **Dorsal artery of the penis**; turns around the ischiatic arch to reach the dorsum of the penis and anastomoses with the middle artery of the penis, branch of obturator artery. iii)**Artery of the bulb**; supplies the bulb of penis. **4b) Artery of the vestibular bulb**; the continuation of the internal pudendal artery in female, passes to the ventral surface of the vulva and gives twigs to the vestibular bulb.
	7. External iliac artery		Arises from the abdominal aorta ventral to the fifth lumbar vertebra. It descends at the side of the pelvic inlet along the tendon of the psoas minor to reach the cranial border of the pubis, beyond which it is continued by the femoral artery. The chief branches of the external iliac artery are:-
		a) Deep circumflex iliac artery	Arises at the origin of the parent trunk. It passes across the iliac fascia toward the coxal tuber to reach the lateral border of the psoas major where it divides into two branches, cranial and caudal. **1) Cranial branch**; gives small branches to the sublumbar muscles, lateral iliac lymph nodes, gluteus medius and tensor fasciae latae. It passes cranially and ventrally in the flank on the dorsal margin of the obliquus internus abdominis to supply the abdominal muscles, fascia and skin of the flank. **2) Caudal branch**; perforates the abdominal wall close to the coxal tuber and descends on the medial surface of the tensor fasciae latae to the fold of the flank. It supplies the obliquus internus abdominis, tensor fasciae latae and iliacus.
		b) Cremaster artery (in male)	Slender flexuous vessel springs just caudal to the latter. It courses extraperitoneally to the inguinal canal to supply the cremaster muscle, vaginal tunic and the other contents of the spermatic cord.

Table (21) Arteries of the abdominal viscera and wall (continued)

Main trunk	Branches	Subdivisions	Distribution
		b)'Uterine artery (in female)	The main arterial supply to the uterus. It has a similar origin as the **cremaster artery** but it is much larger and passes in flexuous manner within the broad ligament of the uterus to the concave border of the uterine horn. It is divided into several branches to supply the horn and body of uterus. It joins with the uterine branch of **ovarian artery** and uterine branch of urogenital **(vaginal)** artery.
		c) Deep femoral artery	A short trunk arises from the external iliac artery at the level of the cranial border of the pubis. It passes caudally under the pubis where it divides into two branches:- **1) Pudendoepigastric trunk**; passes cranially across the edge of the inguinal ligament, then inclines ventromedially to run on its abdominal surface. At the medial part of the deep inguinal ring it is divided into the caudal epigastric and external pudendal arteries. i) **Caudal epigastric artery**; passes along the lateral border of the rectus abdominis to reach the umbilical region where it anastomoses with the cranial epigastric artery, the branch of internal thoracic. Its branches supply the rectus abdominis and obliquus internus abdominis. ii) **External pudendal artery**; descends in the medial part of inguinal canal and emerges at the medial angle of superficial inguinal ring. The distribution of the artery is differing in both sexes. • **In male**; the artery is divided into the caudal superficial epigastric artery and cranial artery of the penis. - **Caudal superficial epigastric artery**; runs on the abdominal tunic near the linea alba and gives branches to the scrotal wall, abdominal rectal sheathes and scrotal lymph nodes.

Table (21) Arteries of the abdominal viscera and wall (continued)

Main trunk	Branches	Subdivisions	Distribution
			- **Cranial artery of the penis**; passes to the dorsum of the penis and ends in the glans penis as the artery of the glans. It gives off collateral branches to the corpus cavernosum penis, prepuce and scrotal lymph nodes. • **In female**; the external pudendal artery divides into the cranial mammary artery and the caudal mammary artery. - **Cranial mammary artery**; gives branches to the mammary lymph nodes and continues superficially near the linea alba to supply the abdominal rectal sheathes and skin. - **Caudal mammary artery**; enters the base of mammary gland, in which it ramifies. **2) Medial circumflex femoral artery**; runs caudally ventral to the pubic bone and supplies the thigh. (described with the arteries of the pelvic limb, page 326)
	8. Lumbar arteries		Six pairs of lumbar arteries; the first five pairs are detached form the dorsal aspect of the abdominal aorta at the level of the corresponding lumbar intervertebral foramen and the last pair from the internal iliac artery at the level of lumbosacral articulation. Each passes across the body of the lumbar vertebra to the intertransverse space to supply the sublumbar muscles and divides into dorsal and ventral branches.
		a) Dorsal branch	Courses dorsally and divides into muscular and spinal branches:- **1) Muscular branch**; to the epaxial muscles of the lumbar region and skin. **2) Spinal branch**; enters the vertebral canal though the intervertebral foramen to supply the spinal meninges and spinal cord of lumbar region. The spinal branches are joined with the ventral spinal artery.
		b) Ventral branch	The lateral continuation of the lumbar artery in the intertransverse space and continues between the transversus abdominis and obliquus internus abdominis, gives branches to these muscles and ends in the obliquus externus abdominis , cutaneous trunci and skin of the flank.

Part III. Nerves of the trunk

Table (22) Nerves of the thoracic wall (thoracic spinal nerves)

Nerve	Branches	Subdivisions	Course and distribution
Thoracic nerves			Eighteen pairs, each arise from the either side of the thoracic spinal segment of the spinal cord. They arranged numerically according to the vertebra caudal to which they emerge from the vertebral canal. For description of the branches, subdivisions and distribution, they could be divided into two groups; eight pairs for each and the last pair is descried alone (the costoabdominal nerves).
I. Thoracic nerves (first to eight pairs)	**1. Dorsal branches**	**a) Medial branches**	Emerge caudal to the levatores costarum, then ascend on the multifidus thoracis and supply the latter, spinalis and semispinalis thoracis.
		b) Lateral branches	Run laterally between the longissimus thoracis and iliocostalis thoracis and pass through the thoracolumbar fascia to ramify in the skin as dorsal cutaneous nerves under the skin of the cranial part of the thorax. In the region of the withers they give branches to the serratus dorsalis cranialis, rhomboideus thoracis, trapezius thoracis, dorsal scapular ligament and skin of the withers.
	2. Ventral branches (intercostal nerves)		<ul><li>The ventral branch of the first thoracic nerve; shares entirely in the formation of brachial plexus, but sends a small branch in the first intercostal space without reaching its distal end.</li><li>The second ventral branch; furnishes a considerable root to the brachial plexus, but its intercostal continuation is typical.</li><li>The remaining intercostal nerves; descend in the intercostal spaces with the dorsal intercostal vessels, between the intercostal muscles at the proximal ends of the spaces and then follow the caudal borders of the corresponding ribs to their sternal ends. Each nerve lies cranial to the accompanied artery.</li><li>The lateral cutaneous branches; emerge through the spaces between the costal cartilages to supply the transversus thoracis, pectoralis ascendens and skin.</li></ul>

Table (22) Nerves of the thoracic wall (thoracic spinal nerves) (continued)

Nerve	Branches	Subdivisions	Course and distribution
II. Thoracic nerves (ninth to seventeen pairs)	**1. Dorsal branches**	a) Medial branches	Emerge caudal to the levatores costarum, then ascend on the multifidus thoracis and supply the latter, spinalis and semispinalis thoracis.
		b) Lateral branches	Run laterally between the longissimus thoracis and iliocostalis thoracis and pass through the latissimus dorsi to the thoracolumbar fascia to ramify in the skin as dorsal cutaneous nerves under the skin of the thorax. They give branches to the iliocostalis thoracis, serratus dorsalis caudalis and latissimus dorsi.
	2. Ventral branches (intercostal nerves)		<ul><li>Descend in the intercostal spaces accompanied by the intercostal vessels. Each intercostal nerve lies caudal to the caudal border with the artery cranial to it.</li><li>They give off muscular branches to the costal part of the diaphragm, pass between the transversus abdominis and obliquus abdominis internus and end in the rectus abdominis.</li><li>The lateral cutaneous branches; ramify in the skin of the dorsal, middle regions of the thoracic wall and ventral region of the abdominal wall cranial to the flank and umbilicus.</li></ul>
III. Last thoracic nerves (eighteen pair)	**1. Dorsal branch**		The course and distribution are closely resembled to the dorsal branches of the second group.
	2. Ventral branch (costoabdominal nerve)		This branch does not course between two ribs. It passes laterally, caudal to the last rib and divides into lateral and medial branches.<ul><li>Lateral branch; runs over the superficial face of the transversus abdominis, perforates the obliquus abdominis externus and ramifies under the skin of the flank.</li><li>Medial branch; descends on the deep face of the obliquus abdominis internus to the rectus abdominis in which it terminates.</li></ul>

Table (23) Nerves of the abdominal wall (lumbar spinal nerves)

Nerve	Branches	Subdivisions	Course and distribution
Lumbar nerves			There are six pairs of lumbar nerves, arise from the sides of lumbar spinal segments. The last pair emerges between the last lumbar vertebra and the sacrum. The ventral branches of the last three lumbar nerves share the ventral branches of the first two sacral nerves in the formation of the lumbosacral plexus.
I. The first, second and third lumbar nerves	**1. Dorsal branches**		Small and ascend between the longissimus lumborum and intertransversii lumborum to supply these muscles, multifidus and skin of the lumbar region.
	2. Ventral branches	**2a. Ventral branch of the first lumbar n. (iliohypogastric n.)**	Passes laterally between the quadratus lumborum and psoas major muscles and divides, at the lateral border of the latter, into lateral and medial branches. 1) **Lateral branch**; descends between the obliquus internus abdominis and obliquus externus abdominis, perforates the latter and runs caudoventrally as **lateral cutaneous branch** to ramify under the skin of the flank and lateral surface of the thigh. 2) **Medial branch**; runs caudoventrally under the peritoneum to the lateral border of the rectus abdominis where it terminates as **ventral cutaneous branch** to the latter muscle and skin
		2b. Ventral branch of the second lumbar n. (ilioinguinal n.)	Connects by a communicating branch with the genitofemoral nerve. It divides into lateral and medial branches. 1) Lateral branch; perforates the obliquus externus abdominis cranial to the coxal tuber and runs ventrally as **lateral cutaneous** branch to the cranial aspect of the thigh and lateral surface of the stifle. 2) Medial branch; supplies the abdominal muscles. It joins a branch of the genitofemoral nerve to form a trunk which descends in the inguinal canal to be distributed to the external genital organs and skin of the inguinal region as **ventral cutaneous branch**.

Table (23) Nerves of the abdominal wall (lumbar spinal nerves) (continued)

Nerve	Branches	Subdivisions	Course and distribution
		2c. Ventral branch of the third lumbar n. (genitofemoral n.)	Passes caudally inside the psoas minor muscle and divides into two branches. 1) Muscular branch; emerges cranial to the deep circumflex iliac vessels and supplies the cremaster and obliquus internus abdominis muscles. 2) Genital branch; emerges caudal to the deep circumflex iliac vessels and runs parallel with the external iliac artery. It descends in the medial part of the inguinal canal and emerges at the superficial inguinal ring with the external pudendal artery. It ramifies in the external genital organs and skin of the inguinal region.
II. The fourth, fifth and sixth lumbar nerves	**1. Dorsal branches**		Emerge through the lumbodorsal fascia near the median plane in the caudal part of the lumbar region. They are constituted the **cranial clunial nerves** which run caudally and ventrally to reach the skin of the gluteal region to the stifle
	2. Ventral branches	**2a. Ventral branch of the fourth lumbar n.**	The majority of its fibers share in the formation of the femoral nerve. The remaining of this branch joins a branch from the third lumbar nerve to form the **lateral cutaneous femoral nerve** which passes laterally and caudally on the iliac fascia. It perforates the abdominal wall ventral to the coxal tuber to the deep face of tensor fasciae latae and descends on its medial face to the skin of the lateral surface of the stifle.
		2b. Ventral branch of the fifth lumbar n.	Share in the formation of the lumbosacral plexus and fully described in tables of pelvic limb.
		2c. Ventral branch of the sixth lumbar n.	

Table (24) Nerves of the rump and tail (sacral and caudal spinal nerves)

Nerve	Branches	Subdivisions	Course and distribution
I. Sacral nerves			Five pairs of sacral nerves are present; arise from the sides of the sacral segments of the spinal cord which usually placed within the lumbar part of the vertebral canal. Each sacral nerve is divided into dorsal and ventral branches. The dorsal and ventral branches emerge from the sacral canal through the separate dorsal and ventral sacral foramina. The ventral divisions of the sacral nerves form the sacral plexus which contribute to the lumbosacral plexus with both somatic and autonomic components.
	1. Dorsal branches	**a) Medial muscular branches**	Supply the dorsal surface of the sacrum and the adjoining part of the tail.
		b) Lateral cutaneous branches	Constitute the **middle clunial nerves** and supply the skin of the sacral region, around the hip and the thigh.
	2. Ventral branches	**2a. Ventral branches of the first and second sacral nerves**	The largest and unite with each other and with those of the last three lumbar nerves to form the lumbosacral plexus.
		2b. Ventral branches of the third and fourth sacral nerves	Are connected with each other and the majority of their fibers go to form the pudendal, perineal and caudal rectal nerves. **1) Pudendal nerve**; passes caudoventrally, partly embedded in the broad sacrotuberal ligament. It accompanies the internal pudendal artery to the ischiatic arch where it gives off the deep perineal nerve, then turns around the arch and continues along the dorsum of the penis as the dorsal nerve of the penis. • **Dorsal nerve of the penis**; pursues a flexuous course to ramify in the glans penis and penile layer of the prepuce (preputial branch). • **Deep perineal nerve**; within the pelvis, it receives connections from the superficial perineal and caudal rectal nerves.

Table (24) Nerves of the rump and tail (sacral and caudal spinal nerves) (continued)

Nerve	Branches	Subdivisions	Course and distribution
			It furnishes branches to the urinary bladder, urethra, terminal part of the rectum, muscles and skin of the anus as well as the perineal musculature. The termination of the nerve differs in both sexes. - In the male, it supplies the ischiocavernosus muscle and gives numerous branches to the corpus cavernosum and spongiosum penis. - In the female, it terminates in the clitoris and vulvas, as well as two slender nerves extend to the caudal part of the udder. **2) Caudal rectal nerve**; passes ventrally and caudally dorsal to the pudendal nerve, detaches the superficial perineal nerves and continues to be distributed in the terminal part of rectum and the sphincter ani externus. • **Superficial perineal nerves**; three to four branches receive connections from the pudendal nerve. Their terminations differ in both sexes. - In the male, give off the **caudal scrotal nerves** to the fascia and skin of the caudal aspect of the scrotum. - In the female, detach the **labial nerves** to the labia of the vulva.
		2c. Ventral branch of the fifth sacral nerve	Small branch joins the first caudal nerve. It gives twigs to the sacrocaudalis ventralis lateralis and the skin of the root of the tail.
II. Caudal nerves			Five pairs, arise from the conus medullaris of the spinal cord. Each divides into dorsal and ventral branches. Their dorsal and ventral branches are connected to form, respectively, **a dorsal and a ventral caudal plexuses** on the corresponding side along the tail. They supply the muscles and skin of the tail.

292

Chapter 3

Thoracic Limb

Part I. Muscles of the thoracic limb

Table (25) Muscles of shoulder girdle (extrinsic muscles of thoracic limb)

Muscle	Origin	Insertion	Action	Innervation
Trapezius cervicis	Funicular part of nuchal ligament, from the level of the second cervical to the third thoracic vertebrae	Tuber of the scapular spine	Elevates the shoulder and draws the scapula cranially and dorsally	Dorsal branch of accessory nerve
Trapezius thoracis	Supraspinous ligament extending between the spinous processes of the thoracic vertebrae from the third to tenth	Tuber of the scapular spine	Elevates the shoulder and draws the scapula caudally	- Dorsal branch of accessory nerve - Dorsal branches of thoracic nerves
Rhomboideus cervicis	Funicular part of nuchal ligament, from the level of the second cervical to the second thoracic vertebrae	Medial surface of the scapular cartilage	Elevates the neck	Dorsal branches of the sixth and seventh cervical nerves
Rhomboideus thoracis	Supraspinous ligament extending between the spinous processes of the thoracic vertebrae from the second to seventh	Medial surface of the scapular cartilage	Draws the scapula dorsally and cranially	Dorsal branches of the thoracic nerves
Latissimus dorsi	Thoracolumbar fascia which attached to the spinous processes of the thoracic and lumbar vertebrae	Teres major tuberosity of the humerus	Flexes the shoulder joint and draws the trunk cranially	Dorsal thoracic nerve, the branch of brachial plexus
Brachiocephalicus	- Mastoid process of petrous part of temporal bone and nuchal crest - Wing of the atlas - Transverse processes of the 2nd, 3rd and 4th cervical vertebrae	Deltoid tuberosity, humeral crest and the fascia of the shoulder and arm regions	Extension of the shoulder joint	-Axillary nerve - Accessory nerve - Cervical nerves

Table (25) Muscles of shoulder girdle (extrinsic muscles of thoracic limb) (continued)

Muscle	Origin	Insertion	Action	Innervation
pectorales	A large fleshy mass occupies the space between the ventral part of the thoracic wall and the shoulder and arm. It is clearly divisible into a superficial pectoral and a deep pectoral muscle. Each can be subdivided into cranial and caudal parts.			
Pectoralis descendens (cranial superficial pectoral)	Short, thick and rounded muscle appears clearly in front of the sternum. It arises from the cartilage of the manubrium	Deltoid tuberosity and humeral crest Fascia of the arm	Adducts and advances the thoracic limb	Cranial and caudal pectoral nerves of brachial plexus
Pectoralis transversus (caudal superficial pectoral)	Wide muscular sheet, arises from the ventral edge of the sternum and the fibrous raphe between the right and left muscles	Fascia on the proximal third of the arm and the humeral crest	Adducts the thoracic limb	Cranial and caudal pectoral nerves of brachial plexus
Subclavius (cranial deep pectoral)	Prismatic, extends along the cranial border of the scapula. It arises from the cranial half of the lateral surface of the sternum	Cranial border of the scapula and the scapular fascia	Adducts and retracts the thoracic limb	Cranial and caudal pectoral nerves of brachial plexus
Pectoralis ascendens (caudal deep pectoral)	Triangular large mass, arises from the ventral surface of the sternum and xiphoid cartilage	Cranial parts of the lesser and greater tubercles of the humerus	Adducts and retracts the thoracic limb	Cranial and caudal pectoral nerves of brachial plexus
Serratus ventralis	Large, fane shaped muscle situated on the lateral surface of the neck and the thorax. It derives its name from the serrated ventral edge.			
Serratus ventralis cervicis	Transverse processes of the last five cervical vertebrae	Cranial triangular area of the costal surface of the scapula (cranial serrated face)	Suspend the cranial part of the trunk like a sling between the thoracic limbs	- Ventral branches of cervical nerves
Serratus ventralis thoracis	Lateral surfaces of the first nine ribs	Caudal triangular area of the costal surface of the scapula (caudal serrated face)		- Long thoracic nerve of brachial plexus

Table (26) Muscles of shoulder region

Muscle	Origin	Insertion	Action	Innervation
Deltoideus	Scapular spine by means of strong aponeurosis which covers the infraspinatus. Proximal part of the caudal border of the scapula	Deltoid tuberosity and the fascia of the arm	Flexes the shoulder joint and abducts the limb	Axillary nerve
Supraspinatus	Supraspinous fossa, scapular spine and the adjacent part of the scapular cartilage	Cranial parts of the greater and lesser tubercles of the humerus	Extends the shoulder joint	Suprascapular nerve
Infraspinatus	Infraspinous fossa and adjacent part of the scapular cartilage	Cranial and caudal parts of the greater tubercle of the humerus	Abducts the limb and rotates it laterally	Suprascapular nerve
Teres minor	Small triangular, covered by the deltoideus and infraspinatus. It arises from the middle of the caudal border of the scapula and infraspinous fossa	Deltoid tuberosity and teres minor tuberosity which lies just proximal to the deltoid tuberosity	Flexes the shoulder joint and abducts the arm	Axillary nerve
Subscapularis	Subscapular fossa on the costal surface of the scapula	Caudal eminence of the lesser tubercle of the humerus	Adducts the limb	Subscapular nerves
Teres major	Caudal angle and adjacent part of the caudal border of the scapula	Teres major tuberosity of the humerus	Flexes the shoulder joint	Axillary nerve
Coracobrachialis	Lies on the medial surface of the shoulder joint. Arises from the coracoid process of the scapula	Small area proximal to the teres major tuberosity	Flexes the shoulder joint and adducts the limb	Musculocutaneous nerve, proximal muscular branch
Capsularis (Articularis humeri)	A very small muscle lies on the caudal surface of the joint capsule of the shoulder. It arises just dorsal to the caudal part of the rim of the glenoid cavity	Caudal surface of the body of the humerus distal to the head	Supports the capsule of the shoulder joint during flexion	Axillary nerve

Table (27) Muscles of arm region

Muscle	Origin	Insertion	Action	Innervation
Biceps brachii	Supraglenoid tuberosity by a tendon which is molded on the intertuberal groove and played over the large intertuberal bursa	Radial tuberosity and medial collateral ligament of the elbow joint Lacertus fibrosis; blends with the fascia of the forearm and tendon of extensor carpi radialis	Flexion the elbow joint	Musculocutaneous nerve (distal muscular branch)
Brachialis	Proximal third of the caudal surface of the humerus	Medial border of the radius	Flexion the elbow joint	Musculocutaneous nerve
Tensor fasciae antebrachii	Caudal border of the scapula and the tendon of insertion of the latissimus dorsi	Olecranon tuberosity and the deep fascia of forearm	Extension of the elbow joint	Radial nerve
Triceps brachii	Constitutes, with the tensor fasciae antebrachii, the large muscular mass which fills the angle between the caudal border of the scapula and humerus. It is divided into three heads; the long head is the longest, largest and triangular in shape. The lateral head is quadrilateral in shape and lies on the lateral surface of the humerus. The medial head is the smallest and lies on the medial surface of the humerus.			
Long head of triceps brachii	Caudal border of the scapula	Lateral and caudal parts of the olecranon tuberosity	Extension of the elbow joint	Radial nerve
Lateral head of triceps brachii	Deltoid tuberosity and humeral crest	Lateral surface of the olecranon tuberosity	Extension of the elbow joint	Radial nerve
Medial head of triceps brachii	Middle third of the caudal surface of the body of humerus, distal to the teres major tuberosity	Medial and caudal parts of the olecranon tuberosity	Extension of the elbow joint	Radial nerve
Anconeus	Small and covers the olecranon fossa, arises from the distal third of the caudal surface of humerus	Lateral surface of the olecranon tuberosity	Extension of the elbow joint and protection of the joint capsule	Radial nerve

Table (28) Muscles of forearm and manus

Muscle	Origin	Insertion	Action	Innervation
A. Extensor group	The extensors of the carpus and digit lie on the cranial and lateral parts of the forearm and their tendons extend to the manus. The group is covered by very strong and tendinous deep fascia of the forearm which is closely adherent to the surface of the muscles. The deep fascia sends intermuscular septa to separate the muscles and attached to the underlying bones. The carpal fascia stretches over the dorsal surface of the carpus between the styloid processes and accessory carpal bones to form the **extensor retinaculum.** The latter bridging over the grooves and binding down the extensor tendons and their synovial sheaths.			
1. Extensor carpi radialis	Lateral epicondyloid crest and coronoid fossa of the humerus	Metacarpal tuberosity	Extension of the carpal joint	Radial nerve
2. Extensor digitorum communis	<ul><li>Humeral head; lateral epicondyloid crest and coronoid fossa of the humerus</li><li>Radial head; lateral tuberosity of the proximal extremity of radius</li><li>Ulnar head; lateral surface of the body of ulna</li></ul>	Tendons of different parts are joined to form the common digital extensor tendon which inserted in <ul><li>The extensor process of the distal phalanx</li><li>Proximal ends of the dorsal surfaces of the proximal and middle phalanges.</li></ul>	Extension of the carpal and digital joints Flexion of the elbow joint	Radial nerve
3. Extensor digitorum lateralis	Lateral tuberosity and lateral border of the radius. Lateral collateral ligament of the elbow joint and body of the ulna	An eminence on the proximal end of the dorsal surface of the proximal phalanx	Extension of the carpal and digital joints	Radial nerve
4. Extensor carpi obliquus (abductor digiti I longus)	Cranial surface and lateral border of the distal half of the radius	The tendon passes medially and distally over the tendon of the extensor carpi radialis and crosses the medial surface of carpus to the head of the second metacarpal bone	Extension of the carpal joint	Radial nerve

Table (28) Muscles of forearm and manus (continued)

Muscle	Origin	Insertion	Action	Innervation
B. Flexor group	The flexors of the carpus and digit occupy the caudal surface of the forearm and their tendons extend to the palmar surface of the manus. The flexor group is covered by the deep fascia of the forearm which is loosely attached to the surface of the muscles and gives the intermuscular septa and finally blends with the periosteum on the medial border of the radius. The carpal fascia is very thick on the palmar surface of the carpus and forms the **flexor retinaculum**. It stretches across from the accessory carpal bone to the medial collateral ligament and proximal extremity of the second metacarpal bone to complete the **carpal canal**. The latter canal contains the superficial and deep digital flexor tendons, carpal synovial sheathes, medial palmar artery and nerve.			
1.Flexor carpi radialis	Medial epicondyle of the humerus	Proximal end of the second metacarpal bone	Flexes the carpal joint	Median nerve
2. Flexor carpi ulnaris	<ul><li>Humeral head; medial epicondyle of the humerus</li><li>Ulnar head; medial surface and caudal border of the olecranon</li></ul>	Proximal edge of the accessory carpal bone	Flexes the carpal joint and extends the elbow joint	Ulnar nerve
3. Ulnaris lateralis	Lies on the lateral surface of the forearm and arises from the lateral epicondyle of the humerus	Lateral surface of the accessory carpal bone and proximal extremity of the fourth metacarpal bone	Flexes the carpal joint and extends the elbow joint	Radial nerve
4. Flexor digitorum superficialis	<ul><li>Humeral head; medial epicondyle of the humerus</li><li>Radial head (superior check ligament); a ridge near the medial border on the distal half of the caudal surface of the radius</li></ul>	Superficial digital flexor tendon is formed on the palmar surface of the carpus, passes through the carpal canal and descends superficially on the palmar surface metacarpus. Near the fetlock it forms a ring through which the deep digital flexor passes. It divides into two branches to insert on the eminences of the proximal extremity of middle phalanx.	Flexes the carpal and digital joints and extends the elbow joint	Ulnar nerve

Table (28) Muscles of forearm and manus (continued)

Muscle	Origin	Insertion	Action	Innervation
5. Flexor digitorum profundus	• Humeral head; medial epicondyle of the humerus • Ulnar head; medial surface of the olecranon • Radial head; middle of the caudal surface of the radius • Tendinous head (inferior check ligament); palmar carpal ligament	The deep digital flexor tendon is formed by the union of the tendons of the first three heads. It descends through the carpal canal to the palmar surface of the metacarpus between the superficial digital flexor tendon and suspensory ligament. At the middle of the metacarpus, it joins the tendinous head and continues through the ring formed by the superficial digital flexor tendon to the sesamoid groove and proceeds beyond the distal sesamoidean ligaments to the flexor surface of the distal sesamoid bone. The deep digital flexor tendon inserts in the semilunar line and adjacent surface of the cartilage of distal phalanx.	Flexes the carpal and digital joints and extends the elbow joint	Median nerve and Ulnar nerve
6. Interosseous medius (suspensory ligament)	Strong tendinous band contains little muscular tissue and situated in the metacarpal groove. It arises from the distal row of carpal bones and the proximal end of the palmar surface of the third metacarpal bone	The insertion is complex and consists of the following branches:- • Sesamoid branches; directed to the abaxial surface of the corresponding proximal sesamoid bone. • Extensor branches; course obliquely to the dorsal surface of the proximal phalanx to join with the common digital extensor tendon.	- Supports the fetlock joint, prevents its deviation and over extension. - the extensor branches limited the palmar flexion of digital joints.	Median nerve

Part II. Arteries of the thoracic limb

Table (29) Arteries of the shoulder, arm and forearm regions

Main trunk	Branches	Subdivisions	Distribution
I. Axillary artery			The direct continuation of the subclavian artery at the thoracic inlet. It winds around the cranial border of the first rib and passes caudoventrally through the axillary space in the axillary loop. At the interval between the subscapularis and teres major muscles it gives off the subscapular artery and continues in the arm region as the **brachial artery**. The axillary artery gives off the following branches:-
	1. External thoracic artery	a) Cranial branch	A short branch divides into several branches to supply the subclavius; omohyoideus, brachiocephalicus, pectoralis descendens and pectoralis transversus muscles.
		b) Caudal branch	Courses in the cutaneous trunci accompanied by the lateral thoracic nerve. It gives branches to the superficial cervical lymph nodes, subclavius, pectoralis ascendens and cutaneous trunci. It terminates in the skin of the ventral abdominal wall.
	2. Suprascapular artery		A small and flexuous arises near the cranial border of the subscapularis and runs dorsally in the furrow between the latter muscle and the supraspinatus accompanying the Suprascapular nerve. It gives branches to the supraspinatus, subscapularis, subclavius, pectoralis ascendens and brachiocephalicus.
	3. Subscapular artery	a) Thoracodorsal artery	Crosses the medial face of the teres major and runs dorsally and caudally on the latissimus dorsi. It gives branches to these muscles, proper axillary lymph nodes, long head of triceps brachii, tensor fasciae antebrachii and cutaneous trunci.
		b) Caudal circumflex humeral artery	Passes laterally caudal to the shoulder joint between the long and lateral heads of triceps brachii, with the axillary nerve. It gives branches to these muscles, the caudal and craniolateral aspects of the shoulder joint and the muscles and skin of the lateral side of the shoulder. It anastomoses with the cranial circumflex humeral artery.

Table (29) Arteries of the shoulder, arm and forearm regions (continued)

Main trunk	Branches	Subdivisions	Distribution
		c) Circumflex scapular artery	Arises dorsal to the shoulder joint, passes cranially between the subscapularis and long head of triceps brachii to be divided into:- 1) **Lateral branch**; gives the **nutrient artery of the scapula** and detaches branches to the supraspinatus, infraspinatus and teres minor. 2) **Medial branch**; courses cranially on the costal surface of the scapula to ramify in the subscapularis.
		d) Muscular branches	Spring along the course of the subscapular artery to supply the teres major, long head of triceps brachii, tensor fasciae antebrachii and subscapularis.
II. Brachial artery	The continuation of the axillary artery after the subscapular artery is given off. It descends on the medial surface of the humerus and continues over the capsule and medial collateral ligament of the elbow joint. After giving off the common interosseous artery, it is continued as the median artery.		
	1. Cranial circumflex humeral artery		Arises at the cranial border of the teres major muscle. It passes cranially, accompanied by the proximal muscular branch of musculocutaneous nerve, between the coracobrachialis and humerus. It gives branches to the latter muscle, subscapularis, teres major, pectoralis ascendens and biceps brachii. It also supplies the medial aspect of the shoulder joint capsule and anastomoses with the caudal circumflex humeral artery.
	2. Deep brachial artery	a) Muscular branches	Large branches supply the long and medial heads of triceps brachii, tensor fasciae antebrachii, anconeus and brachialis muscles.
		b) Collateral radial artery	Descends in the musculospiral groove with the radial nerve to the cranial aspect of the elbow joint. At the level of the lateral epicondyle of the humerus it anastomoses with both transverse cubital and recurrent interosseous arteries.

Table (29) Arteries of the shoulder, arm and forearm regions (continued)

Main trunk	Branches	Subdivisions	Distribution
	3. Collateral ulnar artery		Springs from the caudal aspect of brachial artery within the distal third of the arm. The collateral ulnar artery passes caudodistally along the ventral border of the medial head of triceps brachii under cover of the tensor fasciae antebrachii. It gives branches to these muscles, pectoralis transversus, cubital lymph nodes, cutaneous trunci and skin. At the level of the medial epicondyle of humerus it descends with the ulnar nerve under the ulnar head of flexor carpi ulnaris and continues between the ulnar and humeral heads of the flexor digitorum profundus. In the distal half of the forearm it descends between the flexor carpi ulnaris and ulnaris lateralis. The collateral ulnar artery unites just proximal to the carpus with the lateral palmar artery, the branch of median artery. Along its course it detaches small collateral branches to the preceding muscles and the caudal aspect of elbow joint.
	4. Nutrient artery of the humerus		A short vessel which enters the nutrient foramen of the humerus.
	5. Bicipital artery		Arises from the cranial aspect of the brachial artery opposite to the origin of the collateral ulnar artery. it courses cranially between the coracobrachialis and biceps brachii, accompanying the distal muscular branch of musculocutaneous nerve. it divides into branches to supply the preceding muscles and the brachiocephalicus.
	6. Transverse cubital artery		Descends on the cranial face of the humerus under cover the biceps and brachialis to the cranial surface of the elbow joint. It continues distally on the cranial surface of the radius under the extensor digitorum communis to the dorsal surface of the carpus to concur in the formation of the **dorsal carpal rete** with the **cranial interosseous artery**. The transverse cubital artery supplies branches to the elbow Joint,

Table (29) Arteries of the shoulder, arm and forearm regions (continued)

Main trunk	Branches	Subdivisions	Distribution
			biceps brachii, brachialis and extensors of the carpus and digit. The dorsal carpal rete gives off the **lateral and medial dorsal metacarpal arteries**. The rete and dorsal metacarpal arteries represent the **dorsal set** which supplies the dorsal surface of carpus, digital extensor tendons and skin of the area.
	7. Common interosseous artery		The last branch of the brachial artery and arises at the level of the interosseous space of the forearm. It enters the interosseous space and gives off the following branches:-
		a) Nutrient artery of radius and ulna	Enters the nutrient foramen of the radius and ulna, which present in the distal part of the interosseous space, to supply the bones of the forearm.
		b) Cranial interosseous artery	Leaves the interosseous space and descends on the craniolateral surface of the radius, between the extensor digitorum communis and extensor digitorum lateralis, to the dorsal surface of the carpus and concurs with the transverse cubital artery in forming the **dorsal carpal rete**. The latter rete gives off the **medial and lateral dorsal metacarpal arteries** which descend in the grooves between the third metacarpal bone and the second and fourth metacarpal bones respectively. At the distal third of metacarpus, the medial and lateral dorsal metacarpal arteries perforate to the palmar aspect to anastomose with the corresponding **medial and lateral palmar metacarpal arteries.**
		c) Recurrent interosseous artery	Emerges the interosseous space and ascends on the lateral surface of the ulna. At the level of the lateral humeral epicondyle it anastomoses with the collateral radial artery, the branch of deep brachial artery.

Table (30) Arteries of the manus

Main trunk	Branches	Subdivisions	Distribution
III. Median artery			The direct continuation of the brachial artery beyond the origin of the common interosseous artery. It descends along the caudomedial aspect of the radius on the deep face of the flexor carpi radialis, accompanying the median nerve. At the distal half of the forearm, it is separated from the radius by the radial head of flexor digitorum superficialis. The median artery divides, proximal to the accessory carpal bone by about 2.5 cm. into the **radial artery** which is directed medially, **lateral palmar** and **medial palmar arteries**. The branches of the median artery represent the **palmar set** which supplies the palmar surface of the manus. The chief branches of median artery are:-
	1. Proximal radial artery		A small vessel arises at the distal third of the forearm. It descends on the caudal aspect of radius to the palmar surface of the carpus. It concurs with the branches of the lateral palmar and radial arteries in the formation of the **palmar carpal rete** which ramifies in the caudal surface of the carpal joint capsule.
	2. Lateral palmar artery		Arises just proximal to the carpus and anastomoses with the collateral ulnar artery. It descends with the lateral palmar nerve on the lateral palmar surface of the carpus to reach the proximal extremity of the fourth metacarpal bone. Here it joins with the **radial artery** by a transverse branch forming the **proximal deep palmar arch**, which lies between the deep digital flexor tendon and suspensory ligament and continues its course on the palmar surface of the third metacarpal, under cover of the suspensory ligament and parallel with the fourth metacarpal as the **lateral palmar metacarpal artery**. At the level of the distal third of metacarpus it anastomoses with the **lateral dorsal metacarpal artery** and inclines medially to join with the medial palmar metacarpal artery to constitute the **distal deep palmar arch.**

Table (30) Arteries of the manus (continued)

Main trunk	Branches	Subdivisions	Distribution
	3. Radial artery		Arises from the median artery slightly proximal to the origin of the lateral palmar artery. It passes distally on the medial side of the carpus and embedded in the flexor retinaculum. On reaching the proximal end of the second metacarpal bone it dips between the suspensory ligament and deep digital flexor tendon to join with the **lateral palmar artery** by a transverse branch forming the **proximal deep palmar arch** and descends on the deep face of the suspensory ligament as the **medial palmar metacarpal artery** along the interosseous space between the second and third metacarpal bones. At the level of the distal third of metacarpus, the medial palmar metacarpal artery is connected with the medial dorsal metacarpal artery which traverses the distal end of interosseous space between the second and third metacarpal bones. Finally, the **medial palmar metacarpal artery** joins the **lateral palmar metacarpal artery** to constitute the **distal deep palmar arch**.
	4. Medial palmar artery		Represents the extension of the median artery in the manus. It descends in the carpal canal along the medial side of the digital flexor tendons with the medial palmar nerve and continues in this relation till the distal fourth of metacarpus, where it inclines toward the midline between the deep digital flexor tendon and suspensory ligament. Here, the medial palmar artery connects with the distal deep palmar arch and divides into **medial and lateral palmar proper digital arteries**. The two arteries diverge and pass distally over the abaxial surface of the corresponding proximal sesamoid bone at the fetlock. Each descends parallel with the corresponding border of the deep digital flexor tendon to the solar groove and foramen of the distal phalanx. The two arteries are united inside the solar canal forming the **terminal arch**. The latter arch gives off numerous branches pass through the bone to the parietal surface and ramify in the corium of the wall and sole of the hoof. The medial and lateral palmar proper digital arteries give off the following branches:-

Table (30) Arteries of the manus (continued)

Main trunk	Branches	Subdivisions	Distribution
		a) Artery of the proximal phalanx	A short trunk arises at a right angle about the middle of the proximal phalanx. It divides into dorsal and palmar branches. **1) Dorsal branch**; passes between the proximal phalanx and the common digital extensor tendon and ramifies on the dorsal surface of the digit. It anastomoses with its fellow of the opposite side. **2) Palmar branch**; dips between the digital flexor tendons and the proximal phalanx and joins with the opposite branch between the straight and oblique sesamoidean ligaments.
		b) Branch to the digital cushion	Arises at the proximal border of the cartilage of the distal phalanx and descends along the palmar aspect to ramify in the digital cushion and the corium of the heels and frog.
		c) Dorsal branch of the middle phalanx	Springs proximal to the level of the distal sesamoid bone. It courses dorsally under the cartilage of the distal phalanx and the common digital extensor tendon on the dorsal surface of the middle phalanx, where it anastomoses with the opposite branch in forming an **arterial coronary circle**. It gives branches to the coffin joint and the coronary corium of the hoof.
		d) Palmar branch of the middle phalanx	Is smaller than the dorsal branch and arises opposite to it. It passes above the proximal border of the distal sesamoid bone and joins the opposite branch, gives branches to supply the coffin joint and the deep digital flexor tendon.
		e) Dorsal branch of the distal phalanx	Arises at the deep face of the process of the distal phalanx, passes dorsally though the notch of the process to the groove of the parietal surface. It gives off ascending and descending branches which ramify in the corium of the wall of the hoof.

Part III. Nerves of the thoracic limb
Table (31) Brachial plexus

Nerve	Origin	Branches	Distribution
Brachial plexus			The brachial plexus is formed by the connections established between the ventral branches of the **last three cervical and first two thoracic nerves**. It appears as a thick, wide band which pierces the scalenus medius muscle and is covered by the subclavius and subscapularis muscles. The last two cervical and first thoracic nerves are connected with the cervicothoracic ganglion by the rami communicates. The nerves of the plexus supply the thoracic limb, but some are distributed on the lateral thoracic wall.
1. Suprascapular nerve	The sixth and seventh cervical nerves		A large nerve passes ventrolaterally, accompanied by the suprascapular artery between the supraspinatus and subscapularis muscles, then winds around the cranial border of scapula to reach the infraspinous fossa. It gives branches supply the supraspinatus and infraspinatus muscles.
2. Subscapular nerves	The sixth and seventh cervical nerves		Two primary trunks, run caudally for a short distance and divide into several branches to enter the subscapularis muscle below its middle.
3. Pectoral nerves	The last two cervical and first thoracic nerves	**a) Cranial pectoral nerves**	Three to four branches emanate from the **axillary loop** formed by the musculocutaneous and median nerves. They pass between the divisions of the pectoralis profundus to supply the pectoralis descendens, pectoralis transversus, pectoralis ascendens and brachiocephalicus muscles.
		b) Caudal pectoral nerves	Two in number, extend from the caudal part of the brachial plexus to supply the pectoralis ascendens.

Table (31) Brachial plexus (continued)

Nerve	Origin	Branches	Distribution
4. Long thoracic nerve	The seventh, eighth cervical and first thoracic nerves		Gives off three branches to the serratus ventralis muscle at the junction of its cervical and thoracic parts and passes caudally across the surface of the serratus ventralis thoracis, to which it is distributed.
5. Dorsal thoracic nerve	The eighth cervical and first thoracic nerves		Passes dorsally and caudally across the subscapularis muscle to ramify in the latissimus dorsi muscle.
6. Lateral thoracic nerve	The eighth cervical and first and second thoracic nerves		Arises by a common trunk with the ulnar nerve. It passes caudally and ventrally across the deep face of the cutaneous trunci muscle and continues caudally in company with the external thoracic vein. Its branches innervate the cutaneous trunci and skin of the abdominal wall till the flank.
7. Musculocutaneous nerve	The seventh and eighth cervical nerves		Descends across the lateral surface of the axillary artery, ventral to which a greater part of the nerve unites with the median nerve to form the **axillary loop** in which the axillary artery is suspended. It gives off the following branches:-
		a) Proximal muscular branch	Passes cranially in company with the cranial circumflex humeral artery between the coracobrachialis muscle and humerus. It gives branches to the biceps brachii and coracobrachialis muscles.
		b) Distal muscular branch	Detaches at the middle of the arm, courses between the coracobrachialis and biceps brachii to reach the brachialis in which it ramifies.
		c) Medial cutaneous antebrachial nerve	Descends spiraling around the biceps brachii in the subcutaneous tissue, then along the medial aspect of the lacertus fibrosus and fascia of the forearm and continues distally in the limb. It ramifies on the cranial and medial faces of the forearm, the dorsal and medial aspects of the carpus and metacarpus and in the fetlock region.

Table (31) Brachial plexus (continued)

Nerve	Origin	Branches	Distribution
8. Axillary nerve	The sixth, seventh and eighth cervical nerves		It runs ventrally and caudally across the distal part of subscapularis muscle in company with the caudal circumflex humeral artery. It dips caudal to the shoulder joint and passes laterally in the septum between the teres minor and long and lateral heads of triceps brachii muscles to reach the deep face of deltoideus muscle, where it releases the cutaneous branches. Along its course it gives of the following branches:-
		a) Muscular branches	Supply the subscapularis, teres major, articularis humeri, teres minor and deltoideus muscle
		b) Lateral cranial cutaneous brachial nerves	Descend in the arm between the deltoideus and long head of triceps brachii muscles to innervate the fascia and skin of the craniolateral aspect of the arm.
		c) Cranial cutaneous antebrachial nerve	Passes distally to the cranial aspect of the forearm to be distributed in the fascia and skin of the region.
9. Radial nerve	The seventh and eighth cervical and first thoracic nerves		The largest nerve of the brachial plexus. It passes caudoventrally over the medial surface of origin of the subscapular artery and distal part of teres major. It is curved laterally in the interval between the teres major and the long and medial heads of triceps brachii to the musculospiral groove of the humerus where it gives the lateral caudal cutaneous brachial nerves. It leaves the latter groove to the **flexor surface** of the **elbow joint** and divides into a **superficial** and **deep** branch. Along its course it gives off:-
		a) Lateral caudal cutaneous brachial nerves	Detach from the radial nerve while traversing the musculospiral groove. They ramify in the fascia and skin of the caudolateral aspect of the arm.
		b) Muscular branches	Emanate from the radial nerve at the flexor surface of the elbow joint. They supply the three heads of triceps brachii and anconeus.

Table (31) Brachial plexus (continued)

Nerve	Origin	Branches	Distribution
		c) Superficial branch	Emerges between the lateral head of triceps brachii and extensor carpi radialis, then descends with the transverse cubital artery and pierces the cutaneous muscle. It gives off the **lateral cutaneous antebrachial nerve** to innervate the skin on the craniolateral aspect of the forearm.
		d) Deep branch	Gives off several muscular branches to supply the extensors of the carpus and digit; the extensor carpi radialis, extensor digitorum communis, extensor digitorum lateralis and extensor carpi obliquus. They also ramify in the ulnaris lateralis which morphologically belongs to the extensor group.
10. ulnar nerve	The first and second thoracic nerves		Descends between the axillary artery and vein, crosses the vein and continues along the cranial border of the tensor fascia antebrachii muscle. It inclines under the latter muscle near the elbow and passes distally and caudally over the medial epicondyle of the humerus. It descends in the forearm under the deep fascia on the ulnar head of the flexor digitorum profundus and continues between the flexor carpi ulnaris and ulnaris lateralis. At the level of the **accessory carpal bone** it divides into two terminal branches, **dorsal** and **palmar**.
		a) Caudal cutaneous antebrachial nerve	Arises at the middle of the arm and passes caudally and distally between the tensor fascia antebrachii and pectoralis transversus to become superficial distal to the elbow. It ramifies in the skin of the caudomedial and caudolateral aspects of the forearm.
		b) Muscular branches	Arise at the elbow to supply the flexor digitorum superficialis, ulnar head of flexor digitorum profundus and flexor carpi ulnaris muscles.
		c) Dorsal branch of the ulnar nerve	Emerges between the flexor carpi ulnaris and ulnaris lateralis to ramify on the fascia and skin of the carpus, metacarpus and fetlock.
		d) Palmar branch of the ulnar nerve	A very short branch unites with the **lateral palmar nerve** of **median** under cover the tendon of the flexor carpi ulnaris at the carpus. It shares the median nerve in supplying the palmar surface of manus.

Table (31) Brachial plexus (continued)

Nerve	Origin	Branches	Distribution
11. Median nerve	The seventh and eighth cervical and first and second thoracic nerves		The longest nerve of the brachial plexus. It is joined by a large branch with the **musculocutaneous nerve** to form the **axillary loop** in which the axillary artery is suspended. It descends on the medial aspect of the arm in company with the brachial artery to the medial collateral ligament of the elbow. It inclines caudally and descends with the median artery in the forearm under cover the flexor carpi radialis. The median nerve divides, proximal to the carpus, into **medial and lateral palmar nerves**. Along its course it gives off the following branches:
		a) Muscular branches	Spring at the proximal end of the radius. They pass under the flexor carpi radialis and supply the latter muscle, humeral and radial heads of the flexor digitorum profundus.
		b) Interosseous antebrachial nerve	Passes through the interosseous space of the forearm and ramifies in the periosteum of the radius and ulna.
		c) Medial palmar nerve (medial palmar common digital nerve)	The medial terminal branch of the median nerve. It descends in the carpal canal with the medial palmar artery along the medial border of the superficial digital flexor tendon. Near the middle of the metacarpus, it gives off the **communicating branch** and divides, just proximal to the fetlock joint, into a **dorsal branch** and **medial palmar proper digital nerve.** 1) **Communicating branch**; winds obliquely over the deep digital flexor tendon and joins the lateral palmar nerve distal to the middle of the metacarpus. 2) **Dorsal branch**; ramifies in the skin of the dorsal surface of the digit and corium of the hoof. 3) **Medial palmar proper digital nerve**; descends with the medial palmar proper digital artery and gives several branches to supply the skin of the medial and palmar aspects of the digit and corium of the hoof.

Table (31) Brachial plexus (continued)

Nerve	Origin	Branches	Distribution
		d) Lateral palmar nerve (lateral palmar common digital nerve)	The other terminal branch of the median nerve. At the carpus, it joins the **palmar branch** of the **ulnar nerve**. It descends with the lateral palmar artery in the texture of the flexor retinaculum and continues distally along the lateral border of the deep digital flexor tendon toward the distal end of the metacarpus. It is joined by the **communicating branch** from the **medial palmar nerve** and divides, just proximal to the fetlock, into a **dorsal branch** and **lateral palmar proper digital nerve**. The lateral palmar artery gives off the following branches:- 1) **Deep branch**; is detached distal to the carpus to supply the suspensory ligament. 2) **Dorsal branch**; ramifies in the skin of the dorsal surface of the digit and corium of the hoof. 3) **Lateral palmar proper digital nerve**; descends with the lateral palmar proper digital artery and gives several branches to supply the skin of the lateral and palmar aspects of the digit and corium of the hoof.

Chapter 4

Pelvic Limb

Part I. Muscles of the pelvic limb
Table (32) Sublumbar muscles

Muscle	Origin	Insertion	Action	Innervation
Sublumbar muscles	The muscles of this group are not confined to the sublumbar region, but extend beyond it cranially to the thoracic region and caudally to the pelvic and thigh regions. The group is covered by the iliac fascia which attached medially to the tendon of psoas minor muscle; laterally to the coxal tuber and blends with the deep layer of the thoracolumbar fascia.			
Psoas minor	Fusiform, flattened and pinnate muscle. It arises from the bodies of the last three thoracic and first four lumbar vertebrae.	The psoas tubercle on the body of the ilium	Flexes the pelvis on the loins	Lumbar nerves
Psoas major	Triangular in shape, its base lies caudally and partially covered by the psoas minor. It arises from the ventral surface of the transverse processes of the lumbar vertebrae and vertebral ends of the last two ribs.	The muscle fibers are blended with that of the iliacus on the ventral surface of the sacroiliac articulation a single muscle, **iliopsoas** and inserted by a common tendon on the lesser trochanter of the femur	Flexes the hip joint and rotates the thigh laterally	Lumbar nerves and Femoral nerve
Iliacus	Sacropelvic surface of the ilium lateral to the sacroiliac articulation, wing of the sacrum and the ventral sacroiliac ligaments	The lesser trochanter of the femur, by a common tendon with the psoas major	Flexes the hip joint and rotates the thigh laterally	Lumbar nerves and Femoral nerve
Quadratus lumborum	Thin muscle lies on the lateral part of the ventral surfaces of lumbar transverse processes. It arises from the ventral surface of the vertebral ends of the last two ribs and the lumbar transverse processes.	Ventral surface of the wing of the sacrum and the ventral sacroiliac ligaments	Lateral flexion of the loins	Lumbar nerves

Table (33) Muscles of the hip and thigh regions

Muscle	Origin	Insertion	Action	Innervation
A. Lateral group	This group lies on the lateral surface of the pelvis and thigh. It also includes those which form the caudal contour of the thigh. The lateral group is covered by the gluteal fascia and the fascia of the thigh. The **gluteal fascia** detaches intermuscular septa, which pass between the muscles. It is attached to the sacral spines, sacral tuber and coxal tuber of the ilium. It is continuous cranially with the thoracolumbar fascia and caudally with the tail fascia. The **deep fascia of the thigh** is thick, strong and continuous with the gluteal fascia. It furnishes insertion to the tensor fasciae latae and attached to the patella, lateral and medial patellar ligaments.			
Tensor fasciae latae	Triangular in shape, arises from the coxal tuber at its apex	The fascia lata which attached to the patella, lateral patellar ligament and tibial crest	Flexes the hip joint and extends the stifle joint	Cranial gluteal nerve
Gluteus superficialis	• Cranial head; from the coxal tuber and adjacent part of the lateral border of the ilium • Caudal head; from the gluteal fascia	The two heads are terminated, by a strong flat tendon, into the third trochanter of the femur	Flexes the hip joint and abducts the limb	Cranial and caudal gluteal nerves
Gluteus medius	A bulk of muscular mass which covers the gluteal surface of the ilium and the lateral pelvic wall. It arises from the gluteal surface of the ilium, dorsal sacroiliac ligament and broad sacrotuberal ligament.	Summit and crest of the greater trochanter of the femur Lateral aspect of the intertrachanteric crest of the femur	Extends the hip joint and abducts the limb	Cranial and caudal gluteal nerves
Gluteus profundus	A small quadrilateral muscle and extends over the hip joint. It arises from the ischiatic spine and adjacent part of the body of the ilium.	Convexity of the greater trochanter of the femur	Abducts the femur and rotates it medially	Cranial gluteal nerve

Table (33) Muscles of the hip and thigh regions (continued)

Muscle	Origin	Insertion	Action	Innervation
Biceps femoris	• The long head; from the dorsal sacroiliac ligament and gluteal fascia. • The short head; from the ventral surface of the ischiatic tuber.	• Cranial part; in the cranial surface of the patella and lateral patellar ligament. • Middle part; in the cranial border of the tibia. • Caudal part; in the common calcaneal tendon and calcaneal tuber	• Extends the hip and stifle joints • Extends the hip and flexes the stifle • Flexes the stifle and extends the hock	Caudal gluteal, Ischiatic and Fibular nerves
Semitendinosus	• The long head; from the transverse processes of the first and second caudal vertebrae. • The short head; from the ventral surface of the ischiatic tuber.	• Cranial border of the tibia by a tendinous band • Common calcaneal tendon and calcaneal tuber	Extends the hip and hock joints, flexes the stifle joint	Caudal gluteal and ischiatic nerves
Semimembranosus	• The long head; from the caudal border of the broad sacrotuberal ligament. • The short head; from the ventral surface of the ischiatic tuber.	Medial epicondyle of the femur, caudal to the medial collateral ligament.	Extends the hip joint and adducts the limb	Ischiatic nerve
B. Medial group	This group lies on the medial surface of the thigh. Its deep layer extends to cover the pelvic floor, obturator foramen and lateral pelvic wall. The muscles of the group are arranged in three layers; the first includes the sartorius and gracilis.The second layer includes the pectineus, adductor and semimembranosus. The deepest layer includes the quadratus femoris, obturatorius externus, obturatorius internus and gemelli.			

Table (33) Muscles of the hip and thigh regions (continued)

Muscle	Origin	Insertion	Action	Innervation
Sartorius	Long and narrow muscle, extends from the caudal part of sublumbar region to the medial surface of the stifle. It arises from the iliac fascia and tendon of the psoas minor.	The medial patellar ligament and the tibial tuberosity	Flexes the hip joint and adducts the limb	Saphenous nerve (branch of femoral nerve)
Gracilis	Wide and quadrilateral muscle covers the greater part of the medial aspect of the thigh. It originates from the middle third of the pelvic symphysis and prepubic tendon.	Medial surface of the tibia and medial patellar ligament	Adducts the limb	Obturator nerve
Pectineus	Fusiform in shape, extends from the cranial border of the pubis to the middle of the medial border of femur. It arises from prepubic tendon, accessory femoral ligament and cranial border of the pubis	Middle of the medial border of the femur, near the nutrient foramen	Flexes the hip joint and adducts the limb	Obturator nerve
Adductor	Prismatic in shape, lies caudal to the pectineus and vastus medialis. It arises from the ventral surface of the pubis and ischium.	• Caudal surface of the femur from the level of third trochanter to the groove for femoral vessels. • Medial epicondyle of femur and medial collateral ligament of the stifle joint.	Extends the hip joint and adducts the limb	Obturator nerve
Semimembranosus	• The long head; from the caudal border of the broad sacrotuberal ligament. • The short head; from the ventral surface of the ischiatic tuber.	Medial epicondyle of the femur, caudal to the medial collateral ligament.	Extends the hip joint and adducts the limb	Ischiatic nerve

Table (33) Muscles of the hip and thigh regions (continued)

Muscle	Origin	Insertion	Action	Innervation
Quadratus femoris	Narrow and quadrilateral in shape, lies under cover of the adductor. It arises from ventral surface of ischium.	An oblique line on the caudal surface of femur, near the ventral part of lesser trochanter.	Extends the hip joint and adducts the limb	Ischiatic nerve
Obturatorius externus	Pyramidal in shape, extends across the caudal aspect of the hip joint. It emanates from the ventral surface of the pubis and ischium, and the margin of obturator foramen.	Trochanteric fossa	Adducts the limb and rotates it laterally	Obturator nerve
Obturatorius internus	Arises within the pelvic cavity by two heads:- • Iliac head; from the pelvic surface of the ilium and the wing of sacrum. • Ischiopubic head; from the pelvic surface of the pubis and ischium around the obturator foramen	Both terminate by a flat tendon which passes through the lesser ischiatic foramen to be inserted in the trochanteric fossa	Rotates the femur laterally	Ischiatic nerve
Gemelli	Thin, triangular in shape and may be regarded as the extrapelvic part of the obturatorius internus. It arises from the lateral border of the ischium near the ischiatic spine.	Trochanteric fossa and intertrachanteric crest	Rotates the femur laterally	Ischiatic nerve
C. Cranial muscles of the thigh	Constitute the large muscular mass which covers the cranial, lateral and medial aspects of the femur (quadriceps femoris muscle) as well as a small fusiform muscle (articularis coxae), placed lateral to the hip joint capsule and attached to the cranial surface of the femur.			

Table (33) Muscles of the hip and thigh regions (continued)

Muscle	Origin	Insertion	Action	Innervation
• **Quadriceps femoris**	Consists of four heads, the **rectus femoris** arises from the ilium, while the other **three vasti** arise from the femur. All heads are inserted into the patella. The **patellar ligaments** are regarded as tendons of the quadriceps femoris which communicate the action of this muscle to the tibia and the patella being intercalated as a **sesamoid bone.**			
1. Rectus femoris	Fusiform and rounded, arises by two tendons from two depressions on the body of the ilium cranial and dorsal to the acetabulum.	Base and cranial surface of the patella.	Flexes the hip and extends the stifle joint (biarticular)	Femoral nerve
2. Vastus lateralis	Lateral surface and border of the femur, extending from greater trochanter to the supracondyloid fossa.	Cranial surface of the patella and the tendon of rectus femoris.	Extends the stifle joint	Femoral nerve
3. Vastus medialis	Medial surface of the femur, extending from the neck to the distal third.	Medial border of the patella, patellar cartilage and the tendon of rectus femoris.	Extends the stifle joint	Femoral nerve
4. Vastus intermedius	Cranial surface of the femur, extending from the proximal fourth to the distal fourth. It is entirely covered by the preceding heads.	Base of the patella and femoropatellar joint capsule	Extends the stifle joint and raises the joint capsule	Femoral nerve
• **Articularis coxae (Capsularis coxae)**	A small fusiform muscle, as long as a finger. It arises, by a thin tendon, from the cranial rim of acetabulum.	The muscle passes over the lateral side of the hip joint capsule, then dips between the vastus intermedius and vastus lateralis. It is inserted, by a delicate tendon, into the proximal third of the cranial surface of femur.	Raises the hip joint capsule during flexion	Cranial gluteal nerve

Table (34) Muscles of the leg and pes regions

Muscle	Origin	Insertion	Action	Innervation
A. Craniolateral group	The muscles of this group are extensors of the digit and flexors of the hock. The **fascia of the leg** which covers the muscles of this group is derived from the medial femoral fascia and lateral gluteofemoral fascia. The two layers are fused distally and attached to the medial and lateral patellar ligaments and the cranial border and lateral surface of the tibia. The **deep fascia** of the leg forms sheaths for the muscles and furnishes intermuscular septa. The **tarsal fascia** is strong and tendinous dorsally, fused with the ligaments and bony prominences. It forms three extensor retinacula. **1) Proximal extensor retinaculum**; at the distal end of the tibia and binds down the tendons of the extensor digitorum longus, fibularis tertius and tibialis cranialis. **2) Middle extensor retinaculum**; attaches to the calcaneus and lateral tendon of fibularis tertius, forming a loop around the long digital extensor tendon. **3) Distal extensor retinaculum**; stretches across the proximal extremity of the third metatarsal bone and encloses the long and lateral digital extensor tendons.			
Extensor digitorum longus	Extensor fossa between the lateral condoyle and trochlea of the femur.	Extensor process of the distal phalanx and dorsal surfaces of the proximal extremities of proximal and middle phalanges.	Extends the digit and flexes the hock joint	Fibular nerve
Extensor digitorum lateralis	Fibula, lateral border of the tibia and interosseous ligament of the leg.	The lateral digital extensor tendon is joined with the long digital flexor tendon at the proximal third of metatarsus	Extends the digit and flexes the hock joint	Fibular nerve
Fibularis tertius	A strong tendon which lies between the extensor digitorum longus and tibialis cranialis. It arises from the extensor fossa with the extensor digitorum longus.	The tendon of insertion is perforated for emergence the tendon of tibialis cranialis and divided into dorsal and lateral branches. • Dorsal branch; attaches to the third tarsal and third metatarsal bones. • Lateral branch; bends laterally to be inserted in the calcaneus and fourth metatarsal bone.	Flexes the hock joint	Fibular nerve

Table (34) Muscles of the leg and pes regions (continued)

Muscle	Origin	Insertion	Action	Innervation
Tibialis cranialis	Lateral condyle and lateral border of the tibia	The tendon of insertion emerges between the branches of fibularis tertius and bifurcates into:- • Dorsal branch; being inserted into the third metatarsal bone. • Medial branch (cunean tendon); into the first tarsal bone	Flexes the hock joint	Fibular nerve
Extensor digitorum previs	A small muscle, arises from the lateral tendon of fibularis tertius and lateral collateral ligament of the hock	The tendons of long and lateral digital extensor tendons	Assists the action of long digital extensor	Fibular nerve
B. Caudal group	The muscles of this group are flexors of the digit and extensors of the hock. The **fascia of the leg** which covers the muscles of this group is derived from the medial femoral fascia and lateral gluteofemoral fascia. About the middle of the leg the two layers are fused caudal to the flexor digitorum profundus and form a strong band which passes distally cranial to the common calcaneal tendon to attach the latter with the dorsal and medial parts of the calcaneal tuber. **The tarsal fascia** covers the plantar aspect of the tarsus, becomes very thick and strong and forms the **flexor retinaculum**. The latter stretches from the medial collateral ligament to the long plantar ligament and calcaneus. It converts the plantar groove of the hock into a canal **(tarsal canal)**, through which the deep digital flexor tendon, plantar arteries and nerves pass.			
Gastrocnemius	Forms with the soleus a muscle termed **triceps surae**. It arises by two heads. • Lateral head; from the lateral supracondyloid tuberosity of the femur • Medial head; from the medial supracondyloid tuberosity of the femur	The two heads and the soleus are terminated by a common tendon, the **calcaneal or Achilles' tendon** which inserted into the plantar aspect of the calcaneal tuber.	Flexes the stifle joint and extends the hock joint	Tibial nerve

Table (34) Muscles of the leg and pes regions (continued)

Muscle	Origin	Insertion	Action	Innervation
Soleus	A small muscle lies along the lateral border of the gastrocnemius. It arises from the head of the fibula.	The calcaneal or Achilles' tendon at the distal fourth of the leg.	Assists the action of gastrocnemius	Tibial nerve
Flexor digitorum superficialis	Lies between and under cover of the two heads of gastrocnemius. It has a very small belly arises from the supracondyloid fossa of the femur.	At the distal third of the tibia, the superficial digital flexor tendon winds around the medial surface of calcaneal tendon, then occupies a position caudal to the calcaneal ligament. At the calcaneal tuber, it forms a cap over the tuber and gives two strong bands insert into the sides of the calcaneal tube. The superficial digital flexor tendon descends over the long plantar ligament and is arranged distally as in the thoracic limb.	Flexes the digit and extends the hock joint	Tibial nerve
Flexor digitorum profundus	The belly of the deep digital flexor muscle lies on the caudal surface of the tibia and consists of three muscular and a tendinous heads which finally unite in a common tendon of insertion, the deep digital flexor tendon. The latter is formed caudal to the distal end of the tibia as a strong rounded tendon of **flexor digiti I longus** and received the tendon of **tibialis caudalis**. It descends in the tarsal canal to the plantar aspect of the metatarsus where it joins with the tendon of **flexor digitorum longus** and the **tendinous head**. It continues distally between the superficial digital flexor tendon and suspensory ligament to the sesamoid groove and proceeds beyond the distal sesamoidean ligaments to the flexor surface of the distal sesamoid bone. The deep digital flexor tendon inserts in the semilunar line and adjacent surface of the cartilage of distal phalanx.			

Table (34) Muscles of the leg and pes regions (continued)

Muscle	Origin	Insertion	Action	Innervation
1. Flexor digiti I longus	The largest of the three heads and lies on the flexor surface of the tibia. It arises from the caudal surface of the tibia, lateral and distal to the popliteal line.	Terminates caudal to the distal end of the tibia by a strong round tendon and receives the tendon of the tibialis caudalis to form the beginning of the deep digital flexor tendon.	Flexes the digit and extends the hock joint	Tibial nerve
2. Tibialis caudalis	Has a flattened belly, arises from the lateral condyle of the tibia, just caudal to the facet for the fibula.	Terminated by a flat tendon which fuses with the principal tendon at the distal end of the tibia.	Flexes the digit and extends the hock joint	Tibial nerve
3. Flexor digitorum longus	Has a fusiform belly lies in a groove formed by the other heads and the popliteus. It arises from the caudal edge of the lateral condyle of the tibia.	Terminates by a round tendon which descends in a canal in the medial collateral ligament of the hock to the metatarsal region and joins the deep digital flexor tendon	Flexes the digit and extends the hock joint	Tibial nerve
Popliteus	A thick, triangular muscle, lies on the caudal surface of tibia proximal to the popliteal line. It arises from the lateral epicondyle of the femur close to the articular surface and under the lateral collateral ligament of the stifle joint.	A triangular area on the caudal surface of the tibia, proximal and medial to the popliteal line (popliteal surface).	Flexes the femorotibial joint and rotates the leg medially	Tibial nerve

Part II. Arteries of the pelvic limb

Table (35) Arteries of the pelvic, thigh and leg regions

Main trunk	Branches	subdivisions	Distribution
I. Internal iliac artery			One of the terminal branches of the abdominal aorta. The distribution of the artery has been described in table (21) as one of the arteries which supplies the abdominal viscera and wall. The internal iliac artery detaches the largest branch; the caudal gluteal artery which gives branches to the lateral and medial muscles of the pelvis and thigh (279 – 282).
II. External iliac artery			Arises from the abdominal aorta ventral to the fifth lumbar vertebra and just cranial to the origin of the internal iliac artery. It descends at the side of the cranial pelvic inlet along the tendon of psoas minor and reaches the cranial border of the pubis, beyond which it is continued in the femoral canal as the **femoral artery**. The chief branches of the external iliac artery are:-
	1. Deep circumflex iliac artery	**a) Cranial branch**	Gives small branches to the sublumbar muscles, lateral iliac lymph nodes, gluteus medius and tensor fasciae latae. It passes cranially and ventrally in the flank on the dorsal margin of the obliquus internus abdominis to supply the abdominal muscles, fascia and skin of the flank.
		b) Caudal branch	Perforates the abdominal wall close to the coxal tuber and descends on the medial surface of the tensor fasciae latae to the fold of the flank. It supplies the obliquus internus abdominis, tensor fasciae latae and iliacus.
	2. Cremaster artery (in males) **2`. Uterine artery (in females)**		Slender flexuous vessel in males, supplies the cremaster muscle, vaginal tunic and the other contents of the spermatic cord. It is much larger in females and considered as the main arterial supply to the uterus It anastomoses with the uterine branch of ovarian artery and the uterine branch of urogenital (vaginal) artery.
	3. Deep femoral artery	**a) Pudendoepigastric trunk**	The trunk has been described in tables of the trunk.

Table (35) Arteries of the pelvic, thigh and leg regions (continued)

Main trunk	Branches	subdivisions	Distribution
		b) Medial circumflex femoral artery	The continuation of the deep femoral artery beyond the origin of the pudendoepigastric trunk. It runs caudally ventral to the pubic bone, between the pectineus, iliopsoas and obturatorius externus where it gives off the obturator branch. It pierces the adductor and reaches the semimembranosus and deep surface of the biceps femoris. Along its course, it gives off the following branches:- **1) Muscular branches**; to the pectineus, iliopsoas, obturatorius externus, quadratus femoris, adductor, semimembranosus and biceps femoris. **2) Obturator branch**; a slender vessel, passes toward the obturator foramen and anastomoses with the obturator artery, the branch of caudal gluteal.
III. Femoral artery	The main arterial trunk of the thigh. It descends vertically in the **femoral canal** caudal to the sartorius muscle, in company with the femoral vein and saphenous nerve. It passes over the insertion of pectineus and perforates the adductor muscle to proceed in the vascular groove of the caudal surface of the femur. It continues between the two heads of gastrocnemius muscle as the **popliteal artery**. the chief branches of the femoral artery are:-		
	1. Descending branch of lateral circumflex femoral artery (former; Cranial femoral artery)		Arises from the cranial aspect of the femoral artery at the level of the level of the femoral ring (entrance of the femoral canal). It passes craniolaterally across the deep face of the sartorius, accompanied by the muscular branch of femoral nerve and dips between the rectus femoris and vastus medialis. The descending branch of lateral circumflex femoral artery gives branches to the vastus medialis, rectus femoris and vastus intermedius.

Table (35) Arteries of the pelvic, thigh and leg regions (continued)

Main trunk	Branches	subdivisions	Distribution
	2. Saphenous artery		The most extensive branch of femoral. It arises from the medial face of femoral artery and about its middle. The saphenous artery emerges between the sartorius and gracilis, accompanied by the saphenous vein and nerve, to the medial aspect of the thigh. It descends superficially on the cranial part of gracilis to be divided proximal to the stifle joint into cranial and caudal branches.
		a) Cranial branch	Gives off cutaneous twigs to the fascia and skin of the medial aspect of the thigh and leg.
		b) Caudal branch	The continuation of the saphenous on the deep fascia of the leg. It has been reinforced twice; the first, at the distal third of the leg where it anastomoses with the **descending branch of the caudal femoral artery** and the second, cranial to the calcaneal tuber where it joins the **medial branch (anastomotic branch for saphenous artery) of the caudal tibial artery** which usually forms a double curve. The caudal branch continues distally on the plantar aspect of the hock and, at the level of the **sustentaculum tali,** it divides into medial and lateral plantar arteries. They have been described with the arteries of the pes region as the **plantar set** of this region.
	3. Nutrient artery of the femur		A small branch detaches from the femoral artery at the middle of the thigh and enters the nutrient foramen of the femur.
	4. Descending genicular artery		Arises from the femoral artery at the distal third of the thigh. It passes craniodistally between the sartorius, vastus medialis and adductor toward the patella and the medial aspect femorotibial articulation. It gives branches to the **capsule of the femorotibial joint and its adjoining ligaments.**

Table (35) Arteries of the pelvic, thigh and leg regions (continued)

Main trunk	Branches	subdivisions	Distribution
	5. Caudal femoral artery		Arises from the caudal face of the femoral artery at the proximal end of the gastrocnemius muscle. It forms a short trunk gives muscular branches to the gastrocnemius and flexor digitorum superficialis, then divides into ascending and descending branches.
		a) Ascending branch	Passes proximally between the adductor and semimembranosus. It ramifies in the biceps femoris, vastus lateralis, semitendinosus and semimembranosus muscles. The ascending branch anastomoses with the medial circumflex femoral artery.
		b) Descending branch	Curves between the biceps femoris and semitendinosus, and then passes distally on the lateral head of gastrocnemius. It gives branches to supply these muscles and popliteal lymph nodes. One of the branches descends between the two heads of gastrocnemius with the tibial nerve. At the distal third of the leg, it anastomoses with the caudal branch of saphenous artery.
IV. Popliteal artery	The direct continuation of the femoral artery between the two heads of gastrocnemius beyond the origin of the caudal femoral artery. It courses at first on the caudal surface of the femur, then on the femorotibial joint capsule. The popliteal artery descends trough the popliteal notch deep to the popliteus muscle, inclines laterally to the proximal part of the interosseous space of the leg where it divides into **cranial and caudal tibial arteries**. During its course, it gives off the **genicular branches** to the stifle joint and **muscular branches** to the gastrocnemius, soleus, popliteus and flexor digitorum superficialis.		

Table (35) Arteries of the pelvic, thigh and leg regions (continued)

Main trunk	Branches	subdivisions	Distribution
	1. Cranial tibial artery		Much larger than the caudal one, passes cranially through the interosseous space of the leg and descends with two satellite veins on the lateral surface of the tibia, deep to the tibialis cranialis and deviates cranially at the distal end of the leg. It descends with the long digital extensor tendon through the proximal extensor retinaculum on the dorsal surface of the hock as the **dorsal pedal artery**, representing the **dorsal set** which ramifies the pes region. The cranial tibial artery gives muscular branches to the tibialis cranialis, fibularis tertius, extensor digitorum longus and extensor digitorum lateralis.
	2. Caudal tibial artery		Much the smaller of the two terminal branches of popliteal artery. It lies at first between the tibia and popliteus, and then descends on the caudal surface of the leg between the popliteus, flexor digiti I longus and flexor digitorum longus. The caudal tibial artery proceeds distally along the long digital flexor tendon to the distal third of the leg and divides into the **lateral caudal malleolar artery** and **anastomotic branch for saphenous artery**. The collateral branches of the caudal tibial artery include the **nutrient artery of the tibia** and the **muscular branches** to the popliteus and flexor digitorum profundus.
		a) Lateral caudal malleolar artery	Ramifies the lateral and caudal aspects of the hock joint. It gives a small branch which ascends along the lateral margin of the common calcaneal tendon and joins a branch of caudal femoral artery.
		b) Anastomotic branch for saphenous artery	Forms a double curve cranial to the calcaneal tuber. It anastomoses with the caudal branch of saphenous artery to reinforce it.

Table (36) Arteries of the pes region

Main trunk	Branches	subdivisions	Distribution
The arteries of the pes region are represented by two sets of arteries. The **plantar set** is formed by the **caudal branch of saphenous artery** after its reinforcing twice by the descending branch of caudal femoral artery and the anastomotic branch for saphenous artery of caudal tibial. The **dorsal set** is emanated from the **dorsal pedal artery**; the continuation of the cranial tibial on the dorsal surface of the hock joint.			
I. Saphenous artery (caudal branch)	The caudal branch of saphenous artery descends on the plantar surface of the hock and, at the level of the **sustentaculum tali**; it divides into medial and lateral plantar arteries. The **medial plantar artery** courses distally along the plantaromedial aspect of the tarsus to the proximal end of the metatarsus where it divides into a deep and superficial branch. The **lateral plantar artery** descends deep to the long plantar ligament and the deep digital flexor tendon to the proximal end of the metatarsus where it also divides into a deep and superficial branch.		
	1. Medial plantar artery	**a) Deep branch**	Dips under the deep digital flexor tendon and unites with the **proximal perforating branch** of the dorsal pedal artery and the **deep branch** of lateral plantar artery to assist in forming the **proximal deep plantar arch.**
		b) Superficial branch	Continues distally along the medial edge of the digital flexor tendons as **medial plantar common digital artery**. At the level of the fetlock joint it opens in the **medial plantar proper digital artery**, between the deep digital flexor tendon and suspensory ligament.
	2. Lateral plantar artery	**a) Deep branch**	Dips between the suspensory ligament and deep digital flexor tendon, joins with the **proximal perforating branch** and **deep branch** of medial plantar artery to share in the formation of the **proximal deep plantar arch**. From the latter arch arise **medial and lateral plantar metatarsal arteries** which descend in the metatarsal groove till its distal fourth where they empty in the distal perforating branch forming the **distal deep plantar arch.**
		b) Superficial branch	Continues distally along the lateral edge of the digital flexor tendons as **lateral plantar common digital artery** and, slightly proximal to the fetlock joint, opens in the **lateral plantar proper digital artery.**

Table (36) Arteries of the pes region (continued)

Main trunk	Branches	subdivisions	Distribution
II. Dorsal pedal artery			The direct continuation of the cranial tibial artery on the dorsal aspect of the hock and forms the **dorsal set** of arteries the pes region. The dorsal pedal artery gives small branches, opposite the tarsocrural articulation, to form the **dorsal tarsal rete**. It also detaches the **medial and lateral tarsal arteries** to ramify in the medial and lateral aspects of the hock joint respectively as well as the extensor digitorum brevis. The dorsal pedal artery passes distally in the joint capsule of the hock and gives off the **proximal perforating branch** and continues as the **lateral dorsal metatarsal artery.**
	1. Proximal perforating branch		Arises from the dorsal pedal artery under cover of the extensor digitorum brevis. It passes plantarad through the **vascular canal** of the tarsus to the proximal end of metatarsal groove and unites with the deep branches of the medial and lateral plantar arteries to assist in the formation of the **proximal deep plantar arch**.
	2. Lateral dorsal metatarsal artery		The continuation of the dorsal pedal artery beyond the origin of the proximal perforating branch. It descends obliquely, on the deep face of the extensor digitorum brevis and lateral digital extensor tendon, to the vascular groove on the proximal part of third metatarsal bone. The artery continues distally in the groove formed by the apposition of the third and fourth metatarsal bones, perforates medially between the latter bones to the distal part of the plantar surface of the third metatarsal bone as the **distal perforating branch** which receives **the medial and lateral plantar metatarsal arteries** to form the **distal deep plantar arch**. The distal perforating branch is divided, beyond the arch, into the **medial and lateral plantar proper digital arteries**. They receive, slightly proximal to the fetlock joint, **the medial and lateral plantar common digital arteries** and diverge distally over the abaxial surface of the corresponding proximal sesamoid bone at the fetlock. Each descends parallel with the corresponding border of the deep digital flexor tendon to the solar groove and foramen of the distal phalanx. The two arteries are united inside the solar canal forming the **terminal arch**. The latter arch gives off numerous branches pass through the bone to the parietal surface and ramify in the corium of the wall and sole of the hoof. **The medial and lateral plantar proper digital arteries** give off the following branches:-

Table (36) Arteries of the pes region (continued)

Main trunk	Branches	subdivisions	Distribution
		a) Artery of the proximal phalanx	A short trunk arises at a right angle about the middle of the proximal phalanx. It divides into dorsal and plantar branches. 1) **Dorsal branch**; passes between the proximal phalanx and the long digital extensor tendon and ramifies on the dorsal surface of the digit. It anastomoses with its fellow of the opposite side. 2) **Plantar branch**; dips between the digital flexor tendons and the proximal phalanx and joins with the opposite branch between the straight and oblique sesamoidean ligaments.
		b) Branch to the digital cushion	Arises at the proximal border of the cartilage of the distal phalanx and descends along the plantar aspect to ramify in the digital cushion and the corium of the heels and frog.
		c) Dorsal branch of the middle phalanx	Springs proximal to the level of the distal sesamoid bone. It courses dorsally under the cartilage of the distal phalanx and the long digital extensor tendon on the dorsal surface of the middle phalanx, where it anastomoses with the opposite branch in forming an **arterial coronary circle**. It gives branches to the coffin joint and the coronary corium of the hoof.
		d) Plantar branch of the middle phalanx	Is smaller than the dorsal branch and arises opposite to it. It passes above the proximal border of the distal sesamoid bone and joins the opposite branch, gives branches to supply the coffin joint and the deep digital flexor tendon.
		e) Dorsal branch of the distal phalanx	Arises at the deep face of the process of the distal phalanx, passes dorsally though the notch of the process to the groove of the parietal surface. It gives off ascending and descending branches which ramify in the corium of the wall of the hoof.

Part III. Nerves of the pelvic limb
Table (37) Lumbosacral plexus

Nerve	Origin	Branches	Distribution
Lumbosacral plexus	The lumbosacral plexus is formed by the connections established between the ventral branches of the **last three lumbar and first two sacral nerves**. It gives origin to the nerves of the pelvic limb.		
1. Femoral nerve	The fourth and fifth lumbar nerves	A large nerve passes ventrally and caudally between the psoas minor and major, then crosses the deep face the tendon of insertion of psoas minor and descends between the sartorius and iliopsoas. Here, it divides into a small saphenous nerve and a large muscular branch.	
		a) Saphenous nerve	Gives a branch to the sartorius and descends with the femoral vessels in the femoral canal. About the middle of the thigh it divides into several branches which emerge between the sartorius and gracilis to the medial aspect of the thigh. They descend superficially to ramify in the skin of the cranial and medial surfaces of the thigh and leg. One of these branches proceeds distally to supply the skin and fascia of the mediodorsal aspect of the metatarsus as far as the fetlock joint.
		b) Muscular branches	Dip between the rectus femoris and vastus medialis, in company with the descending branch of lateral circumflex femoral artery, to innervate the quadriceps femoris muscle.
2. Obturator nerve	The fourth, fifth and sixth lumbar nerves	Courses ventrally and caudally with the external iliac vein, then inclines medially to pass through the cranial part of obturator foramen. It continues ventrally through the obturatorius externus and divides into several branches to supply the obturatorius externus, pectineus, adductor and gracilis.	
3. Cranial gluteal nerve	The fifth, sixth lumbar and first sacral nerves	The nerve is divided into four or five branches which emerge through the greater ischiatic foramen with the branches of the cranial gluteal artery to supply the gluteal muscles, tensor fasciae latae, iliacus and articularis coxae.	

Table (37) Lumbosacral plexus (continued)

Nerve	Origin	Branches	Distribution
4. Caudal gluteal nerve	The first and second sacral nerves		The caudal gluteal nerve is divided into dorsal and ventral trunks which leave the lumbosacral plexus above the ischiatic nerve.
		a) Dorsal trunk	Passes caudally on the dorsal part of the broad sacrotuberal ligament and divides into branches which ramify in the biceps femoris, caudal part of gluteus medius and long head of gluteus superficialis.
		b) Ventral trunk	Passes ventrally and caudally on the broad sacrotuberal ligament and divides into:- 1) **Caudal cutaneous femoral nerve**; passes caudally through the biceps femoris, emerges between the latter and semitendinosus at the level of the ischiatic tuber. It gives of the **caudal clunial nerves** which ramify in the lateral and caudal surfaces of the hip and thigh. 2) **Muscular branches**; supply the semitendinosus.
5. Ischiatic nerve	The sixth lumbar, first and second sacral nerves		The largest nerve in the body leaves the plexus as a broad, flat band. It emerges though the greater ischiatic foramen and passes ventrally and caudally on the ventral part of the broad sacrotuberal ligament. The nerve turns ventrally in the space between the greater trochanter and ischiatic spine, and then descends in the thigh on the deep face of the biceps femoris. Along its pelvic and extrapelvic course, it gives off the **muscular branches** and terminates at the middle of the thigh into **fibular and tibial nerves**.
		a) Muscular branches	• Pelvic part of the ischiatic nerve releases small muscular branches to supply the obturatorius internus, gemelli and quadratus femoris muscles. • Extrapelvic part of the ischiatic nerve detaches a large muscular branch at the caudal aspect of the hip joint to ramify in the semimembranosus and the short heads of biceps femoris and semitendinosus.

Table (37) Lumbosacral plexus (continued)

Nerve	Origin	Branches	Distribution

		b) Fibular nerve	Descends with the parent trunk to the origin of the gastrocnemius where it deviates laterally and cranially across the lateral face of the gastrocnemius under cover of the biceps femoris. It divides at the origin of the extensor digitorum lateralis into superficial fibular and deep fibular nerves. The chief branches of the fibular nerve are:-
			1) **Lateral cutaneous sural nerve**; emerges between the middle and caudal parts of the biceps femoris about the level of the stifle joint and ramifies under the skin.
			2) **Superficial fibular nerve;** furnishes branches to the extensor digitorum lateralis and descends in the furrow between that muscle and extensor digitorum longus. It perforates the deep fascia of the leg and ramifies under the skin of the dorsal and lateral faces of tarsus and metatarsus.
			3) **Deep fibular nerve;** large and dips between the extensor digitorum longus and lateralis, gives branches to these muscles, tibialis cranialis and fibularis tertius. It proceeds distally under cover the long digital flexor tendon and divides on the dorsal surface of the hock joint into medial and lateral dorsal metatarsal nerves.
			  i. **Medial dorsal metatarsal nerve;** descends under the skin on the dorsal surface of tarsus and metatarsus. It supplies the extensor digitorum brevis, joint capsule of hock, fascia and skin of the medial aspect of the metatarsus.
			  ii. **Lateral dorsal metatarsal nerve;** gives twigs to the extensor digitorum brevis and passes distally with the medial nerve to ramify in the skin of the lateral face of metatarsus and fetlock.

Nerve	Origin	Branches	Distribution
		c) Tibial nerve	The direct continuation of the ischiatic nerve at the middle of the thigh. It descends between the two heads of gastrocnemius along the medial surface of the flexor digitorum superficialis. The tibial nerve continues distally under cover the common deep fascia of the leg, situated in the space between the flexor digitorum profundus and medial border of common calcaneal tendon, to the distal third of the leg. Slightly proximal to the level of the calcaneal tuber, the tibial nerve is divided into **medial and lateral plantar nerves**. They pass on the plantar surface of the hock and descend in the tarsal canal, caudal to the deep digital flexor tendon, in company with the medial and lateral plantar arteries. The tibial nerve gives off the following branches:- 1) **Lateral plantar cutaneous sural nerve;** separates from the tibial nerve at its origin and receives a fascicle from the fibular nerve. It descends on the lateral face of gastrocnemius to the distal third of the leg. Here it perforates the deep fascia and ramifies under the skin of the lateral and plantar aspects of tarsus and metatarsus. 2) **Muscular branches;** pass between the two heads of gastrocnemius and radiate to supply the gastrocnemius, soleus, flexor digitorum superficialis, popliteus and flexor digitorum profundus. 3) **Medial plantar nerve (medial plantar common digital nerve);** descends along the medial border of the digital flexor tendons. Near the middle of the metatarsus it releases a **communicating branch** which crosses obliquely the plantar surface of digital flexor tendons and joins the lateral plantar nerve at the distal third of the metatarsus. The medial plantar common digital nerve proceeds distally to be divided, proximal to the fetlock, into the **dorsal branch** and **medial plantar proper digital nerve.**

Table (37) Lumbosacral plexus (continued)

Nerve	Origin	Branches	Distribution
			i. **Communicating branch**; winds obliquely over the digital flexor tendons and joins the lateral plantar nerve distal to the middle of the metatarsus. ii. **Dorsal branch**; ramifies in the skin of the dorsal surface of the digit and corium of the hoof. iii. **Medial plantar proper digital nerve**; descends with the medial plantar proper digital artery and gives several branches to supply the skin of the medial and plantar aspects of the digit and corium of the hoof. 4) **Lateral plantar nerve (lateral plantar common digital nerve)**; deviates laterally between the superficial and deep digital flexor tendons, continues distally along the lateral border of the deep digital flexor tendon toward the distal end of the metatarsus. It is joined by the **communicating branch** from the **medial plantar nerve** and divides, just proximal to the fetlock, into a **dorsal branch** and **lateral plantar proper digital nerve.** The lateral plantar common digital artery gives off the following branches:- i. **Deep branch**; is detached distal to the tarsus to supply the suspensory ligament (middle interosseous muscle). ii. **Dorsal branch**; ramifies in the skin of the dorsal surface of the digit and corium of the hoof. iii. **Lateral plantar proper digital nerve**; descends with the lateral plantar proper digital artery and gives several branches to supply the skin of the lateral and plantar aspects of the digit and corium of the hoof.

References

1. Dyce, K. M.; W.O. Sack and C.J.G. Wensing (2018): Text Book of Veterinary Anatomy. Fifth edition, W.B. Sounders Company, Philadelphia, London.
2. Evans (1993): Miller's Anatomy of the dog. Third Edition. W.B. Sounders Company, Philadelphia. Pennsylvania.
3. Evans, H.E. and Delahaunta (2004): Guide to the dissection of the dog. Sixth edition, W.B. Sounders Company, Philadelphia, London.
4. Getty, N.G. (1975):Sisson and Grossman's The Anatomy of the Domestic Animals. Vol. I & II, fifth edition, W.B. Sounders Company, Philadelphia.
5. Habel, R.E. (1975): Applied Veterinary Anatomy. Ithaca, N.Y.R.E. Habel.
6. Nickel, R., Schummer, A., Seiferle, E. and Sack, W.O. (1973): The Viscera of the Domestic Animals. New York. Springer Verlag.
7. Nomina Anatomica Veterinaria (2017): Sixth Edition. prepared by the International Committee, Hannover, Columbia, Gent.
8. Papesko, P. (1979): Atlas of the Topographical Anatomy of the Domestic Animals. Third edition, W.B. Sounders Company, Philadelphia, London.
9. Schummer, A., H. Wilkens,B. Vollmerhaus and Habermehl K.H. (1981): Anatomy of the Domestic Animals. New York, Springer Verlag.
10. Sisson, S. and Grossman, J.D. (1967): The Anatomy of the Domestic Animals. Fourth edition, W.B. Sounders Company, Philadelphia

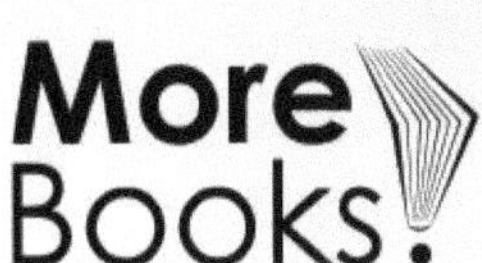

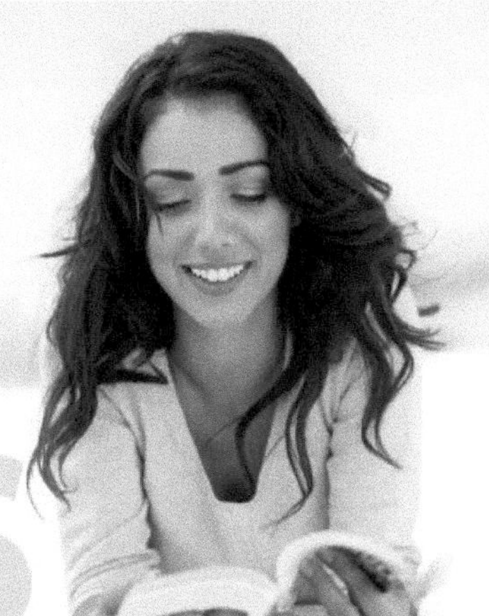

Buy your books fast and straightforward online - at one of world's fastest growing online book stores! Environmentally sound due to Print-on-Demand technologies.

Buy your books online at
www.morebooks.shop

Kaufen Sie Ihre Bücher schnell und unkompliziert online – auf einer der am schnellsten wachsenden Buchhandelsplattformen weltweit! Dank Print-On-Demand umwelt- und ressourcenschonend produzi ert.

Bücher schneller online kaufen
www.morebooks.shop

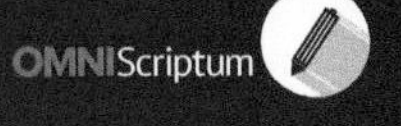

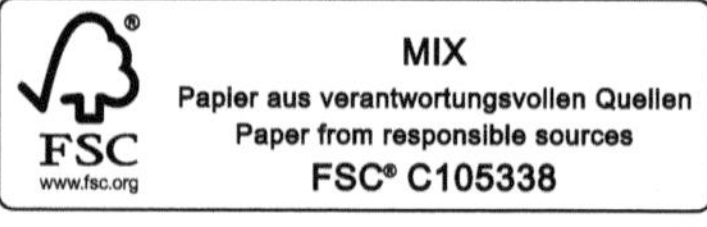

Printed by Books on Demand GmbH, Norderstedt / Germany